D1085121

FAMILY LIFE

The Jones and Bartlett Series in Nursing

FAMILY LIFE
PROCESS AND PRACTICE

ELLEN JANOSIK, M.S.
Alfred University

ELTA GREEN, M.S.S., A.C.S.W.
University of Rochester Medical Center

JONES AND BARTLETT PUBLISHERS

BOSTON

Editorial, Sales, and Customer Service Offices

Jones and Bartlett Publishers
20 Park Plaza
Boston, MA 02116

Library of Congress Cataloging-in-Publication Data

Janosik, Ellen Hastings.
    Family life : process and practice / Ellen Janosik, Elta Green.
        p.   cm.
    Includes bibliographical references and index.
    ISBN 0-86720-318-8
        1. Family—United States.   2. Family services—United States.
    3. Family—Health and hygiene—United States.   I. Green, Elta.
    II. Title.
    HQ536.J36   1991
    306.85—dc20   91-26282
                                                                   CIP

Cover art: "Manhattan Beach" by Edward Potthast. From the Ann and Merrill J. Gross Collection. Reprinted by permission.

Printed in the United States of America
95   94   93   92   91   10   9   8   7   6   5   4   3   2   1

Dedicated to the loving memory of our sisters
MAUDE BLAIR HASTINGS
and
PATRICIA OLD BROWN

CONTENTS

FOREWORD

Family Life: Process and Practice is a highly useful textbook for students preparing to be physical and mental health care providers. In each chapter, the book summarizes volumes of theoretical and research-based literature on the family, often summarizing a whole area of thinking under one chapter subheading. The authors invariably choose the kind of information that can be translated into, and is needed for, direct practice. Indeed, leaving nothing to chance, each chapter ends with careful guidance on how to use the material just presented, including an actual case vignette. The tight integration of theory and practice, as well as the carefully drawn up, detailed charts of both the theoretical material and the intervention steps, will appear heaven-sent to students who are overwhelmed by too much diverse material and look for concise and structured summaries.

Another strength of the book is the authors' double focus on the impact of internal and external forces on family systems, mindful of the interactions of family members and subsystems within the family as well as the constraints and opportunities presented by the larger society. A fine chapter on homosexual families and a very helpful chapter on the diverse family patterns and life-styles of ethnic families illustrate the authors' conviction that health professionals need to be open to, and prepared for, many different kinds of family systems. The authors' writing reflects at all times the nonjudgmental values prevalent in the health care field. The clear and unpretentious language and style of the book will make it accessible to students at any level of learning. It should fill an important educational need.

Sophia Freud, A.C.S.W., Ph.D.
Simmons College
School of Social Work
Boston

PREFACE

This book is intended for health professionals in practice, for students entering the health care field, and for counselors and crisis workers trying to promote family health and healing. Consultation and collaboration among members of different health care disciplines are increasing, as are trends toward providing care that is meaningful to families and communities as well as individuals. Recognizing this movement, we present individuals within a family context, and families within a community context.

Family theory has benefited from contributions drawn from many disciplines, aside from the major health professions of medicine, nursing, psychology, and social work. Sociologists, historians, epidemiologists, and anthropologists have expanded the scope of family theory and revealed broader aspects of family life. In addition to including such contributions, we present selected theoretical frameworks that can be applied to family work by health care professionals.

Every health care professional committed to comprehensive service needs basic knowledge of family theory. No individual exists in total isolation, for each of us has been shaped by a family system of one kind or another. Regardless of our preferences or our resistance, our families largely determine what we are. It is the family that transmits genetic and biological inheritance, that nurtures or fails to nurture us, that preserves or discards customs across generations.

No family exists in isolation, for every family interacts with larger social institutions in its own unique fashion. The social order surrounding the family influences it in countless ways, and the family in turn influences the larger social order. Thus the family is both cause and consequence of social change. As economic, political, religious, and cultural conditions alter over time, so do the family arrangements that coexist under these conditions. The continuous interaction of families with larger social institutions makes it necessary to include significant internal and external factors that affect family arrangements and operations from day to day and year to year.

Promoting positive change in families is not a simple matter, even when a family consists of only two members. Health care professionals, regardless of their discipline or orientation, soon realize that many influences intrude on family life. Often what is happening in a family is incomprehensible to outsiders and to the family members themselves. Because family life contains so many forces and counterforces, a simple, linear cause-and-effect relationship is seldom apparent. Even in the simplest family interaction, so much is happening that even experienced professionals are apt to feel overwhelmed by what they observe. As a result, their objectivity tends to be lost in a maelstrom of opposing currents, emotions, opinions, and actions.

The best way to remain objective in dealing with the complications and contradictions of family life is to become familiar with theory and acquire a conceptual understanding of family dynamics. One of our primary goals is to present theoretical constructs clearly and accurately so that health care professionals can impose organization, order, and rationality on family assessment and intervention.

Despite appearances to the contrary, family life is seldom altogether chaotic. This can be said even of dysfunctional families. Almost always there are recurring rhythms and patterns that are observable and identifiable. Knowledge of family theory enables practitioners to assess families and formulate strategies that mobilize the healing potential that exists even in troubled families.

Family theory utilizes a number of theoretical approaches, each of which has particular strengths and limitations. A distinctive feature of this book is the inclusion of various theoretical approaches and the development of a single comprehensive model showing interdependent relationships within the family, and between the family and society. The contributing theories in this book are developmental, structural, functional, psychodynamic, communication, and learning. They are linked to a tool, developed by us, entitled the *integrated systems model*. According to this model, families are social systems in which internal and external factors continually interact. The model views families as social systems in which patterned relationships exist that are based on structure (position) and function (roles). A further advantage of the model is that it is dynamic, not static, and is therefore useful in analyzing family responses to a changing social environment.

Theory building is a prolonged, difficult process, and there is a tendency among theorists to limit themselves to descriptions of phenomena without formulating therapeutic strategies. This is a limitation that clinicians working with real families cannot afford. The *integrated systems model* is not limited to descriptive assessment. Rather, it has a dual purpose: first, to direct the assessment process, and, second, to guide the intervention process.

The book consists of seven parts and fourteen chapters. Part One deals with major theories and concepts that examine family life from different vantage points. A historic overview looks at changes in family life over time, with current family diversity emphasized. Chapters in this section and throughout the book present therapeutic guidelines for clinicians dealing with particular family problems.

Part Two contains two chapters dealing with internal and external issues affecting contemporary families; Part Three concerns itself with family tasks and is divided into two chapters. One deals with the tasks and responsibilities of expanding families, and the other with the tasks and responsibilities of contracting families. Erikson's explanation of a critical period of ascendance in which individual developmental tasks should be accomplished is combined with Duvall's conceptualization of family developmental tasks. Often there is conflict between the readiness of individual members and the readiness of the family to proceed to the next developmental stage, and compromise must be negotiated. This part begins with the marital dyad establishing a family and moves through the arrival, rearing, and launching of children. Remarriage and stepparenting are included, as are the return of adult children to the parental home and the burden of caring for aged parents and grandparents. The contracting period of family life centers on losses: separation, divorce, decline, and death as the family moves through its life cycle.

Family patterns are the subject of Part Four. One chapter is concerned with patterns and variations in heterosexual families, and another chapter is devoted to patterns and variations in homosexual families. Part Five comprises two chapters, one describing adaptation to physical illness in a family and a second discussing adaptation to psychiatric illness in a family. Here attention shifts from developmental tasks to confronting unusual events that threaten the integrity and well-being of the family system. Severe physical or psychiatric illness in a family member may strain and deplete the resources of a family that previously functioned well. Distinctive features of acute, chronic, and terminal illness are contrasted, and characteristic problems are identified.

Part Six explores special problems arising in family life. One chapter looks at abuse and violence in the family, and notes the impact of abuse and violence on victims and perpetrators. Another chapter explores the effects of alcoholism and other forms of substance abuse on families. The last part of the book, entitled "Family Perspectives," describes healthy family coping. It discusses interactions in healthy families and examines discrepancies between functional and dysfunctional families. It also emphasizes the importance of recognizing strengths in apparently dysfunctional families, and of mobilizing those strengths that exist.

ACKNOWLEDGMENTS

The authors are indebted to Peter Ziarnowski, Ph.D., for contributing Chapter Eleven on psychiatric illness in the family. We are also indebted to James Keating for his commitment, enthusiasm, and availability. Edward Kobayashi contributed greatly to the authenticity of the text by describing the vicissitudes of wartime internment. Finally, we would like to thank family members and colleagues who expressed interest in this project and offered encouragement along the way.

PART
ONE

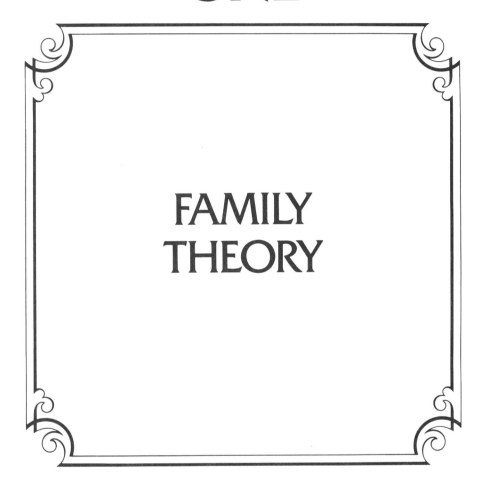

FAMILY
THEORY

CHAPTER ONE

Basic Family Theory: Contributing Theories and Concepts

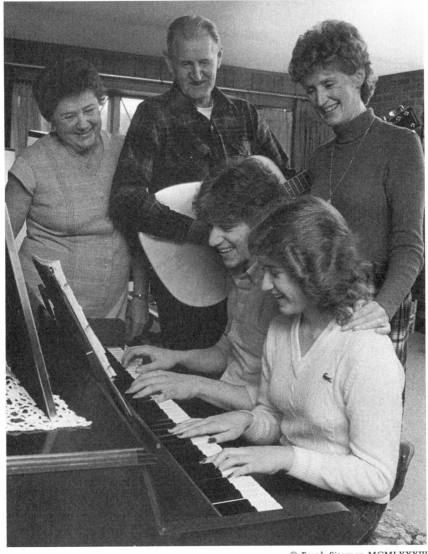

© Frank Siteman MCMLXXXIII

No matter how many communes anybody invents, the family always creeps back.

Margaret Mead

The family into which we are born is the first and most meaningful group we ever join, even though most of us leave it at some point in our lives. It is this nuclear family that is the primary group of society, for it not only shapes us as individuals but, by joining with other families, forms the communities in which we live. No family exists in isolation, for there is an ongoing exchange of energy in the form of transactions between the family and the surrounding community. Just as the values and standards of the family are a reference point for individual members, so the values and standards of the community are a reference point for its families. It is the community that specifies the norms to which its families conform, either wholly or in part.

In exchange for a measure of conformity, the community confers on its families approval, acceptance, and a sense of neighborhood. When the family is part of a stable community where a wholesome life-style prevails, the transactions between family and community are usually beneficial for everyone concerned. A compatibility exists that sustains both family and community. In a mobile, pluralistic society, however, many different kinds of communities may be found. As a result, some families find themselves living in communities whose customs they find unacceptable. An example of this is the plight of an elderly couple living on a fixed income and residing in a deteriorating neighborhood that is a locale for drug traffic and other criminal activity. Families whose values do not coincide with those of the surrounding community suffer a loss of identity and growing alienation.

When those families who reject the values of the community become a majority, they may act as a powerful force for change. A community can survive as it is only as long as its standards are accepted by the majority of its families. Thus, the relationship between the family and the community may be both cause and consequence of change.

The influence of the family on its own members is durable and persuasive. Whether we accept or reject family values, we continue to be influenced by them. Our experience of family life affects us from the moment of birth, and when we choose to renounce family customs and patterns, we must find other groups and other patterns to fill the void in our lives. We may decide to adopt a new life-style, but the memories persist in one way or another. The Irish writer James Joyce, for example, became an expatriate but carried Dublin in his heart as long as he lived and recreated its streets and its people in much of his work.

EARLY FAMILY STUDIES

The origin and nature of human families have been studied by historians, anthropologists, and sociologists, among others. Their findings are invariably interesting but, like family life itself, are sometimes contradictory and confusing. Frederick Engels (1902) contended that the monogamous family is based not on natural conditions but on economic considerations. Engels, a fervent Marxist, contended that the nuclear family based on monogamy was instituted to preserve private property. In a partisan essay, Engels wrote that the monogamous family upholds male supremacy, subjugates females, and guarantees to men that only their true and legitimate offspring will inherit the father's possessions. The institution of the monogamous family confines the sexuality of wives to one man — the husband. Beyond controlling and certifying the parentage of children, Engels asserted the monogamous family has no merit.

Engels regarded the monogamous nuclear family as a burden primarily for women because it imposes fidelity on women who for economic reasons must accept the lifelong restrictions of monogamy. He also regarded the monogamous nuclear family as irksome for men, and he cited the ancient Greeks, who barely tolerated the monogamous family and found it "a burden to them, a duty to the gods, the state, and their own ancestors" (p. 45). In the classless, communist society that Engels hoped for, divorce would be easily available, for "if marriage founded on love alone is moral, then it follows that marriage is moral only as long as love lasts" (p. 46). Because he believed that the preservation of the monogamous nuclear family depended on private property, Engels assumed that the abolition of private property would lead inevitably to the demise of the family as we know it. In the absence of the family, the state would be responsible for child rearing. Freed from the task of child rearing and no longer subject to economic pressure to marry, women would be socially and sexually liberated, bestowing their favors freely on the men of their choice. With women free of conventional restraints, prostitution and, indeed, all commerce in sexual transactions would also disappear.

The family theories of Engels and other Marxists contributed to the official disfavor felt by families in postrevolutionary Russia. For a time divorce and abortion were to be had for the asking, but the Soviet state soon realized that it was unequal to the child-rearing responsibilities discharged by the family. By 1936 the ideas of Engels had been discarded, and commitment to family stability became the official Soviet position. Although the Soviet state has remained influential in the education and socialization of children, the nuclear family continues to perform a crucial role in the USSR.

Another viewpoint is that of George Murdock (1949) who stated that the nuclear family is not a form of exploitation, but is natural and universal. He studied 250 preindustrial societies and found three organizational patterns. The most common form is nuclear, comprising a man and woman living with their children. In most societies this family is affiliated with other nuclear families to which it is joined by ties of blood or marriage. These affiliations of nuclear families make up the extended family. The third identified family organization is the polygamous family, which unites several nuclear families by means of plural marriage in which one father (or mother) produces children with more than one mate. While identifying three distinct patterns, Murdock claimed that because of its utility the nuclear family is both universal and inevitable. In support of this claim, he noted:

> There are societies which permit sexual gratification in other relationships but none that deny it to married spouses. There may be in exceptional cases little social disapproval of child birth out of wedlock, and relatives, servants, nurses, and pediatricians may assist in child care, but the primary responsibility for rearing children ever remains with the family. . . . No society, in short, has succeeded in finding an adequate substitute for the nuclear family to which it might transfer these functions. It is highly doubtful whether any society will ever succeed in such an attempt, utopian proposals for the abolition of the family notwithstanding. (p. 44)

For generations the economic skills, religious practices, and political institutions approved by society were acquired in the context of family life. As economic, religious, and political needs changed over time, so did the family arrangements that supported them. Murdock (1949) attributed four essential functions to the family: sexual, economic, reproductive, and educational. Levy and Fallers (1968) proposed that education and socialization are the primary family task, with reproduction and regulation of sexual activity the secondary task. The third task, the economic function of the family, is distinct and separate from the first two. It is clear that there is little agreement regarding family functions, perhaps because a primary function in one family is of secondary importance in another. Without differentiating their importance, the major family functions today are partnering, nurturing, communicating, adapting, and providing respite for members.

Some Major Functions of Present-Day Families

- *Partnership Functions*
  A family usually begins as a dyad in which each partner hopes to have certain needs gratified by the other. Accepting and sharing emotional and instrumental (task) responsibilities are aspects of marital function.

- *Nurturing Functions*
  This includes the basic care of family members, especially children, who require protection, socialization, education, and security.

- *Communication Functions*
  Intrafamily communication should be clear, consistent, and nonthreatening. Extrafamily communication should be congruent and acceptable to the prevailing expectations of the community surrounding the family.

- *Adaptation Functions*
  Family members accept and adapt appropriately to the critical tasks of each family member, and to the changing family life cycle stage. The entry and departure of any family member requires adaptation from the parents and siblings still in the home.
  Recurrent adjustment to individuation, separation, expansion, and contraction is inherent in family life.

- *Respite Functions*
  A family offers its members an environment where they may relax, rest from the demands of life in the outside world, and safely regress on occasion.

Family tasks that once persisted across generations have changed markedly. One significant change is the transformation of the family from a unit of production to a unit of consumption. Contemporary families produce very few of the products they use, but not too many generations ago most families were fairly self-sufficient. Today it is the individual, not the family, that constitutes the work unit. Production and distribution are removed from the family sphere and are controlled by vast corporations. The mobility of the work force is another fact of life, as are frequent relocations of families from one geographic area to another. As a consequence of these uprootings, many families experience a feeling of loneliness and anomie. Having lost contact with old friends, extended families, and familiar neighborhoods, present-day families tend to turn inward for security and psychological support. This produces more intensity and emotional involvement, as family members rely largely on each other. Such intensity and involvement may be comforting for a time, but eventually prove detrimental, especially if family members have unrealistic expectations of one another (Astrachan, 1986).

It is not just the economic function of the family that has changed. Family control of sexual activity and of reproduction has lessened, perhaps because these are less closely linked than they once were. The period of adolescence is a time when young people are sexually mature but still financially dependent on the family. Not many years ago teenagers were apt to be sexually frustrated, and their parents were likely to be anxious concerning this issue. This is less true today because dependable contraception now permits sexual activity without procreation. The availability of contraception has weakened prohibitions against premarital and extramarital sex for teenagers, their older siblings, and their parents as well. The threat of AIDS (acquired immune deficiency syndrome) has led to an emphasis on "safe sex," but it is not yet known whether sexual practices will be significantly or permanently altered.

FAMILY THEORY

Sometimes family investigation can be a means of understanding the behavior of an individual. In this book, however, it is the family itself rather than any individual member that draws our attention. Family theory begins with the premise that the problems of any individual often originate or are perpetuated by interactions with the family. The difficulties of individual members reflect family dysfunction; therefore, family issues should be addressed. In addressing family issues, care providers often turn to a series of interrelated questions. First, does the family in question exist in harmony or in conflict? In other words, what is happening to make some families engage in continual warfare while other families go to great lengths to preserve peace at any price? Second, why do some families manage to cope under adverse conditions, while others cannot manage even in very favorable circumstances? Moreover, why do some harmonious families seem unable to solve problems or make decisions, whereas other families that are always in conflict somehow reach a consensus on what should be done, and proceed to do it? Along the same line of inquiry, why do some seemingly conflicted families survive while apparently harmonious ones do not?

These are complicated questions, and the answers are not immediately apparent. Searching for answers to such questions is facilitated by familiarity with family theories and concepts that explain aspects of family life. The point has been made that families are part of the community around them, just as individuals are part of the family to which they belong. Families and communities share the characteristics of reciprocal interaction and interdependence. These characteristics are basic to general systems theory and validate the application of systems theory to family life. The general systems approach presented in this chapter provides a broad focus that may be used advantageously with a majority of families.

Pioneers in the field of family theory had to invent new terminology to explain the processes they found in families with whom they worked. During the 1950s family theorists were chiefly concerned with interactional patterns in families of schizophrenic persons, especially if the identified client was young. There were several reasons for this interest. To begin with, families with a schizophrenic member offered an accessible laboratory for study, because the disorder is usually of long duration with a course interspersed with periods of remission and relapse. Additionally, young persons with schizophrenia were usually at a developmental point where family factors that might mitigate or worsen the disorder could be identified. Biological research in psychiatric disorders was just beginning and had not been clearly linked to schizophrenia. In the absence of definitive research, it was hoped that studying the families of young persons with schizophrenia might uncover certain risk factors, besides helping the families to cope with this disabling, often chronic disorder (Cohen, Younger, & Sullivan, 1983).

Although family theory was initiated by clinicians working with psychiatric clients, many concepts derived from their work proved applicable to families in which no member suffered from a diagnosable psychiatric disorder. Even without evidence of a psychiatric disorder, many dysfunctional families seemed to demonstrate similar interactional patterns. Discovery of certain interactional patterns and of the interdependent quality of these interactions led some theorists to believe in a cause-and-effect relationship between family interactions and the problems of the identified client. These beliefs led to the scapegoating of some families and the use of the pejorative term *schizophrenogenic*. This term is less often used today, partly because the biological genesis of schizophrenia is being sought with some success. Present-day family theorists assert that family interactional patterns may increase a client's dysfunction without necessarily causing it (Weiner, 1985; Foley, 1974).

FAMILY THERAPY

As a formal treatment modality, family therapy is relatively new. It is an accepted but complex treatment modality that requires graduate preparation and supervised clinical experience from those who practice it. *Family theory* rests on the premise that a client's problems may reflect the family's problems. *Family therapy* carries this premise even further, dealing not merely with the family *of* the client, but with the family *as* the client. It is a multidisciplinary treatment mode, and practitioners are drawn from medicine, nursing, psychology, social work, and counseling. Any health professional who is engaged in family therapy needs in-depth knowledge of normal family development in order to recognize deviations. In 1978 the Department of Health, Education and Welfare recognized the American

TABLE 1.1. Forms of Family Therapy	
Form of Therapy	**Characteristics of Therapy**
Conjoint family therapy	The family meets with one therapist or a pair of cotherapists. This is the most usual form of family therapy, especially for marital counseling or nuclear family meetings that include parents and children.
Multiple-impact family therapy	The family or subgroups of the family meet with several therapists simultaneously or concurrently. In this form of family therapy, the impact of treatment is increased by the teamwork of a group of therapists working with the family.
Network family therapy	A nuclear family is joined by the extended family group and by significant friends and neighbors to meet with a therapist or a pair of cotherapists. This form of therapy reduces the isolation of a small family unit and mobilizes a strong supportive network.
Multiple family therapy	A number of families meet together with one or two therapists. Families with common problems or shared interests profit from this form of therapy, in which the therapists use group leadership tactics.

Association for Marriage and Family Therapy as the accrediting body for family therapy programs. The National League for Nursing is the accrediting body for graduate nursing programs, most of which have a family theory and practice component.

Health professionals undertaking family therapy should be aware that this is a demanding field, and they should not exceed the limits of their competence. Whenever indicated, families should be referred by generalist practitioners to clinical specialists with sufficient expertise. Although family therapy per se is beyond the scope of most generalists, this is not true of family assessment and planning. If a generalist has the ability and experience to provide family intervention beyond assessment and planning, the interventions should be fairly straightforward and should deal with social and environmental modification rather than intrinsic change. Throughout the therapeutic encounter, even the most experienced family therapist will soon discover that families are unlikely to change unless they are willing to do so.

Family therapy may be offered in one of several ways, depending on the needs of the family, the expertise of the therapists, and the policies of the agency under whose auspices care is given. Family therapy frequently utilizes an interdisciplinary model, in that cotherapists may represent more than one health care discipline. The gender of the therapist is thought to be significant; many practitioners prefer cotherapy where a male and female work in tandem. For example, a female therapist working with a single woman raising adolescent boys might promote family comfort by inviting a male therapist to join the sessions.

Table 1.1 summarizes the general forms of family therapy.

DEFINITIONS OF FAMILY

Any health professional adopting a family approach must first determine what constitutes a family. Making this determination is more difficult than it sounds, for there is considerable disagreement on the subject. One reason for the difficulty is that *family* is an emotionally charged word that means different things to different people. For decades sociologists, anthropologists, and historians neatly labeled nuclear and extended families by means of two criteria: *consanguinity* (blood ties) and *marriage* (legal ties). Nuclear and extended families with these characteristics still exist in great numbers, but they have been diluted by the proliferation of single-parent families, foster-parent families, stepparent families, and cohabiting couples who may or may not be heterosexual. Added to these family variations are arrangements whereby a residence is shared by a group of individuals, unrelated by blood or marriage, who consider themselves a family. Not too long ago communal living was largely the province of young people, but many senior citizens have found the arrangement practical and rewarding. When one looks at the enormous variety in families living in the United States and elsewhere, it is apparent that the trend toward diversity is increasing, not diminishing.

In New York City alone, only 43 percent of the households conform to the traditional norm. A 1988 federal census report noted that only 27 percent of the nation's households followed the pattern of two parents living with their children, down from 40 percent in 1970. In 1989 the New York Court of Appeals ruled that any homosexual couple who had lived together for a decade or more was a family, at least for rent control purposes. The ruling stated that protection from eviction depended not on fictitious legal distinctions or genetic history, but instead should find its foundation in the reality of family life. Family, according to this ruling, should be defined by the presence of several factors, such as "exclusivity and longevity" and the "level of financial and emotional commitment." The ruling further stated that "It is the totality of the relationship as evidenced by the dedication, caring, and self-sacrifice of the parties which should, in the final analysis, control." Earlier that year the same court overturned a prohibition against four unrelated people living in a single-family zone, ruling that rejecting a "functional family" was unconstitutional. San Francisco, Los Angeles, Seat-

---

TABLE 1.2. Variations in Family Composition

- *Natural or biological family:* Family into which the individual is born or is related by consanguinity.

- *Adoptive family:* Family to which an individual belongs through adoption, usually by legal means.

- *Family of origin:* Family into which an individual was born.

- *Nuclear family:* Family created by a marital or ongoing relationship between two individuals and their offspring, if any.

- *Family of procreation:* Family created by individuals entering a relationship into which children are born.

- *Extended family:* Family group that includes one or more nuclear families plus other individuals related by blood or marriage.

- *Intact family:* Family that includes two parents and their natural or adopted children living in one household.

- *Single-parent family:* Family consisting of children and one parent, either father or mother, living in one household.

- *Stepparent family:* Family created by the remarriage of one or both parents; this family may include children of the present marriage as well as children from previous marriages of one or both spouses.

---

tle, and Madison, Wisconsin, are other cities that have moved or are moving in the direction of recognizing nontraditional family forms (Gutis, 1989).

There are a number of explanations for the diversity of present-day families. High divorce rates, the tendency of divorced persons to remarry, the decisions of unmarried mothers to keep their children, cohabitation without marriage, and more tolerance of homosexual partnerships have had an effect (Polman, 1989). Elderly persons whose spouses have died may react to loneliness and lowered incomes by living with other senior citizens. Evidence of family diversity is all around us and one need only watch television a few times to realize that the traditional families of "Ozzie and Harriet" have virtually disappeared.

Nontraditional families make conservative observers uneasy, and many people deplore the recognition now being granted to new family forms. Others assert that family diversity results from efforts to fulfill individual needs within a family structure. Without taking sides, one may state that the composition of today's families is a response to overwhelming social forces. Families mirror the changes occurring in society. Once established, nontraditional families claim the legal recognition that was previously denied them. The granting of legal rights to nontraditional families ensures their continued existence and promotes diversity. The family is an active, responsive system operating within the larger social system; historical as well as contemporary perspectives offer concrete examples of how deeply and reciprocally the family reacts to changes in the social order (Frazer, 1985; McNally, 1980). Table 1.2 lists some of the variations in family composition.

FAMILY SYSTEMS THEORY

A broad definition of family is that it is a system of interdependent members possessing two fundamental system attributes: *structure*, or membership, and *function*, or interaction. Here the term *function* is used in a generic sense to denote that families are not static entities but are dynamic systems engaged in interaction within and across their borders. Understanding the family as a system begins by considering who belongs in the family (structure) and how they relate to one another (function). Defining the family as an interacting social system helps shed light on the complexities of family life.

The family is a system whose components (members) engage in continual interaction according to rules and norms that evolve over time and make it possible for the family to survive. Borders or boundaries are indispensable aspects of the family system. Boundaries surround each individual member, and boundaries surround the entire family unit. Individual boundaries help family members preserve their individuality or selfhood. Family boundaries determine how, when, and with whom members may interact outside the family.

Depending on the nature of family boundaries, a family system may be fully open, entirely closed, or somewhere in between. All families, functional or dysfunctional, contain some degree of tension generated by the emotional connections between members. Family boundaries should be somewhat open (permeable) so that internal tension can be discharged rather than held within the family system. Undischarged tension may rise to unbearable levels if the family is a closed system with no mechanisms for tension release.

An example of a closed family system is one that tries to make crucial decisions without obtaining information from reliable outside sources. A family might decide that a daughter should attend college at her father's alma mater, without finding out whether the college is equipped to meet the needs of the daughter. Without adequate information, the family may jeopardize the daughter's success and happiness. Although excessive tension may cause strain among family members, a family without any tension would not be a viable system. In a sense, it is tension within the family that helps supply the energy needed to sustain the interdependent operations of the system.

Homeostasis

In order to operate appropriately, families need stability, or *homeostasis*, a steady state of balance that allows families to respond to internal and external conditions. Stability does not imply stagnation, for a family's ability to react to changing conditions is necessary for survival. Family boundaries that are too permeable promote a climate of instability. An illustration of this is the upwardly mobile family that abandons its old habits too quickly in order to copy mindlessly the behaviors of a higher, more affluent socioeconomic group. Family stability may be impaired just as easily by refusal to permit the entry of any influence from outside the family. This might occur in an immigrant family, where parents fear the influence of the mainstream culture and cling to old habits in the face of opposition from the community and from some of its own members. The term *equilibrium* is often used as a synonym for homeostasis.

Feedback

Feedback is an important concept in systems theory. By means of feedback, the family transmits output to the community through verbal and nonverbal messages. The community, through various institutions such as church, school, or the workplace transmits responses to the family. These responses then become input to the family system. Feedback is a continuous process of input and output exchanges between families and the community that surrounds them. Sometimes the feedback from the community is informal and represents community reaction to the family's actions. An example is neighborhood gossip about family quarrels, or criticism of the family for not measuring up to community standards in caring for their home. A more formal kind of feedback would consist of complaints from the children's school or a summons issued by the police.

 Feedback is not a series of linear events but, rather, a circular process in which components of the system (members) reciprocally influence one another. In circular feedback the action of A influences the actions of B and C. Thereupon B and C react toward each other and also toward A, who instigated the circular events. Figure 1.1 shows the feedback process.

 By analyzing feedback processes it is possible to identify the family's boundary characteristics and assess family stability. When transactions between the family and the community are dysfunctional, the health professional may try to increase the family's awareness of their actions and of community norms. When input from the community indicates that a family should modify its behavior, the community feedback is negative. When input from the community indicates that the family should continue its present behavior, the feedback is positive. Whether positive or negative, feedback promotes adaptive family functioning.

FIGURE 1.1. Circular Feedback: The action of A influences the actions of B and C, who then interact with each other and with A, who initiated the circular feedback.

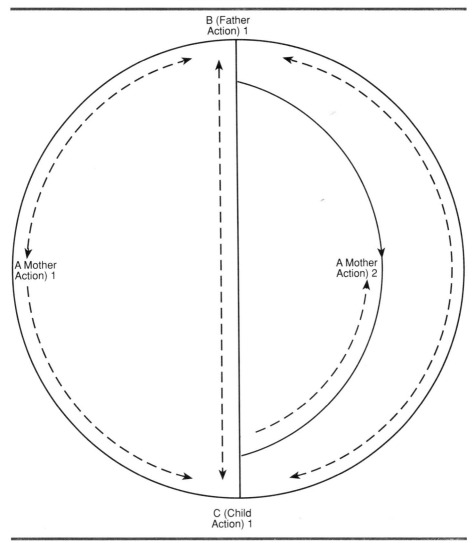

An advantage of applying systems theory to families is that it prevents heaping blame on any single member. Approaching the family as a system in which parents, children, extended family members, and the community influence each other in reciprocal ways means that whatever occurs is a shared responsibility. Systems theorists contend that alterations in one part of the family inevitably lead to alterations in other parts of the family.

Adopting a systems approach helps health care professionals to recognize family strengths as well as weaknesses. Systems theory may be used to reinforce the confidence and competence of all family members, especially the parents, so that a family climate is promoted in which every member flourishes and no member is exploited.

Basic Assumptions of Systems Theory

Assumption: Living systems are organized in a hierarchy wherein complex, higher level systems emerge from simpler, lower level systems. Every system is contained within boundaries that are more or less permeable. Individuals make up family systems that are organized into larger systems such as communities. Within families various members are organized into subsystems.

Assumption: A change in one family member or subgroup creates changes in all other family members and subgroups. When a family member becomes dysfunctional, for whatever reason, there is a shift that affects everyone in the family. Conversely, restoration of functionality in a member also creates a shift. Families that coped well with the maladaptiveness of a member may prove reluctant to readjust in order to allow the improved member to function adaptively again.

Assumption: Family equilibrium is not static but involves a constant search for balance among the internal and external forces impinging on families. Family balance may be disrupted periodically, and the balance regained after disruption may not be the same as that which previously existed. The state of balance may be stronger or more fragile than the one before.

Assumption: Family behaviors are not linear but circular. Linear behaviors are said to occur in a certain sequence. (Mother cooks dinner, the children set the table, Dad gets home from work and reads the newspaper. After dinner, Dad cleans up.) Described in this fashion, the behaviors are linear.

In a circular behavior pattern, the actions are described differently. (Mother is a teacher's aide in the morning but is free in the afternoon. Her schedule permits her to relax for a few hours before starting dinner. The children help with predinner preparations so they can do their homework later. Dad needs to unwind after a full working day, so the rest of the family gets dinner ready while he recuperates. His awareness of the family's consideration makes him willing to help later in the evening.)

Identifying circular behavior patterns means that there is no search for a victim or a culprit, and no single nugget of truth to be discovered. What is explored is the meaning of events to the various family members.

Assumption: Families have the ability to monitor themselves internally and externally, regulating the interactions between members and with larger systems by means of positive and negative feedback. Feedback is simply a response to events and actions: Positive feedback tends to maintain or increase whatever is happening; negative feedback tends to modify or decrease whatever is happening.

FAMILY DIMENSIONS

Visualizing the family as an active, interdependent system facilitates our understanding of family dynamics. In one important respect family life entails modification of the systems approach. In general, a systems approach is limited to what is currently happening in the family. Every family, however, lives not only in the present but in the past and the future as well. Past events influence family reactions to what is happening now and to what may happen in the future. The experience of success and failure influences family coping ability in both subtle and not so subtle ways. Whenever the resources of the family are depleted, family dysfunction follows even if the family has been able to cope in the past. Disproportion between the needs of the family and its resources impair role enactment. Families that try to cope by engaging in appropriate but inadequate role enactment are called *marginal*. Families that attempt to cope by engaging in distorted or inappropriate role enactment are termed *disorganized.*

When family resources are insufficient for family needs because of illness or misfortune, marginality is more frequent than disorganization. This is due to the fact that appropriate role enactment continues to be respected even if it is difficult to maintain. Many women functioning as wage earners and as single parents struggle to enact family roles to which the family was once accustomed. In a marginal family suitable role enactment is attempted and barely maintained, whereas in disorganized families suitable role enactment is rarely attempted and never maintained. Dysfunction is more obvious in disorganized families; functionality may be present in marginal families, but their appropriate role enactment is fragile and tenuous. As a result, marginal families are quite vulnerable when additional stress is imposed.

Marginality is a descriptive rather than a pejorative term. Any change makes new demands on individuals and families. Because marginal families lack discretionary resources in the form of time, energy, or money, their equilibrium is always precarious. One factor contributing to the marginality of contemporary families is mobility, which transforms extended families into nuclear households. Small nuclear families lack the capacity of extended families for mobilizing their resources and for deflecting or absorbing the anxieties and inadequacies of individual family members. When the family confronts adverse conditions that are severe or long-lasting, few relatives are available to lend a hand. Nuclear households have few peripheral members to neutralize family stress or discharge family responsibilities during periods of stress or extreme need.

The efforts of marginal families to enact roles appropriately may limit their access to community assistance. All families differ in their willingness to accept help from outside sources, but marginal families often hesitate to reveal their straits. These relatively closed families discourage intrusion and self-disclosure, preferring to make great demands on family members in the form of self-sacrifice and self-discipline. Such behavior is particularly unfortunate in families whose resources are already meager; their privacy is protected, but at considerable cost.

Disorganized families are less likely to be sensitive about seeking outside help. Because their problems take more dramatic forms, these families are often known to community agencies, either through receiving aid or through experiencing official supervision of one kind or another.

The categories of marginality and disorganization are not fixed or permanent. Under stress, marginal families may become disorganized, just as they may become truly functional under favorable conditions. In some circumstances a period of stress may be growth-producing if new coping behaviors are adopted. Therefore, it is not enough for health professionals to assess the family as it now presents itself. Family recollections of the past and expectations of the future also require careful exploration. Howell (1975) formulated a comprehensive assessment guide that is not systems-oriented but looks at a family's memories of the past and expectations of the future to explain the present. This assessment guide and its application are presented in Figure 1.2.

FIGURE 1.2. **Family Assessment Tool**

	Past	Present	Future
I. *Characteristics of individual members:*			
1. What members make up the nuclear family?			
2. What members make up the families of origin?			
3. Which member is the identified patient or patients?			
4. What signs of equilibrium or disequilibrium are apparent in the identified client?			
5. What signs of equilibrium or disequilibrium are apparent in other members?			

	Past	Present	Future
6. What signs of equilibrium or disequilibrium are apparent in the family system?			
II. Characteristics of internal family communication:			
1. How does each family member communicate and interact with other members of the nuclear family?			
2. How does each family member communicate and interact with members of the families of origin?			
3. How are decisions made in the family?			
4. How is conflict handled in the family?			
5. What are the prevailing communication patterns in the family? Specific? Consistent? Ambiguous? Tangential? Contradictory? Placating? Blaming? Confusing?			
III. Characteristics of external family communication:			
1. Are family boundaries open or closed to external influence?			
2. Is the family integrated into the social mainstream?			
3. Is the family isolated from the social mainstream?			
4. How does the family relate to larger systems, such as school, church, or community?			
5. How do individual family members relate to external systems?			

FIGURE 1.2. (continued)

	Past	Present	Future
IV. *Psychological characteristics of the family:*			
1. Whose needs are being met in the family?			
2. Whose needs are being ignored in the family?			
3. Where is the locus of power in the family?			
4. Who is the task leader in the family?			
5. Who is the emotional leader in the family?			
6. Is leadership invested in both parents, one parent, or neither parent?			
7. Are family alliances based on natural distinctions of age, gender, and generational roles?			
8. Are family alliances based on coalitions that transcend age, gender, and generational roles?			
V. *Socioeconomic/environmental characteristics of the family:*			
1. Are family and socioeconomic resources sufficient for basic needs?			
2. Is there harmony between material resources and family expectations?			
3. Are the hopes and expectations of family members realistic?			
4. Are the hopes and expectations of family members unrealistic?			
5. Are conditions present that are likely to promote social class advancement?			
6. Are conditions present that are apt to promote social class slippage?			

	Past	Present	Future
7. Are external socio-economic resources available to the family? 8. Are external socio-economic resources acceptable to the family?			

Source: Adapted from Howells (1975).

CLINICAL EXAMPLE: ASSESSING PAST, PRESENT, AND FUTURE CHARACTERISTICS IN COUNSELING A TROUBLED COUPLE

Sheila Colby is a 24-year-old married woman who requested an appointment for marital counseling for herself and Matt, her husband. When making the appointment, Sheila said that she believed her husband was a manic depressive who was now in a depressed phase of his illness. When questioned, she explained that her husband had never been diagnosed and that she based her opinion on his current behavior. She stated that Matt had lost the ability to enjoy life and had no drive or enthusiasm. An appointment was made for the couple to be seen together.

They are an attractive couple, well dressed and well spoken; they have been married for two years and live with Sheila's parents. Sheila is the only daughter of a successful businessman and his socially active wife. Also living in the family home is Sheila's brother Dick. Dick is 16 years old and attends a private prep school. He is a fine athlete and a better than average student. The family home is comfortable, even luxurious. Sheila's parents are delighted to have Sheila live with them. Her father is especially pleased to be able to provide so well for his family. Matt's parents are less affluent, and the young couple seldom see Matt's family. Although Matt was reluctant to live with Sheila's parents after marriage, he was persuaded to do so in order to save money for a home of their own. Before and after marriage Matt had been able to do little more than make ends meet. Sheila graduated from a prestigious university and works two or three days a week as a substitute teacher. Matt is a college dropout who has never held a steady job. He is, however, a competent house painter and earns adequate money when he can obtain work.

In the initial interview the marriage counselor saw that the marriage was in trouble. Sheila is more articulate than Matt, and it was she who expressed the most dissatisfaction. Her major complaint was that Matt had no ambition and no pride.

"He lets everybody take advantage of him, including my father. Daddy insults Matt all the time and Matt never defends himself," said Sheila angrily.

When questioned by the counselor, Matt agreed that Sheila was proba-bly right. His acceptance of her criticism seemed to make Sheila even angrier. Moving from generalizations to specific examples of Matt's behav-ior, Sheila expressed the following complaints.

"Matt lets my father and brother belittle him and never says a word."

"Matt has no ambition. He enjoys painting houses but the man he works for doesn't need him all the time. When Matt isn't working he stays in our room and sleeps."

"Matt refuses to work for my father even though Daddy offered to make a job for him."

"Matt won't socialize with my friends but he has no friends of his own. As a result we don't see anyone."

"Matt never makes love to me anymore unless I initiate it. And I get tired of making the first overture."

After listening to Sheila's litany of complaints against Matt, the coun-selor tried to draw him out. Matt was reluctant to disclose his feelings, but when the counselor gently asked what it was like for Matt to live with Sheila's family, the young man's eyes filled with tears. "It's hard living there," he said. "I know they mean well but I don't fit in. I love Sheila and want to stay married to her even though we don't do much anymore except argue. I wish we had our own place but we can't afford it. Right now I feel I don't have the right to stand up to Sheila's father. After all, I live under his roof and eat at his table."

Observing the couple together, the counselor realized that genuine affection and strong physical bonds exist between Sheila and Matt. Matt does not lack ambition, but his failure at college lowered his self-confi-dence. He enjoys working as a house painter and considers himself good at it. He expressed a wish to work as an independent contractor someday.

The counselor suspected that Sheila did not altogether object to Matt's choice of occupation, but was sensitive to the reactions of her family and friends. In a nondirective way the counselor asked if Sheila could help Matt realize his desire to set himself up in a business specializing in exterior and interior painting. Until that point, Sheila had not heard Matt talk about going into business for himself, but she supported the idea. Since she had some understanding of the arrangements for a small business enterprise, she offered to help Matt obtain a bank loan, make estimates, and set up a bookkeeping system. It was obvious that Sheila liked the idea of being married to an independent contractor rather than a part-time employee. For Matt, Sheila's enthusiasm and involvement were very gratifying, especially since his work performance was unchanged.

As the couple moved ahead with their plans, the counselor encouraged Matt to verbalize his feelings and Sheila to listen. In time Sheila realized that it was not easy for Matt to live in her parents' home. She gradually became more aware of Matt's sensitivity. Instead of remaining silent when her father and brother made Matt the target of their half teasing, half serious jibes, Sheila began to align herself with Matt. Although her family ridiculed the idea of Matt becoming an independent contractor, the couple did not give up their efforts. Along with their business venture, the couple established the goal of moving to their own apartment as soon as possible instead of waiting until they had money to buy a house. The prospects for the young couple were brighter as a result of their common goals, although their different backgrounds indicated that compromise and counseling might be necessary to resolve future issues.

Characteristics of Individual Members

Sheila is an intelligent but impatient young woman, indulged by her family and fond of having her own way. She loves her husband but is reluctant to give up the comforts of her parents' home. She has always been surrounded by assertive, affluent people and desperately wants Matt to be more successful so that he will fit into her social circle. She wants Matt to be self-confident like her father, but she does not seem to realize his uncomfortable position. Instead of being sympathetic and understanding, Sheila has behaved in ways that further undermine Matt's confidence. Sheila is very sensitive to the opinions of her family and her friends. She knows that Matt is a nonachiever in their eyes, and she would like to change this, but she does not know how.

Matt is an easygoing but sensitive young man who wants to make Sheila happy but has begun to doubt his ability to do so. In their two years of marriage Matt has made many concessions. He dislikes living with his wife's family but has not told her how much he dislikes it. Sheila wants to continue living with her family until she and Matt have enough money for a house. Matt thinks this goal is at least five years away; the prospect of continuing the present living arrangement is very discouraging for him. Since his marriage Matt has seen very little of his family of origin. Sheila seldom accompanies him on his rare visits to his own parents. He is tired of making excuses for her absence and would like to tell Sheila this. But here again, he hesitates to express his feelings.

Characteristics of Internal Communication

Sheila can tell Matt what she wants and how she feels, but she behaves in ways that do not encourage him to do the same. The rude teasing her father aims at Matt does not upset Sheila because she is accustomed to her father's ways. For a long time she did not see the effect on Matt, especially when Matt did not tell her. Perfectly comfortable at home, Sheila saw no point in moving to a small apartment. Although she tried to be accepting of Matt's choice of occupation, she was embarrassed by his limited earning power. She loved Matt too much to say this directly, but she betrayed her feelings in subtle ways, such as suggesting Matt return to college or take a job with her father.

Characteristics of External Communication

Sheila cannot understand Matt's refusal to socialize with her friends, nor does she realize the extent of his feelings of inadequacy. Even before marriage Matt was guarded and uncommunicative until he knew people well. He deeply resents being the butt of jokes by Sheila's father, but thinks he has no right to defend himself. Although Matt was never very close to his own parents, he misses the familiar, down-to-earth atmosphere of his old home. Some of his reluctance to socialize with Sheila's friends stems from his lack of confidence; some of his reluctance is due to resentment at Sheila's refusal to accompany him on visits to his parents. When Matt first came to live with Sheila's family, he anticipated becoming part of her family, but he no longer has hopes on that score. Partly from a sense of obligation and partly as a form of self-protection, Matt has withdrawn from everyone—Sheila, her family and friends, and his own family of origin.

Psychological Characteristics of the Family

Sheila is an outgoing and somewhat pampered young woman. Initially she was attracted to Matt's gentleness and sincerity, but she now wants him to be more self-assured. Many aspects of her personality complement those of Matt, and this may be the reason for their mutual attraction. She is emotional where Matt is rational, bold where he is timid, voluble where he is inarticulate. Even though her marriage is in trouble, Sheila is able to appreciate Matt's qualities of steadiness and dependability. When Matt makes a commitment or gives his word, he lives up to his promises. In the frivolous, sophisticated world that she grew up in, these were rare qualities. Although she doesn't acknowledge it often, Sheila admires traits in Matt that she never found in her ambitious father, whom Sheila resembles in many ways.

In the working-class neighborhood where Matt grew up, he was liked and respected just for being himself. Financial accomplishments were not the measure of success. What was valued was physical presence, loyalty, and a talent for friendship; these were qualities that earned Matt the acceptance of peers and parents in his old neighborhood. The easy acceptance Matt had experienced from childhood on did not equip him to deal with Sheila's father or her friends.

Socioeconomic/Environmental Characteristics of the Family

Sheila belonged to a privileged family and objected to giving up the life-style she had always enjoyed. With Matt's intermittent work and her substitute teaching, their income was sufficient to afford a modest apartment. Sheila, however, did not want to relinquish the luxuries she loved even though she knew that Matt was unhappy. Matt's reticence in expressing his feelings made it easy for Sheila to overlook his reactions and concentrate on her own. One goal of counseling was to enable Matt to verbalize more easily, and he was able to do this with encouragement. He was delighted when Sheila agreed to move with him to their own apartment as soon as possible. Starting his own business made Matt anxious, but he drew courage from Sheila's self-confidence. Because Matt grew up in modest circumstances, the prospect of economizing for a time did not dismay him. Therefore, he was able to reassure Sheila when she worried about leaving her parents' home. She also derived satisfaction from Matt's newfound ability to deflect her father's ridicule.

SUMMARY

Early family theorists disagree on the inevitability and universality of the nuclear family, but Murdoch has insisted that because of its usefulness, the nuclear family is irreplaceable. Family theory and family therapy are based on the premise that individual dysfunction originates within the family and may be aggravated by interactional patterns. This does not imply, however, that the family is the *cause* of dysfunction. Family therapy requires advanced preparation of its practitioners, but family approaches are within the scope of any health professional with knowledge of normal growth and development and of basic family theory. Even the most experienced family therapist cannot alter family interactional patterns unless the family is willing to change. When there is disagreement between family and therapist regarding goals, negotiation is needed to resolve areas of disagreement. Unless specific goals are agreed upon, neither the family nor the therapist has a sense of direction or criteria by which to evaluate progress.

This introductory chapter examines some divergent family forms that have emerged in contemporary life. General systems theory is presented as a conceptual tool that may be used in assessing various family forms. Systems theory contends that alterations in one part of the family lead to alterations in all parts. Using a systems theory approach enables health professionals to identify both strengths and weaknesses without assigning blame.

Because families possess a remembered past and an anticipated future, they do not live only in the present. Therefore, family assessment should include the exploration of past memories and future expectations of the family members. A tool is provided to facilitate exploration of these three dimensions of family experience.

REFERENCES

Astrachan, A. (1986). *How Men Feel: Their Response to Women's Demands for Independence, Equality and Power.* New York: Anchor/Doubleday.

Cohen, M. W., Younger, R., & Sullivan, J. M. (1983). "Treating the Family of Chronically Impaired Adults." *The Family Therapist*, 4(1): 2–12.

Engels, F. (1902/1968). *The Origin of the Family: Private Property and the State*, trans. Ernest Untermann. Chicago: Charles Kerr. Reprinted in N. W. Bell & E. F. Vogel (Eds.), *A Modern Introduction to the Family.* New York: Free Press.

Foley, V. D. (1974). *An Introduction to Family Therapy.* New York: Grune and Stratton.

Frazer, A. (1985). *The Weaker Vessel.* New York: Random Vintage.

Gutis, P. S. (1989). "Family Redefines Itself and Now the Law Follows." *New York Times*, May 28.

Howells, J. G. (1975). *Principles of Family Therapy.* New York: Brunner/Mazel.

Levy, M. S., & Fallers, L. A. (1968). "The Family: Some Comparative Considerations." In M. A. Sussman (Ed.), *Source Book of Marriage and the Family.* Boston: Houghton Mifflin.

McNally, S. (1980). "Historical Perspectives on the Family." In J. R. Miller & E. H. Janosik (Eds.), *Family-Focused Care.* New York: McGraw-Hill.

Murdock, G. (1949). *Social Structure.* New York: Macmillan.

Polman, D. (1989). "Partners in Love but Not in Law." *Philadelphia Inquirer*, July 30.

Weiner, H. (1985). "Schizophrenia: Etiology." In H. I. Kaplan & B. J. Sadock (Eds.), *Comprehensive Textbook of Psychiatry*, 4th ed. Baltimore, MD: Williams and Wilkins.

CHAPTER TWO

Expanded Family Theory: Contributing Theories and Concepts

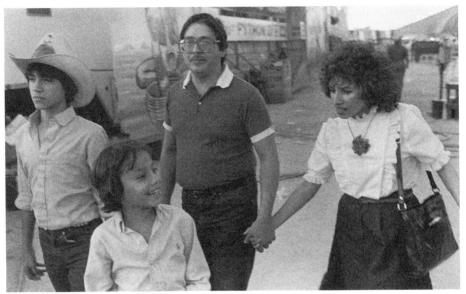

© Frank Siteman MCMLXXXII

Traditions are group efforts to keep the unexpected from happening.

Mignor McLaughlin

In order to understand family dynamics, one must look at family life from several vantage points and draw from several contributing theories. Each contributing theory contains concepts that focus and clarify data. Although generally assigned to a specific framework, the concepts often overlap and reinforce one another. Therefore, concepts drawn from various theoretical frameworks may be used to increase the health professional's assessment and intervention skills. Any theoretical framework may be used to provide a focus, but restricting oneself to a single framework is limiting because each tends to emphasize some aspects of family life at the expense of other aspects. In this chapter the following theoretical frameworks are described and applied to family life:

Developmental
Structural
Functional
Psychodynamic
Communication
Learning

Concepts related to each theoretical framework are placed within the framework within which they were developed, although some concepts might correctly be placed in any of several frameworks. In organizing this chapter, the preferences of contributing theorists were followed even though arbitrary distinctions were sometimes necessary. What is important for health professionals working with families is to understand the nature and implications of various concepts, regardless of the theoretical framework that claims them, and to apply the concepts accurately so as to assess family interaction and promote healthy change (Constantine, 1986).

FAMILY DEVELOPMENT

Developmental theory helps in assessing the family as it exists over time, moving from one chronological stage to the next. Each stage introduces new

[28]

tasks and responsibilities for individual members and for the family as a system. Inherent in developmental theory is the idea that each life cycle task is best completed within a critical time period if succeeding tasks are to be accomplished successfully (Erikson, 1963). The impetus for family development is the growth and maturation of individual members as they move from one life stage to the next. Individual maturation and development result from the convergence (meeting) of three important factors operating on the individual: (1) physical maturation, (2) social and cultural expectations, and (3) individual values and aspirations. These three powerful factors induce the individual to confront the life cycle task of a particular stage. Erikson described the convergence of these factors as a period of "ascendance" when circumstances are most favorable for completion of the critical task. Table 2.1 shows Erikson's eight individual critical tasks.

Beyond the life cycle tasks of individual members, the family has its own developmental transitions to make. Family transitions, like those of individuals, are chronological and sequential. A major contributor to family developmental theory is Evelyn Duvall (1977) who formulated an eight-stage model of the family life cycle similar to the individual life cycle model proposed by Erikson. In explaining the time period during which conditions

TABLE 2.1. Comparison of Duvall's Family Critical Tasks and Erikson's Individual Critical Tasks

Family Stages and Critical Tasks	Individual Critical Tasks
Marital stage: Establishing a marriage	Trust versus mistrust
Childbearing stage: Adjusting to parenthood and maintaining a home	Autonomy versus shame and doubt
Preschool stage: Nurturing children	Initiative versus guilt
School-age stage: Socializing and educating children	Industry versus inferiority
Teenage stage: Balancing teenagers' freedom and responsibility	Identity versus role confusion
Launching stage: Releasing children as young adults; developing postparental interests	Intimacy versus isolation
Middle-aged stage: Reestablishing the marital dyad; maintaining links with older and younger generations	Generativity versus stagnation
Aging stage: Adjusting to retirement, aging, loneliness, and death	Ego integrity versus despair

Source: Adapted from Duvall (1977) and Erikson (1963).

are most favorable for accomplishing a life cycle task, Duvall applied the term "teachable moment." Duvall divided family development into two broad phases: (1) the expanding phase and (2) the contracting phase. The expanding phase lasts from the joining of the marital pair until children are reared, launched, and leave home. The contracting phase begins when the first child leaves home and ends with the death of the surviving spouse. Figure 2.1 shows the family life cycle as conceptualized by Duvall.

By contrasting the eight stages of the family life cycle with the eight stages of the individual life cycle, it is possible to foresee potential difficulties. In the best circumstances the family provides a wholesome, suppor-

FIGURE 2.1. **Developmental Directional Guidelines**

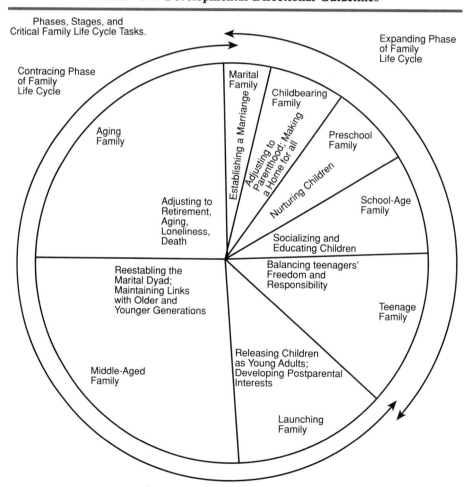

Source: Adapted from Duvall (1977).

tive environment where each member has ample opportunity for growth and receives needed material, physical, and emotional support. Sometimes, however, families are unwilling or unready to adjust to the changing needs of members, and resist the completion of individual critical tasks. For example, the critical task of a teenager is to begin to separate from parental influence. The separation process may proceed at a rate too rapid for parents to accept, perhaps because they are reluctant to exchange the characteristics of a school-age family for those of a teenage family. Similar resistance may be seen in a younger couple moving from the relatively carefree habits of a marital family to the responsibilities of a childbearing family. Many such couples require assistance and reassurance as they make this transition. If they fail to accomplish the transition successfully, their young children may not move toward trust and autonomy, the first individual tasks in Erikson's scheme of things.

A health professional using the developmental approach to assess families might begin by identifying the family's life cycle stage and then note the progress of individual members in achieving their critical tasks. If the family is inflexible and resists change, assessment should include a search for the source of resistance. Sometimes merely teaching families the importance of stage-appropriate critical tasks reduces their anxiety about change and thereby reduces family resistance. It must be noted that a usual family life cycle consisting of phases of expansion and contraction is experienced differently by persons who confront successive stages of estrangement, separation, divorce, single parenting or coparenting, remarriage, and stepparenting. Less traditional family life stages are shown in Figure 2.2.

FIGURE 2.2. Life Cycle Model of Marriage, Divorce, and Remarriage

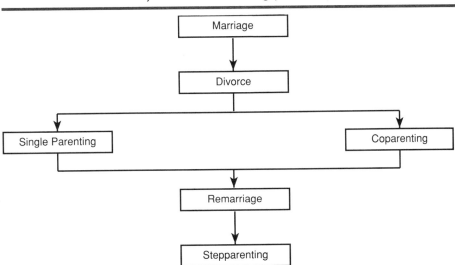

According to Carter and McGoldrick (1980), family development is more than the current relationships between adults and children who happen to be connected by ties of blood, marriage, or commitment. Beyond the different life cycle stages of its members, the family itself engages in an interdependent process of task and emotional change over time. Not all families manage to move easily from one transitional stage to the next. Usually some members move willingly, even eagerly, from one stage to the next, but other members are reluctant to give up customary behaviors that are no longer necessary or appropriate. In addition to the ever-changing needs of individual members within the family, the entry or departure of any member may create conditions of stress.

Stage One Tasks: The Marital Family

For organizational purposes, the families discussed in this chapter are assumed to follow heterosexual, marital norms. In later chapters variations of family forms are discussed at length. When a couple decides to establish a new family, they bring with them customs and habits learned in their respective families of origin. An early task of the couple is to relinquish some ingrained habits learned in their original families and negotiate new ways of thinking and interacting. As new allegiance develops, attachment to the family of origin changes, causing shifts within the original families of both partners. The couple must make decisions about the quantity and quality of transactions with their original families, and about maintaining old friendships that are meaningful to only one of the partners. If the new relationship is to be mutually rewarding, compromise is essential. If one partner is more committed to the original family than to the new one, or if one original family resists the weakening of previous ties, conflict may result. Forging strong allegiance to the new family does not require either partner to break ties with the family of origin; it does mean that the ties will be maintained in a different way. Much depends on the attitudes of the original families, particularly if they are very intrusive. Ideally, the original families should not believe that they have lost a son or daughter, but that they have eased their children through life cycle stages and released them to responsible adulthood.

In these days of working women and dual-career marriages, the allocation of household responsibilities is another sphere that must be negotiated in new families. The structural family theorist Salvador Minuchin (1974) suggests that all obligations concerning household duties, job demands, and recreational choices be considered and regulated early in a marriage.

Stage Two Tasks: The Childbearing Family

In the second family developmental stage, the marital couple become parents. This stage begins with the birth of the first child and lasts until the child is about three. There is some overlap in the developmental stages of a family when there are several children, but it is the first child who is considered the pathfinder and who introduces family transitions. With subsequent children the family tends to repeat its adjustment patterns, although these may be modified according to the resources of the family and the needs of different children.

The birth of a child drastically changes a couple's life-style and interactions. Some studies indicate a decrease in marital satisfaction after the birth of a child, even when the child is planned and welcome (Tomlinson, 1987). In some families the role of spouse becomes subordinate to the role of parent. When this happens, parents may have to be reminded that the parental role needs to be combined with the marital role. Especially for women, the period immediately after the birth of a child may be very stressful, and attention and solicitude from the father are crucial. It is important for the father to be included in making decisions and planning daily routines. Fathers, as well as mothers, need to bond with the infant; sharing in the care of the infant facilitates bonding between father and child.

Stage Three Tasks: The Preschool Family

Fathers are more involved in parenting activities than was once the case, but generally it is the mother whose life is most changed by the arrival of children. Beginning with pregnancy and throughout the early years of child care, mothers find that their lives are restricted. Even working mothers find that their attention and energy center on children and the home. One result of this is that mothers tend to expect more from family relationships. Because they are so invested in family life, they look to their husbands and children for emotional compensation. When the father is detached and uncommitted to the family, resentment may arise in the mother. Eventually the mother comes to feel unappreciated and unhappy. She may then establish family arrangements that reinforce her overinvolvement with the children and her husband's detachment from the family.

Stage Four Tasks: The School-Age Family

The entry of a child not only alters the relationship between the partners, but also alters the interactions between the nuclear and the extended family. New roles evolve for which norms and patterns are established. Siblings of the parents become aunts and uncles; parents of the couple become grandparents, who may approve or criticize the way a grandchild is being raised. As the first child enters school, the parents usually engage more actively in community life. Again, this requires adjustments on the part of the parents and the extended family, who may worry that their influence is diminished by community input. The way families deal with the school years of their children may contribute or detract from the children's sense of competence and mastery. Thomas and Chess (1977, 1980) state that children flourish when the child-rearing practices of the family are compatible with the values upheld by the school and the community. Unless family arrangements reflect school and community standards, children must repeatedly adapt to conditions at home that are not encountered elsewhere.

Stage Five Tasks: The Teenage Family

This family stage begins when the oldest child enters the teens. During the preceding years the family has experienced many changes. New siblings have probably entered the family. Aunts and uncles may have moved away; grandparents may have retired, relocated, or died. Inevitably there have been recurring periods of adjustment and reorganization. As teenagers struggle with their task of establishing identity, parents struggle with the dilemma of granting independence to teenagers for whom they still feel responsible. By this time parents are accustomed to guiding and nurturing their children and find it hard to give up control. In many families this is a stage of conflict and upheaval as parents and teenagers search for a balance between dependence and independence. The teenage period may usher in a new freedom for parents, some of whom will embrace this freedom while other distrust it. The physical care of teenagers is less arduous, but their psychological needs continue. In functional families parents deal with the outward movement of children by finding new outlets or by strengthening the marital relationship.

Stage Six Tasks: The Launching Family

This stage begins when the oldest child leaves the family home and lasts until the youngest child leaves. In families with several children, this is a prolonged period during which parent–child relationships gradually change. At this point children may be physically mature and yearn for independence but must still look to their parents for financial support. Parents are used to giving to their children but also to exerting control over their actions. It is obviously harder to relinquish control if the giving continues. The task of launching parents is to foster the physical and psychological strengths that enable children to leave the family home and cope reasonably well with adult life. Family observers describe the parenting role at this stage as one of standing on the sidelines, watching but not actively participating, and being interested and available to their adult children only when help is really needed. Many launching parents deal with the launching stage by drawing closer to one another. The "first fine careless rapture" of the early marital partnership may have dissipated, but the parents now have time to replenish their relationship if they are so inclined. Reinvesting in the marital relationship is a useful way of handling the separation and individuation of the children.

Stage Seven Tasks: The Middle-Aged Family

Families enter middle age when the last child leaves home, and they continue in this stage until one or both partners retire from active employment. This was once considered a period of great trial for women, but as more women have become part of the labor force or embarked on careers, this period often is marked by excitement and productivity. A number of investigators have found this stage to be one of increased personal and marital satisfaction, although there are notable exceptions (George, 1980; Lauer & Lauer, 1987).

At this time new roles are likely to be imposed on the partners as they become in-laws and grandparents. Just as their own children have become independent, the partners see new needs emerge as their own parents enter the declining years. The partners then must respond as the oldest generation looks to the middle-aged partners for assistance. The term *sandwich generation* has been coined for middle-aged people who must care for elderly parents just when they look forward to more leisure and less responsibility. Even so, this is a period marked by fairly high levels of satisfaction (Ryff, 1986; Neugarten, 1973).

Stage Eight Tasks: The Aging Family

Beginning with the retirement of one or both partners, this stage continues until both have died. Loss is a frequent theme at this stage of family life. For individuals who found satisfaction in the work role, retirement means a partial loss of identity. Almost always retirement means a less active, more limited life, as the strength of work associations lessens over time. After retirement many persons search for new outlets and new interests, but this is not always the case. There are two points of view on the aging process: the activity theory and the disengagement theory. In the activity theory, elderly people are urged to continue the activities of middle age as long as possible and to find substitute activities for those that are no longer within their ability to perform. Advocates of the disengagement theory believe that society inevitably makes fewer demands on elderly persons and gives them fewer opportunities for self-expression and productivity. Therefore, the disengagement of the elderly is not unilateral but is a response to the way they are treated. This does not mean that disengagement should be forced upon elderly persons, but they should have a choice in the matter. It should be remembered that there are many elderly people who found little satisfaction in the work role and gladly renounce the demands of the labor market. For these persons detachment may be a pleasure not available to them during their younger, hard-working lives. Some elderly people may appreciate continued activity and involvement but others are content with quiet lives and find contentment in solitude and inactivity (Kermis, 1986; Baltes & Brim, 1980).

Evers (1985), in a study of elderly women, identified two distinct groups: passive responders and active initiators. The active initiators either began new interests late in life or maintained old ones, and felt a sense of purpose and involvement. The passive responders reported a lack of purpose and control in their lives. Most of them were women who had worked hard all their lives but received little monetary or social reward. This lack of recognition in earlier years adversely affected their enjoyment of life and involvement later on.

FAMILY STRUCTURE

Every family is organized in a structural fashion that governs how family members relate to one another, when they relate, and with whom. Family structure reflects family function by controlling space and closeness between members. The organizing structure of the family establishes consistent interactional patterns that help control tension levels. Family structure makes some amount of stability and predictability possible. At times the organizing structure of the family causes resentment in some members. For example, if one child is the mother's favorite, the other members know how the mother and this child are likely to interact. Recognizing the interactional pattern may frustrate the less preferred children but may also help them cope with the extremely strong bonds between the mother and the favorite child. One reaction of the siblings might be to exclude the favorite child, thus reinforcing that child's closeness to the mother. Like other aspects of family life, structure is not a constant but is subject to modification as members enter or leave the family unit. Even when the composition of the family remains the same, structure changes as various family members progress through their individual life cycles.

Families begin with two partners who make a formal commitment to each other. Every person is protected by boundaries that surround the self. When partners form a family, the boundaries that mark and protect their individuality must be flexible enough and open enough to admit another person. The formation of a family unites the partners and transforms separate people into a marital system. As children arrive, the marital system becomes a parental subsystem, with the children forming a sibling subsystem. Together the two subsystems constitute the family. If there are several children in the family, there may be more than one sibling subsystem based on age or gender. In some families the males may constitute one subsystem and the females another. Usually each family member belongs to more than one subsystem. In families where gender differences are very important, the mother may be part of the marital subsystem but also part of the female subsystem in the household. Subsystems are usually formed by naturally occurring differences, and in functional families they help members relate in an orderly way. In dysfunctional families natural boundaries tend to be less respected. Instead of subsystem structure, dysfunctional families rely on alliances and coalitions based on contrived or artificial divisions. An illustration of this is a coalition consisting of mother and children that excludes the father.

Natural boundaries uphold family and subsystem well-being. Boundaries surrounding the family, its subsystems, and individual members should be strong enough to be protective but permeable enough to permit exchange and feedback between members and subsystems, and between the family and the community. When boundaries between family members are diffuse (weak), excessive closeness develops so that separation and individuation are threatened. Family members then become enmeshed or overly involved with one another. This may be comfortable for some family members, but it threatens the autonomy and freedom of individual members. When boundaries around the family and between the family and the community are so rigid that they cannot be penetrated, the result is disengagement from each other and isolation of the family from the community that surrounds it.

Structural Therapeutic Guidelines

Minuchin (1974) is a prominent advocate of structural family theory. He believes that active therapeutic intervention makes it possible to restructure maladaptive families. The following guidelines are based on structural concepts formulated by Minuchin:

Restructuring Operations	Therapeutic Guidelines
Guiding family transactional patterns	Listen but do not accept the family's verbal descriptions of their interaction. Observe ways the family operates to resolve conflict, make decisions, support or attack each other. Note alliances and coalitions that support some members at the expense of others.
Recreating communication channels	Minimize the role of the health professional as referee. Insist that members speak only for themselves, and talk directly to each other rather than talk about each other.

Restructuring Operations	*Therapeutic Guidelines*
Manipulating space	Use seating arrangements to strengthen natural subsystem boundaries and challenge dysfunctional coalitions and alliances. If an older son, for example, has replaced father in the marital subsystem, arrange seating in the therapeutic session so that mother and father must interact directly rather than through the son. If the health professional wants to inhibit interaction between members of an alliance or coalition, the professional might take a seat between them or break up the alliance by seating family members along natural boundary lines.
Marking boundaries: Individual and subsystem	Family boundaries should be flexible, not rigid, protective but penetrable. Differentiate family members according to their roles and position in the family. Emphasize the right of individual members to be different. Strengthen partners in their parental functions. Help parents make demands and grant privileges appropriate to the developmental level of each child. Challenge the inappropriate placement of any member in a subsystem where he does not naturally belong. Work selectively with different family subsystems to improve boundaries and boundary management.
Relabeling problem behaviors	Recognize the tolerance of family members for stress and confrontation. Relabel behavior that the family considers negative so that positive aspects can be identified. A father's excessive attention to his job, for example, might be in-

Restructuring Operations	*Therapeutic Guidelines*
	terpreted as an expression of love and caring for his family rather than a sign of neglect.
Assigning tasks and homework	Within the therapeutic session a monopolizing member may be asked to be silent, or a silent member to speak. At home the family might be forbidden to argue during the dinner hour and to discuss only noncontroversial subjects. Emphasis on task assignment depersonalizes friction and exchanges positive activity for blaming tactics.

FAMILY FUNCTION

Family structure refers to how a family is organized; family function refers to how a family operates. Structure and function are interdependent and influence each other in many ways. For example, in families where there is a male subsystem and a female subsystem, tasks are likely to be differentiated according to gender. In functional families where most of the needs of members are being met, natural family boundaries are maintained, and the parental subsystem consists of two partners with strong ties to one another. Closeness between the partners is a structural concept that contributes to effective family functioning. In a sense, boundaries enforce rules concerning subsystems, who belongs in the system, and how subsystems interact with other subsystems. Boundaries also monitor exchanges of information and interaction between the family and larger social systems in the community. Extremely rigid boundaries inhibit exchanges between family members or across subsystems. This means that there is little caring in the family because members disengage from each other. At the other extreme, families with diffuse boundaries are characterized by excessive involvement and intrusiveness. Thus, boundaries maintain balance in the family and promote adaptation to change unless they are overly rigid or diffuse. They regulate exchanges of energy and information according to the families' ability to cope. In stressful situations, families may be able to tolerate little interaction with the surrounding environment and reduce input from outside sources. This might occur just after the death of a member, when the family withdraws in order to grieve. When there is illness in the family, however, input from outside sources may be needed. When boundaries are too rigid, the family may not receive needed help simply because the extent of need is not known outside the family.

A triangle is another structural concept that influences family function. According to Murray Bowen, the triangle is the basic molecule of the family. Whenever relationships between two family members become difficult, one of them will propel or "triangle" a third person into the relationship to reduce tension. A wife who feels unappreciated may turn toward a son to fulfill her needs. This impairs the development of the son but reduces the distress of the mother, allowing the father to continue his behaviors. Often the father is content to leave things as they are, but sometimes the father becomes aware of his isolation and moves toward the son, thus compounding the problem by becoming his wife's rival for the son's affection. Ideally, the father would react to feelings of isolation by moving closer to his wife, but in dysfunctional families this rarely happens without outside intervention.

Triangling is not confined to interactions between two human beings. The classic triangle consists of a husband, a wife, and a lover, but the spouse who is totally preoccupied with a career or develops a drinking problem creates a different kind of triangle. In the first instance the third part of the triangle is the job; in the second instance alcoholism is part of the triangle. The solution to a dysfunctional triangle is known as *detriangulation*. Often this is a complex, prolonged process for which therapeutic guidelines are presented later in the chapter.

Functional aspects of family life are the concern of Bowen (1971, 1974, 1976), whose work centers on the emotional life of families. Among Bowen's concepts dealing with assessment of family function are nuclear family emotional system, differentiation of self, multigenerational transmission, family constellation, family projection, and societal regression.

Nuclear Family Emotional System

In some families the members do not see themselves as separate individuals but as persons emotionally joined or fused together. The result of family fusion is that members do not think, speak, or act for themselves. Thoughts, words, and actions are not individualized; even feelings are not attributed to a single member but are experienced by everyone. Family fusion creates a shared or "undifferentiated" ego which makes it difficult for family members to identify clearly what they think and how they feel. Confusion arises between what an individual member actually thinks and feels about an issue and what other members think and feel. Family thoughts and feelings that are always shared and never individualized then become confusing and distorted. Confusion and distortion further hinder the ability of individual members and of the whole family to handle decisions and problems.

Emotional Cutoff

This term is used to describe the detachment from the family of origin that should occur when a nuclear family is formed. When deep attachment to the original family continues after a new family is established, conditions of emotional dependency persist. Prolonged or profound attachment to the family of origin can become a source of contention in the new family. Only when the partners are committed to each other and moderate their emotional dependency on their original family can they move toward autonomy and maturity.

Differentiation of Self

Self-differentiation is a process that requires individuals to separate emotionally from their families of origin. In some respects self-differentiation is similar to emotional cutoff, but it is a far broader concept. Self-differentiation does not bar interaction with families of origin, but it expects the emotional forces in the original family not to dominate the adult members who have left the home. Bowen distinguished between the "solid self" and the "pseudoself." He formulated a differentiation of self scale, with the solid self at one extreme and the pseudoself at the other, as shown in Figure 2.3. One's place on the continuum is determined by the degree of self-differentiation that has been attained. Bowen believes that one's extent of self-differentiation is not fixed but may move in either direction over the life cycle.

The solid self is composed of ingrained, rational principles that evolve gradually and change as an individual learns or fails to learn from life experiences. Because the solid self is rational and intrinsic, it does not submit easily to outside pressures. The pseudoself, on the other hand, is neither rational nor intrinsic, and depends on outside sources. A simpler explanation is that the solid self is internally directed, whereas the pseudoself is externally directed. Persons who remain dominated by the emotional climate of their family of origin usually occupy a place near the pseudoself end of the self-differentiation scale. Such persons tend to react more on emotional than on rational levels. In determining relative degrees of solid selfhood or pseudoselfhood, the health professional notes whether an individual is operating primarily on a thinking or on a feeling level. This does not mean that all emotional reactions must be suppressed but, rather, that feelings should be integrated and regulated by cognitive processes.

The self-differentiation scale is not a precise measure, but it provides impressionistic data to guide assessment and planning. The nuclear family emotional system and self-differentiation are complementary. Every person brings to new relationships remnants of behaviors and attitudes learned in the original family. Out of habit, one partner may choose to enact a domi-

FIGURE 2.3. Comparison of Pseudoself and Solid Self

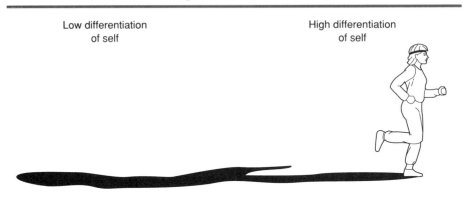

Low differentiation of self   High differentiation of self

Pseudoself:	Solid self:
Automatic responses	Self-directed
Subjective reactions	Objective reactions
Emotional dependence	Rational
Low self-identity	Flexible
High vulnerability to stress	High self-identity
High incidence of illness	Good coping skills
Prone to recurrent crisis	Lower incidence of illness

Source: Adapted from Bowen (1971, 1974, 1976).

nant role and the other a subservient role. A balance may exist for a while, but it is a fragile one. For instance, the illness of the dominant partner may cause disorganization when the subservient partner cannot discharge new responsibilities. When both partners are competitive, they may vie for dominance and conflict may ensue. Conflict may take the form of open hostility between the partner or emotional distancing between them, or in the projection of conflict onto one or more children. In utilizing the concept of self-differentiation, the health professional works on a cognitive level to promote self-awareness, emotional separation from the original family, and the substitution of reason for unbridled emotion.

Multigenerational Transmission

Multigenerational transmission is the means by which certain family values, attitudes, and behaviors persist across generations. Multigenerational transmission helps explain the devotion of certain families to specific occupations or pursuits, such as politics or music. Bowen connects intergenerational transmission to self-differentiation, explaining that families can move toward or away from self-differentiation from one generation to another. After several generations of decreasing self-differentiation in families, dysfunctional patterns such as triangling or projection become dominant. Eventually the psychological development of some family members is so impaired that they are at risk for psychiatric disorders of one kind or another.

Family Constellation

It is generally accepted that sibling rank and order in the family have an effect on achievement and personality. Toman (1976) suggests that sibling positions, gender differences, and family configurations influence the personality traits and social tendencies of children. In addition to being an only child or one of twins, Toman listed these significant family positions:

Oldest brother of brother(s)
Youngest brother of brothers(s)
Oldest brother of sister(s)
Youngest brother of sister(s)
Oldest sister of sister(s)
Youngest sister of sister(s)
Oldest sister of brother(s)
Youngest sister of brother(s)

The concept of family constellation makes certain assumptions about behavior and personality development. One assumption is that oldest siblings tend to be more directive and responsible, whereas youngest siblings tend to be more dependent and willing to take direction. Family constellation is a very broad concept and one that should be applied with care. It may be useful as part of a provisional assessment, but it does not take into account relevant family history. Therefore, assumptions should be validated in order to note exceptions to generalizations about sibling positions and family constellation (Hoopes & Harper, 1987).

Family Projection

In family projection the parents deal with conflict and anxiety by unconsciously transmitting or projecting their feelings to a selected target, usually a child. The child then becomes a magnet drawing attention from one or both parents. Frequently one parent is very involved with the child, and this involvement may cost the child the affection of the second parent and arouse the jealously of siblings. When parental feelings are projected to a target child, the parents can avoid the need to deal with problems that exist between them. Problem solving is avoided but at the expense of the child. In some instances the target child is self-selected. A child who is dimly aware of problems between the parents may begin to engage in aggressive or withdrawn behavior that is unacceptable to the parents. The parents then join forces to deal with the child's behavior, without addressing their own conflicts that are the underlying cause of the child's behavior. In dealing with the child, one parent usually remains overly involved but is joined by the parent who was previously uninterested.

Societal Regression

Just as families must strive for rationality, so society at large must strive to avoid regressive, dysfunctional behavior. Stressful conditions contribute to family breakdown, and stressful conditions such as crop failure, economic fluctuation, war, and catastrophe contribute to social breakdown. When this happens, political and social decisions are made for emotional reasons that worsen the problems. One example of societal regression is the massive internment of Japanese Americans during World War II, when the civil rights of a minority group were abruptly suspended. The concept of societal regression is important because all families reflect the conditions of the society that surrounds them. Poverty, crime, and industrial obsolescence are a few of the negative forces that contribute to societal regression.

Roles and Role Enactment

Role theory utilizes structural and functional concepts. If roles are defined as family positions determined by closeness and distance between members, then roles are part of family structure. When role performance or role enactment is being assessed, then role theory is part of family function. This ambiguity means that role theory is a bridge between family structure and family function. Role enactment in families may be assigned or ascribed to family members because of who they are, irrespective of family preferences or individual abilities. The husband/father role is assigned to the male who is the marital partner and has sired the children. Not too many years ago, the husband/father was expected to be the chief breadwinner, the head of the household, and the major decision maker, but this is less true today. In contemporary families both parents are likely to work outside the home and to share earning responsibilities and decision-making powers. When the husband/father is absent from the family, whatever the cause, the role enactment expected of him is carried out by the mother, perhaps with the help of one or more children. When role enactment is carried out by family members not usually associated with that role, this is called *achieved* rather than assigned or ascribed role performance (Parsons, 1951; Lambert & Lambert, 1984).

Structural variations in contemporary families have reduced enactment of assigned roles in favor of enactment of achieved roles. In other words, role performance in present-day families depends more on who is able and available to perform family tasks than on who should be performing them. Many families operate largely through achieved role performance, but there are hazards to this. A single parent trying to fulfill both parental roles may often feel overwhelmed. Children in the family may be expected to assume parenting responsibilities for which they are unprepared. Maturation, aptitude, readiness, and experience are factors that affect role performance. However, in dual-career families, single-parent families, and stepparent (remarried) families there may be few choices. Here the survival of the family may depend almost entirely on the enactment of achieved rather than assigned roles.

Functional Therapeutic Guidelines

The following therapeutic guidelines are based on the assessment of family function and suggest interventions designed to redistribute family functions so as to foster adaptive change.

Functional Redistribution	*Therapeutic Guidelines*
Promoting detriangulation	Identify any family triangle that has replaced the marital relationship. Encourage the removal of any third person or object that triangles the marital dyad.
Supporting the nuclear family emotional system	Assess the attachment of each partner to his or her original family. Note the results of excessively close ties to the family of origin. Reinforce attachment and commitment to the nuclear family. Reassure partners that emotional separation from the family of origin does not mean total separation.
Differentiating the self	Analyze the degree of self-differentiation of the partners and the extent to which self-differentiation is tolerated in family members. Use the more rational behavior of self-differentiated members to decrease the emotional behavior of the others.

Functional Redistribution	*Therapeutic Guidelines*
Examining multigenerational transmission	Explore cross-generational patterns that set the tone of family life. Note any customs present in the original families that have been transmitted to the nuclear family. Are the transmitted customs intact or modified? If they are modified, the nuclear family has moved toward differentiation.
Tracing the family constellation	Examine sibling rank and order; note how these influence family functioning. Determine whether operational patterns based on the family constellation enhance or inhibit the development of any member.
Redirecting family projection	Assess the interactions between the parents and a child who is the object of excessive concern, either favorable or unfavorable. Explore the function served by a child who absorbs the emotion generated between parents. Look for reasons that a target child has been selected.
Monitoring societal regression	Uncover social factors that may support or adversely affect family functioning. Help the family mobilize internally to deal with regressive social forces. Discourage tendencies of family members to blame themselves for circumstances beyond their control.
Promoting effective role enactment	Compare assigned role performance and achieved role performance in the family. Does current role performance facilitate family functioning? Determine whether current role enactment is rigid and inflexible or diffuse and vague. Encourage cooperation and negotiation on how family roles are performed. Use specific rather than general terms when discussing role performance.

FAMILY PSYCHODYNAMICS

To understand family dynamics it is necessary to explain several concepts derived from psychoanalytic theory and apply them to family life. Essential to the psychoanalytic framework is the conflict between the desires of individuals to belong and yet remain separate. The struggle most people experience in relating to others without sacrificing their own identity is intensified in many families. Freud (1949) described opposing desires for nurture and for independence as instinctual drives. Actually, it does not matter much whether these opposing drives originate in instinctual forces or not. What matters in family theory is that opposing drives exist in many people, and their presence complicates family interaction.

Functional families nurture their members but accept separateness and individual differences. Dysfunctional families do not tolerate differences and expect conformity from all members. Wynne et al. (1958) described a type of interaction in which a surface harmony was preserved even if this denied identity and selfhood to family members. A family characterized by false harmony, or pseudomutuality as Wynne called it, values compliance more than individuality and may stifle the free expression of its members. Similarly, the term *pseudohostility* is applied to families that bicker and wrangle in order to avoid intimacy and involvement. Even though argument is frequent in such families, they rarely deal with genuine issues, but use arguments to avoid authentic conflict resolution. Pseudomutuality and pseudohostility are destructive but are beyond the conscious awareness of families who need help in changing these interactional patterns.

The concepts of pseudomutuality and pseudohostility are useful in assessing families, and help health professionals analyze family interaction and develop working hypotheses. A health professional might first identify the prevailing style of family interaction and then ask certain questions. If the family appears harmonious but has many problems, one might ask oneself whose rights are being sacrificed to maintain peace. In quarrelsome families one might ask oneself what the real problem is and what the real goals of the contenders are. Are family members confronting each other honestly, or are side issues being used to sidestep the real problem? The answers to these questions enable the health professional to construct hypotheses that facilitate therapeutic planning and intervention.

An example of pseudohostility is evident in the actions of a mother who resents her husband's indifference to the substance abuse of their son. She berates her husband for his indifference, but when he tries to intervene, the wife shelters and protects the son. By isolating the father from the son, the wife gains the favor of the son. Because she is truly worried about the son's behavior, she alternately rescues the son and complains about him to the father. At the same time she blames her husband for not being a better father and attributes the son's delinquency to the father's shortcomings. Anger rages in the family, but the mother's inconsistency and interference are the crux of the problem. If this were a family where harmony was highly valued, mother, father, and son might join in a pretense that substance abuse was not present. In another family the substance abuse of the son might unite the parents in a common cause, so that the son's actions, while personally destructive, would benefit his parents who have little to keep them together except shared concern for their son.

Rubber Fences

Though considered part of psychodynamic family theory, the concept of "rubber fences" has structural and functional overtones. Rubber fences are unreliable, elastic boundaries that surround an emotional field in which family rules and actions continually change. As a result, family members never know what is acceptable or unacceptable to the family. The emotional climate within the family is one of secrecy, disorder, and bewilderment, so that members have little sense of stability (Wynne, 1978).

Psychodynamic Therapeutic Guidelines

The following therapeutic guidelines are based on the assessment of family psychodynamics and suggest interventions that challenge dysfunctional psychodynamic patterns in the family.

Family Psychodynamics	Therapeutic Guidelines
Challenging pseudohostility and pseudomutuality	Observe the collective emotional life of the family. Determine if family interaction is characterized by pseudohostility or by pseudomutuality.
	Analyze the nature of family quarreling and of family harmony. What family problems are avoided by constant confrontation or by refusal to confront?
	Which family member is pivotal to the preservation of harmony or the eruption of hostility in the family?
Reshaping rubber fences	What rules and values are sometimes upheld and sometimes ignored in the family? Which member(s) contribute most to family inconsistency and confusion?
	Point out inconsistencies in the family's values and attitudes. Encourage the family to move toward stability and consistency in adhering to certain rules and values.

FAMILY COMMUNICATION

All family interactions and transactions depend on communication patterns. In using communication patterns to assess families, the health professional observes the process by which messages are sent, received, validated, and answered. The therapeutic goal is to improve communication so that messages are clear and meaningful to all family members. Communication theorists conceptualize family operations in terms of communication patterns. The process of communication (how messages are sent and received) is just as important as the content of communication (what messages are sent and received).

Communication patterns consist of a message and a response. It is impossible not to respond to a message, but the response need not be verbal. Silence is a response to a message, as is refusal to answer the ring of a phone. Though not verbalized, such responses denote an emotional or cognitive message. In some families communication patterns are strong and durable. For example, some children rarely make direct requests of the father but prefer to use the mother as an intermediary.

Communication theorists emphasize that the messages sent are not always the same messages that are received. Three modifying factors that intrude on communication have been identified: (1) cognition, (2) power and (3) emotion.

Communication and Cognition

Jackson and Lederer (1967) state that family communication is governed by norms and standards that operate within certain limits. Theirs is a cognitive analysis of how families communicate. One concept identified by Jackson and Lederer is *equifinality*, which explains that the same family assessment will be made regardless of its timing. As an illustration, consider a family in which the wife is a worrier and the husband a happy-go-lucky person. Over the years the husband and wife may reverse their behaviors, but the outlines of family communication are unchanged because the partnership still contains a worrier and a nonworrier. The worrying of one partner frees the other from a need to worry; equifinality thus demonstrates the reciprocal, interlocking nature of family communication and interaction.

A cognitive therapeutic strategy often used is *relabeling* or reframing, as it is sometimes called. Relabeling takes behavior that the family considers negative and emphasizes its positive aspects. For example, the unacceptable actions of a youngster might be presented as a cry for love, or the controlling behavior of a husband might be interpreted as an expression of caring.

Communication and Power

Power is a troublesome issue in many human relationships, especially when power is unequally distributed. Haley (1971) referred to unequal relationships between people as *complementary* and to equal relationships as *sym-*

metrical. When a relationship is complementary, one person occupies a superior position and one occupies an inferior position, with the person in the superior position having more power. Relationships between teachers and students or between employers and workers are usually complementary. Power tends to be shared by persons who are in symmetrical relationships, but occasionally a struggle for dominance occurs. Haley does not blame either member of a symmetrical relationship for a power struggle but suggests that the entire family is involved. A health professional adopting Haley's approach would guide and teach the family about power struggles in the family, and help members negotiate an equitable sharing of power among themselves.

Communication and Emotion

Satir et al. (1977) direct attention to how family members feel about one another, and contend that the causes of family dysfunction are to be found in the marital relationship. Assessment therefore starts with the marital dyad. At one time both partners believed their needs could be met in their relationship. Because they are no longer sustained by this belief, it is important to review family events so as to understand what happened. Taking a family history or chronology has two advantages. It reminds the partners of what they once found in each other and it compares two different sets of expectations and memories.

A fundamental belief of Satir is that low self-esteem is the chief obstacle to family happiness. Where the self-esteem of one or both partners is deficient, rising levels of tension and anxiety surface. Relationships can only be healthy when the participants think well of themselves. In order to develop adequate self-esteem, people need reassurance that they are valued for themselves. Unless they were loved and nurtured in their original families, they are unlikely to offer love and acceptance to members of their nuclear family. Satir does not discount the importance of cognition, but insists that to understand thinking one must also understand what oneself and others are feeling.

Three ideas are important in Satir's approach to family assessment:

1. Everyone wants to be valued and to be close to significant people. All behavior is aimed at achieving these ends.
2. Behavior that seems bizarre or "crazy" is usually an attempt to transmit distress signals to others.
3. Thoughts and emotions are closely connected; to understand thoughts, one must get in touch with what oneself and others are feeling.

Satir considers it essential for family members to be able to express their needs and feelings honestly, but with consideration for the needs and feelings of others. She identifies several dysfunctional forms of family communication. Dysfunctional communication forms are described as follows:

Communication Form	Rationale
Blaming	Family members fear being blamed and therefore assign blame for error or failure to someone else.
Placating	Family members pretend to be inadequate but well-meaning in order to preserve peace at any price.
Generalizing	Family members make general statements using terms like *always* and *never* instead of dealing with specific issues.
Computing	Family members emphasize cognitive and intellectual matters, ignoring emotions in order to seem in control and fully reasonable.
Distracting	Family members introduce irrelevant side issues in order to avoid solving problems.

Satir contends that the husband and wife are the architects of the family and that the source of dysfunction may be found in their relationship. Assessment and intervention therefore are concentrated on the marital dyad.

Double Binds

The concept of double binds was formulated by Bateson, who distinguished between situations that present alternative choices and situations where no choices are available (Bateson et al., 1956). In a double bind situation, a primary command or message is given followed by another command or message that contradicts the first. The message sender tells the recipient, "Do this or you will suffer consequences," but also adds, "Do not do this or you will suffer consequences." When double bind messages are sent repeatedly, the recipient tries to escape the situation and feels frustrated and trapped.

The double bind communication pattern was first identified in the families of schizophrenic persons, but the phenomenon is present in other families as well (Wynne, 1978). Children are often the recipients of double bind messages, although any family member may be victimized by the double bind. The secondary message in the double bind may be nonverbal. A parent might tell a child she has free choice about what to wear, and then show disapproval of how a daughter has dressed. A father might indicate to a son that playing the game is more important than winning but express displeasure when his son's team loses.

People who are frequently subjected to double binds are flooded by mixed feelings. When they fail to comprehend the message, they suspect that something mysterious is going on and try to figure it out. When their bewilderment continues, they may get angry with themselves or with others. They may adopt the attitude that since nothing makes sense, why try to understand? Some react by becoming careful and literal as they try to follow every command, no matter how contradictory. Others simply withdraw from interpersonal involvement in order to reduce their anxiety. Double bind communication is usually beyond the conscious awareness of the message senders, who do not realize the effect their messages have on the recipients. Health professionals are in a good position to identify these contradictory messages and try to teach better modes of communication to family members.

Communication Therapeutic Guidelines

The following therapeutic guidelines are based on the assessment of family communication patterns and suggest interventions and actions aimed at improving dysfunctional family communication.

Family Communication	Therapeutic Guidelines
Analyzing communication patterns	Note preferred communication patterns. Determine whether messages are transmitted directly or indirectly. Identify the family spokesperson or interpreter of family messages. Assess presence and effects of double bind messages.
Replacing control (power) with cooperation	Identify prevailing communication patterns of complementarity and/ or symmetry. Teach family how each prevailing pattern influences communication.
Balancing thinking (cognition) and emotional processes	Help family members separate thought from feeling. Establish communication rules and norms that regulate strong emotion and impose constraints.

Family Communication	*Therapeutic Guidelines*
	Demonstrate how family communication can influence members' self-esteem.
	Promote positive, rational communication by focusing on problem solving and decision making, rather than blaming.
Redirecting communication channels	Teach clear, direct ways of communication by enforcing new rules. Allow no member to speak for another or interpret for another.
	Model respectful listening.
	Acknowledge every member's right to be heard.
	Permit divergent opinions to be heard.

FAMILY LEARNING

Social learning is an ongoing process within families that teaches members how to interact. Within the family, social learning depends on a reward-and-punishment system that may be subtle but is very powerful. A husband, for example, who sees himself as the competent head of the household may complain that his wife is frivolous and immature but may actually prefer that she act like this. He actually needs a childish, dependent mate to reinforce his own self-image. Whenever his wife moves toward autonomy, he resists her, but when she behaves in a scatterbrained manner he is tolerant and indulgent. The result is that the wife continues to behave in ways that please her husband, and their complementary interaction is maintained. The stability of the family is threatened only when one of the partners becomes unwilling or unable to continue to act in the accustomed way.

A great deal of human behavior is learned in the family of origin and transferred to the nuclear family. If conditions in the newly established family are such that the old behavior is valued and rewarded, the behavior will persist. If, however, the old behavior is neither valued nor rewarded, change must ensue; the change may occur in the behavior that is no longer rewarded or in the operations of the nuclear family. For example, a young woman who was the mainstay in her family of origin, who was looked up to and depended on, may continue to act the part of family executive or manager, especially if she is rewarded for this by her husband and children. If, on the other hand, her managing skills are construed as "bossiness" and resented in the nuclear family, she is likely to feel angry and confused. This may induce her to examine her own behaviors and modify them. More often, family managers try to continue their executive behaviors, creating mounting tension. Only if family members can express their feelings and be heard will the manager reduce the behaviors that the nuclear family deems inappropriate. In this instance, the young woman and the nuclear family were, in a sense, victimized by the social learning that had taken place. Because each partner brings to the nuclear family social learning experiences of their original families, exploration and comparison of these experiences may be fruitful. Even partners who have spent years together may not have shared early experiences that markedly influence current interactions. Timidity in one partner and rashness in the other are explainable in terms of social learning. When differences are explained in terms of social learning, partners often become more accepting of each other's actions. The most powerful reinforcers of behavior in family life are social and intangible, for families cannot control factors like pay raises or promotions. A smile, an embrace, or praise may be very effective in producing social learning. Single episodes of reinforcement do not have great impact, but repeated ones have strong effects on human expectations and behavior. Difficulties arise when socially learned behaviors cease to be highly regarded or rewarded, and require modification.

Family Learning Therapeutic Guidelines

Therapeutic guidelines may be formulated and implemented on the basis of the assessment of rewards, modifiers, and extinguishers of social learning in the family. Families are frequently unaware of connections between behaviors and dysfunctional reinforcement of questionable actions.

Family Learning	Therapeutic Guidelines
Exploring social learning in the families of origin	Contrast the divergent experiences of the two partners.
	Point to similarities in social learning.
	Point to differences in social learning.
	Examine ways in which early social experiences influence current behaviors.
Reinforcing social learning of the families of origin	Identify positive attitudes and behaviors that enhance nuclear family life.

Family Learning	*Therapeutic Guidelines*
	Explore ways these positive aspects might be strengthened (rewarded).
Modifying social learning of the families of origin	Identify negative attitudes and behaviors that threaten nuclear family life.
	Explore ways these negative aspects might be modified (extinguished).
Teaching learning theory concepts	Demonstrate use of rewards and punishment in family interactions.
	Promote awareness of connections between rewards, punishment, and family behavior.

INTEGRATED SYSTEMS MODEL

Health professionals working with families are urged to utilize some of the concepts presented in this chapter, depending on their suitability for the family in question. To assist health professionals in developing an integrated method in counseling families, a systems-oriented model is offered that contains an assessment component and an intervention component. For less experienced clinicians or those working with complex family systems, the integrated systems model is likely to be helpful. It is a versatile model that lends itself to appropriate modification. Because the integrated systems model suggests intervention guidelines in addition to assessment guidelines, it leads health professionals beyond assessment into planning and implementation activities.

Integrated Systems Model: Assessment Component

Contributing Theory	Focus	Assessment Questions for the Health Professional
1. Family development	Tasks and transitions	What is the family's life cycle stage?
		What are family members' life cycle tasks at this time?
2. Family structure	Positions and boundaries	What subgroups, alliances, and coalitions exist in the family?
		Are family positions based on natural boundaries and differences?

Integrated Systems Model: Assessment Component (continued)

Contributing Theory	Focus	Assessment Questions for the Health Professional
3. Family function	Roles and behaviors	What roles are present in the family?
		How are roles assigned and enacted?
		Does family role enactment limit or exploit any member?
		Which family member has the most to gain or lose by changed behaviors and role enactment?
4. Family psycho-dynamics	Individuation, interdependence, attachment, separation	Do family attachments permit members' individuation and growth?
		Is separation encouraged, tolerated, or thwarted?
		What attributes of members are highly valued in the family? Conformity? Creativity? Self-expression?
		What is the prevailing emotional climate in the family?
		Who is the most powerful family member?
		Who is the least powerful family member?
5. Family communication	Verbal messages Nonverbal messages	Are verbal messages direct and specific?
		What nonverbal messages are sent?
		Are verbal and nonverbal messages congruent?
		Is there a family spokesperson?
		Whose messages are unheard or disregarded?
6. Family learning	Stimulus-and-response conditioning Rewards	What functional behaviors are rewarded in the family?
		What dysfunctional behaviors are rewarded in the family?

Integrated Systems Model: Intervention Component

Contributing Theory	Therapeutic Guidelines for the Health Professional
1. Family development	Promote family awareness of members' life cycle tasks.
	Call attention to the family's life cycle stage.
	Emphasize the cyclical nature of family life and the need to adapt to change.
2. Family structure	Encourage appropriate psychological space between members.
	Strengthen the marital or parental dyad.
	Reinforce natural boundaries between subgroups.
	Question blurring of natural boundaries.
3. Family function	Encourage consistent, appropriate behavior.
	Question inconsistent, inappropriate role enactment.
	Identify power and control issues. Promote power redistribution, if indicated.
	Foster role enactment consistent with individual and family needs.
4. Family psychodynamics	Encourage awareness of family interdependence.
	Encourage acceptance of individual differences, autonomy, separation, and individuation.
5. Family communication	Question evasion, distortion, and secrecy.
	Teach active listening and sharing.
	Encourage clear, direct, open communication.
	Promote congruence between verbal and nonverbal messages.
6. Family learning	Teach ways of rewarding desirable behaviors and reducing undesirable behaviors.
	Employ learning and behavioral concepts at the family's level of understanding.

The integrated systems model draws on the contributing theories described in this chapter. An overview of these theories and their significant concepts, presented as follows, will assist the health care professional in applying the integrated systems model to assessment and intervention.

Overview of Contributing Theories

Contributing Theory	Concepts	Health and Healing Processes
Developmental theory	Individual life cycle tasks	Identify stage-specific individual tasks.
	Family life cycle tasks	Identify stage-specific family tasks.
		Recognize obstacles to achievement of individual and family tasks.
		Help families negotiate regarding obstacles to achievement of life cycle tasks.

Structural theory	Boundaries:
	  Clear
	  Rigid
	  Diffuse
	Alliances
	Coalitions
	Disengagement
	Enmeshment
		Identify boundary characteristics.
		
		Promote clear boundaries.
		
		Strengthen natural boundaries of subsystems.
		
		Restructure family positions so parents form a parental dyad and children form a sibling subsystem.

Functional theory	Triangles
	Family emotional system
	Emotional cutoff
	Differentiation of self
	Multigenerational transmission
	Family constellation
	Family projection
	Societal regression
	Role enactment
	  Assigned
	  Achieved
		Promote emotional separation from family of origin.
		
		Strengthen emotional ties to nuclear family.
		
		Identify any target child used to absorb parental emotion.
		
		Encourage self-differentiation and toleration of individual differences.
		
		Modify dysfunctional family triangles.
		
		Teach the effects of age, gender, and rank order on various family members.
		
		Discourage regressive family behaviors arising in response to negative social forces.
		
		Encourage rational rather than emotional responses in the family.

Contributing Theory	Concepts	Health and Healing Processes
Psychodynamic theory	Pseudohostility Pseudomutuality Rubber fences	Differentiate genuine harmony from surface harmony. Differentiate conflict around real issues from conflict used to avoid real issues. Identify significant family attitudes and values. Note inconsistencies in family attitudes and values. Promote consistency in family attitudes and values, so as to reduce confusion and instability.

Communication theory	Equifinality
	Complementarity
	Symmetry
	Double binds
	Dysfunctional patterns:
	  Blaming
	  Placating
	  Generalizing
	  Distracting
	  Computing
		Help families recognize complementary and symmetrical interaction.
		Show how one type of interaction maintains another type of interaction, neither of which aids family functioning.
		Encourage specific, clear messages.
		Decrease dependence on a family interpreter or spokesperson.
		Encourage members to speak for themselves.

Learning theory	Rewards and punishment Reinforcement Extinguishment Modification	Utilize stimulus–response interactions to demonstrate how social learning occurs. Help families use reward and punishment techniques to reinforce appropriate behaviors and modify behaviors that are no longer appropriate.

CLINICAL EXAMPLE: THEORY APPLICATION FOR A TROUBLED FAMILY

Jason is a bright little boy enrolled in second grade. Shortly after the start of the school year, Jason's father lost his job as a car salesman and his mother began working as a secretary. Before Joe, Jason's father, became unemployed, this had been a traditional family where the father was the primary provider and Sue, his wife, was a homemaker. Jason is an only child. Both parents are devoted to him, but Jason is especially close to his mother. The role reversal of the parents continues to create problems in the family. Jason goes to sleep hearing his parents quarreling and wakes up to the same sounds. Sometimes Jason thinks that his parents do not sleep at all but spend the nights arguing. Sue's mother is very critical of Joe, insisting that he could get a job if he really tried. She has often said that it is a disgrace for a married woman with a child to work outside the home.

When this situation had gone on for a few weeks, Jason began to resist going to school. Although his father or grandmother was available to care for Jason during the day, he began to cling to his mother, crying and begging her not to go to work. After trying to reason with Jason, Joe would storm out of the house. By this time Jason was hysterical, retching, and out of control. His mother would then stay home from the office in order to stay with Jason. She missed so many days that she was threatened with dismissal. This increased the quarrels between the parents, which in turn made Jason more upset and increased his fears of leaving his mother. In desperation, Sue arranged a joint interview with the school counselor, the school nurse, and Jason's teacher.

In working with this troubled family, a health professional could turn to a number of theoretical approaches, all of which contribute to resolving some aspect of the problem, which Sue and Joe define simply as their son's refusal to go to school.

Developmental Theory

According to Erikson's psychosocial model, Jason is at the stage of resolving conflict between initiative and guilt. As long as his family life was untroubled, he showed initiative and competence at home and at school. Now he misses his mother, who is less available to him, and he has heard his grandmother criticize his jobless father. Jason is unhappy but does not know how to change the situation. His solution is to cling to his mother more than ever, fearing that if he goes to school and she goes to work, he might lose her altogether. The family is at the school-age stage of its expanding period. It is a traditional family whose developmental progress is impeded by Joe's unemployment and the role reversal of the parents.

Psychodynamic Theory

Psychodynamic theory explains Jason's predicament in terms of his strong wish for nurture and his fear of independence. Jason also resists giving up his close attachment to mother in order to identify with father. The quarrels between his parents and the criticisms his grandmother expresses make Jason distrustful of his father. So much has changed at home that Jason is frightened and anxious. As a consequence, his behavior has regressed to infantile levels that cause his mother to hover over him. In the family the collective expectation of all members is that roles should be enacted in traditional, accustomed ways. When this became impossible, Sue and Joe also regressed. Emotional outbursts prevented them from working out their problems. The parents' behaviors perpetuated and exacerbated Jason's anxiety. Staying home from school solves Jason's dilemma temporarily but adds to family tension.

Structural Theory

Jason has always been very close to his mother, but he has been brought up to love and respect his father as well. His fear of going to school stems from his wish to hold on to his mother, but is also an attempt to keep his parents together. However, the result of his behavior is to keep his mother at home but drive his father from the house. The absence of his father is less upsetting to Jason than the absence of his mother, since father's absence has been the usual pattern. Over the years Jason's mother has been overly involved (enmeshed) with him; his father has been underinvolved (disengaged). In effect, Jason was an intruder in the marital subsystem; this structural arrangement was not disruptive until it became necessary for the parents to behave differently with one another and for Jason to accept the family position appropriate for him, a position equidistant from both parents.

Functional Theory

In their respective families of origin, Sue and Joe were accustomed to sex role differentiation. When their roles were reversed, they responded emotionally to the changes that were necessary. The fact that Jason was an only child contributed to the fusion between him and his mother. Because Sue was still emotionally connected to her own mother, she was influenced by her mother's criticism of Joe. The family's problems are complicated because the marital dyad is not a functioning subsystem. It has been adversely affected by Jason's actions, which have made him part of a family triangle that includes him, his mother, and his father. Jason's parents blame each other for their problems, partly because their traditional background make them view Joe's joblessness as a disgrace rather than a misfortune.

Communication Theory

Losing his job robbed Joe of his self-esteem and his image of himself as a breadwinner. When Sue obtained a job, she did not consider this an accomplishment but a sign that she had made a poor choice in marrying Joe. As long as Sue was able to be a full-time homemaker and mother, she gave Joe the respect that she thought was due him. After Joe lost his job, Sue gave him no emotional support. Her chief concern was her son's welfare and her embarrassment at having to work as a secretary. Joe was so preoccupied with his feelings of inadequacy that he did not acknowledge his wife's efforts to keep the family solvent. Neither partner reached out to the other, and the result was bitterness and arguments that impeded real communication. Instead of dealing with their situation as a family problem, both parents thought only of their own needs and sent double messages to Jason. Jason was told that he must go to school; yet he knew that his mother resented working and preferred staying home. Sue gives one message verbally and another message behaviorally. Jason's resistance to going to school is a primitive response to dysfunctional communication in the home.

Learning Theory

Even if family problems were minimal, Jason and his mother would probably have had problems with separation. As an only and well-loved child, Jason was very dependent on his mother and was unprepared to handle the changed circumstances of his family. He was not accustomed to having his father act as caretaker and fought against his father's efforts to assume tasks that had always belonged to his mother. Jason's behavior concerning school attendance is a learned response that is reinforced by parental behavior. Although Joe is able and willing to care for his son, Jason prefers the companionship of his mother. He recognizes that once Sue has decided not to go to work, she eventually is in a good humor. With his angry father out of the house, Jason and his mother can spend a pleasant day together.

Planning

Regardless of the theoretical approach used by the health professional, the following questions facilitate planning:

What does the family see as the major problem?
What are the developmental tasks of the family at this stage, and what are the developmental tasks of individual members?
What changes occurred in the family shortly before the present problem emerged?
What other problems exist in the family that seem to be connected to recent changes?
What tasks and responsibilities are assigned to members?
What is the nature of interactions between the family members and their respective families of origin?
How are disagreements resolved in the family?
How are decisions made in the family?
What has the family done so far to deal with the identified problem?

Implementation

A health professional using an integrated approach might use some of the following strategies:

Ask the parents to describe their early relationship, including how they met and why they married.
Ask the parents to contrast their present relationship with the earlier one.
Permit each member to speak only for himself or herself. Encourage them to speak directly to one another.
Draw attention to nonspecific statements that include words such as *always* or *never.*
Help members be less positive that they are always right. Suggest that they begin controversial statements with "I think" or "It seems to me." This will reduce resentment and opposition.
Support the self-esteem of every family member.
Restructure the family by strengthening the marital subsystem.
Identify the problem as a family problem rather than an individual one.

Evaluation

Outcome evaluation is possible only if goals are clear, attainable, and acceptable to the family. For Jason's family, goals were established that addressed his behavior directly and the parents' behavior indirectly. The health professional and the family reached a consensus that the marital problems were situational, even though they undoubtedly instigated Jason's behavior.

The agreed-on goals were outlined as follows:

Sue will go to her job every day unless she herself is ill.
Jason will go to school every day unless seen by a physician. If he is sick or upset in the morning, his father will take him to school as soon as he recovers. Lateness will be excused by his teacher, but not absence.
Joe will take responsibility for Jason on school days and will not leave the house when Jason complains of being too upset to go to school.
Joe will acknowledge Sue's contribution to the household and express appreciation for her help.
The parents will refrain from yelling and arguing so that Jason's sleep is not disturbed.
Two evenings a week will be devoted to inexpensive activities that all three family members enjoy, such as making popcorn or watching television.
One evening a week will be spent by Jason and his father on an activity of their choosing, such as playing ball or building a model airplane.
Sue will strongly discourage her mother's criticisms of Joe.
Sue and Joe will unite in their responses to Jason's unacceptable behaviors, and not disagree on this issue in the presence of their son.

Once the parents accepted the goals that were established, they became more willing to alter their own behavior. Both were committed to each other and to the welfare of their son, so they were motivated toward change. When the parents united in their reaction to Jason's manipulation, his tactics were no longer effective. No direct attention was given to the marital relationship, but the counseling sessions caused them to become closer. Jason's growing involvement with his father attenuated his enmeshment with mother. There was some family restructuring as Jason and his father found common interests. As Joe spent more time with Jason, he became less critical of the way Sue treated Jason, and this improved the marital relationship. Because Sue was used to family organization in which male members formed a subsystem, she was comfortable with Jason and Joe spending time together. Eventually Joe found another job and Sue was able to stop working. She discovered that Jason and Joe's new friendship gave her leisure to pursue her own interests, all within the context of traditional roles to which the family was committed.

SUMMARY

Theories that help organize the assessment of family interactions are presented in this chapter. A working knowledge of family theory directs observations that become the basis of hypotheses that promote planned change. The use of any theoretical approach helps transform discrete observations into meaningful data. The application of theory introduces order and organization to family assessment, planning, implementation, and evaluation.

Each theoretical framework presented here has its advantages and disadvantages. Developmental theory looks at family tasks over the life cycle and contrasts family maturation with individual maturation. An advantage of this framework is its longitudinal perspective; a disadvantage is that family task achievement can be assessed only in an impressionistic way. Structural theory looks at family positions and at emotional space between various members. Minuchin, who formulated the structural framework, gives specific suggestions about reinforcing the marital relationship and strengthening natural subsystems. Functional theory, whose most prominent exponent is Bowen, advocates differentiation of family members and separation from the family of origin. This is a cognitive approach to family work that may not be suitable for every family. The intellectual challenge of Bowen's concepts might be difficult for nonverbal families to comprehend.

Every family interaction has psychodynamic overtones, but psychodynamic family theory is concerned with the emotional climate of family life. Family harmony and family hostility are not accepted at face value, but are explored to discover what issues, if any, are avoided by the prevailing emotional climate of the family. Communication theory proposes that the self-esteem of all family members is the essential ingredient of effective communication. When family communication is used to attack or belittle any member, dysfunction almost surely follows. Effective communication requires the integration of thought with feeling and the maintenance of every member's self-esteem. Learning theory is related to family dynamics in that social learning perpetuates certain behaviors even when the behaviors are no longer desirable or appropriate. The psychodynamics of family life engender internal responses such as pseudomutuality or pseudohostility that must be carefully analyzed. Social learning produces outward behaviors that are more easily recognized. Learned behaviors often respond to modification provided the participants acknowledge their influence and are willing to change.

Chapter One introduced the concept of interdependence among family members. Just as there is interdependence among family members, so there is interdependence among the contributing theories discussed in this chapter. Boundaries may exist between the theories, but the boundaries are permeable. Eclecticism means taking the best, most usable parts of the various theories. Consigning concepts to different frameworks is an organizational strategy that makes it easier for health professionals to consider all possibilities and select those most relevant for a particular family.

Chapter One viewed the family as a dynamic, interacting system. Chapter Two presents an integrated systems model with an assessment and an intervention component. This integrated systems model draws upon the six contributing theories described in this chapter as appropriate frameworks in family counseling.

REFERENCES

Baltes, P. B., & Brim, O. G. (1980). *Life Span Development and Behavior.* New York: Academic Press.

Bateson, G., Jackson, D. D., Haley, J., & Weakland, J. (1956). "Toward a Theory of Schizophrenia." *Behavioral Sciences,* 1(3): 251–264.

Bowen, M. (1971). "The Use of Family Theory in Clinical Practice." In J. Haley (Ed.), *Changing Families.* New York: Grune and Stratton.

Bowen, M. (1974). "Toward the Differentiation of Self in One's Family of Origin." In F. Andres & J. Loria (Eds.), *Georgetown Family Symposia: Collection of Selected Papers.* Washington, DC: Georgetown University Press.

Bowen, M. (1976). "Theory in the Practice of Psychotherapy." In P. Guerin (Ed.), *Family Therapy.* New York: Gardner.

Carter, E. A., & McGoldrick, M. (Eds.) (1980). *The Family Life Cycle.* New York: Gardner.

Constantine, L. L. (1986). *Family Paradigms: The Practice of Theory in Family Therapy.* New York: Guilford Press.

Duvall, E. (1977). *Marriage and Family Development,* 5th ed. Philadelphia: Lippincott.

Erikson, E. H. (1963). *Childhood and Society.* New York: Norton.

Evers, H. (1985). "The Frail Elderly Woman: Emergent Questions in Aging and Women's Health." In E. Lewin & V. Oleson (Eds.), *Women, Health and Healing: Toward a New Perspective.* New York: Tavistock Press.

Freud, S. (1949). *Outline of Psychoanalysis.* New York: W. W. Norton.

George, L. K. (1980). *Role Transition in Later Life.* Monterey, CA: Brooks/Cole.

Haley, J. (1971). *Changing Families.* New York: Grune and Stratton.

Hoopes, M. M., & Harper, J. H. (1987). *Birth Order, Roles, and Sibling Patterns in Individual and Family Therapy.* Rockville, MD: Aspen Press.

Jackson, D. D., & Lederer, W. (1967). *The Mirages of Marriage.* New York: W. W. Norton.

Kermis, M. D. (1986). *Mental Health in Later Life: The Adaptive Process.* Boston/Monterey, CA: Jones and Bartlett.

Lambert, V. A., & Lambert, C. E. (1984). "Role Theory and the Concept of Powerlessness." *Journal of Psychosocial Nursing,* 11(1): 11–14.

Lauer, J. C., & Lauer, R. (1987). *Till Death Do Us Part: How Couples Stay Together.* New York: Haworth Press.

Minuchin, S. (1974). *Families and Family Therapy.* Cambridge, MA: Harvard University Press.

Neugarten, B. L. (1973). *Middle Age and Aging.* Chicago: University of Chicago Press.

Parsons, T. (1951). *The Social System.* New York: Free Press.

Ryff, C. D. (1985). "The Subjective Experience of Life Span Transition." In A. S. Rossi (Ed.), *Gender and the Life Course.* New York: Aldine and Graytor.

Satir, V., Stachwiak, J., & Taschmen, H. (1977). *Helping Families to Change.* New York: Jason Aaronson.

Thomas, A., & Chess, S. (1977). *Temperament and Development.* New York: Brunner/Mazel.

Thomas, A., & Chess, S. (1980). *The Dynamics of Psychological Development.* New York: Brunner/Mazel.

Toman, W. (1976). *Family Constellations.* New York: Basic Books.

Tomlinson, P. S. (1987). "Spousal Differences in Marital Satisfaction During Transition to Parenthood." *Nursing Research,* 36(3): 239–243.

Wynne, L. (1978). *Beyond the Doublebind.* New York: Brunner/Mazel.

Wynne, L., Rykoff, I., Day, J., & Hirsch, S. I. (1958). "Pseudomutuality in Family Relations of Schizophrenics." *Psychiatry,* 21: 205–220.

CHAPTER THREE

Applied Family Theory:
Setting the Stage for Change

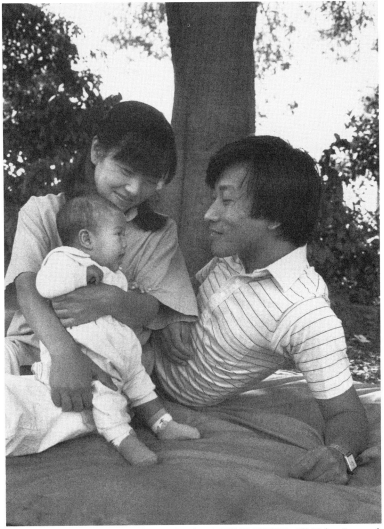

*The turning points of lives are not the great moments.
The real crises are often concealed in occurrences so
trivial in appearance that they pass unobserved.*

George Washington

Family theory and family therapy are complex fields in which clinical and laboratory investigation are ongoing. Many family theorists have formulated concepts that help practitioners understand what is happening in the families with whom they work. In addition to numerous concepts, family theorists have developed various tools and methods designed to facilitate family assessment and intervention. These tools and methods are a means of organizing family data so that understandable patterns emerge. Once certain patterns are identified, clinicians can develop working hypotheses that eventually lead to realistic goal setting and positive changes.

This is a practical chapter describing assessment strategies, some of which are more helpful than others. The content expands on material introduced in Chapter Two. It demonstrates how conceptual formulations are used to build appropriate tools and methods. The chapter is eclectic in that the strategies discussed here are drawn from several sources. No strategy is all-inclusive; many can be used in conjunction with each other, based on the clinical situation and the skills of the health care professional.

The closing section of the chapter describes the longitudinal progress of family work. This stage-related description lends direction to health care professionals as they move from introductory family sessions to working sessions, and eventually to termination sessions. Depending on the family's needs and motivation, family work may be of long or short duration. Regardless of time factors, however, the efforts of a health care professional in an early family session differ from the efforts of the same practitioner in later sessions. In some respects the actions of family and practitioner are reciprocal and are likely to evolve over time.

FAMILY MAPS

The family map is a tool that enables the practitioner to assess family organization and relationship patterns by means of diagrams and mapping legends or keys (Minuchin, 1974). The mapping legend presents symbols that depict the positions of various family members in relation to other members. Mapping these structural arrangements allows the practitioner to make inferences about family life and develop hypotheses about possible changes. In Figure 3.1 the family map implies that leadership in the family is shared between the parents, both of whom appear to interact equally with the children. In Figure 3.2 the family map indicates a hierarchical organization in which the father is dominant. The map also permits the inference that mother is closer to the children than father is, and that she does perform some leadership functions.

Family mapping uses various structural concepts—boundaries, subsystems, coalitions or alliances, dyads, and triangles or triads—to diagram the positions and relationship patterns of family members. Some of these concepts were introduced in Chapter Two, but they are briefly defined as follows:

- Boundaries are unwritten rules that regulate family relationships and establish limits between individual members or subsystems, and between the family and other systems.
- Rigid boundaries are impermeable and inflexible, thereby encouraging isolation and poor communication.

FIGURE 3.1. **Structure in Which the Leadership Is Shared**

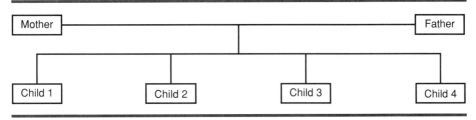

FIGURE 3.2. **Structure in Which the Father Is Dominant**

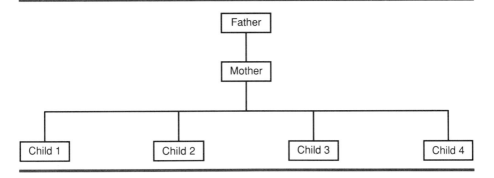

- Diffuse boundaries are weak and indistinct, thereby encouraging overinvolvement between family members.
- Clear boundaries are consistent and appropriate, thereby encouraging functional family relationships.
- Disengagement and underinvolvement among family members results from rigid boundaries.
- Enmeshment or overinvolvement of family members results from diffuse boundaries.
- Subsystems are psychosocial arrangements within families based on natural divisions of age, gender, or role.
- Alliances or coalitions are psychosocial arrangements within families not based on natural divisions of age, gender, or role.
- Dyads are groups of two family members; dyads may be subsystems or coalition/alliances depending on who constitutes the dyad. Mother and father form a dyad that is a subsystem; father and daughter form a dyad that is a coalition/alliance. The latter is based not on natural boundaries but on special bonds that exclude other family members.
- Triangles consist of three family members or of two members plus a third entity such as father's job or mother's alcoholism. Triangles are seldom equilateral. Usually there is greater closeness between two persons or between one person and the specific entity, with the third person placed at a distance.
- Detours are family patterns of handling conflict by shifting it to a chosen member, who then becomes the identified family problem.

The symbols used in family mapping are uncomplicated and understandable. They are essential to the interpretation of the map and are widely used. Figure 3.3 shows the mapping symbols devised by Minuchin (1974).

Family mapping can be applied to both functional and dysfunctional families. It can also be used to show changes in structure and relationship patterns that occur as a result of family intervention. For example, a troubled family may consist of mother, father, an adolescent son, and two daughters. The son is doing poorly in school, is a habitual truant, and has been picked up by the police for minor vandalism. The two girls are apparently well adjusted and have formed a strong subsystem where they offer each other mutual support. This reduces their awareness of being overlooked by their parents. When the son gets in trouble, mother excuses his actions and rescues him from the consequences. If possible, she conceals his misdemeanors from his father, even if this means lying and dissembling. At the same time she complains about father's lack of involvement in family life. The mother is the more powerful parent, protecting the son and preventing direct communication between father and son. Figure 3.4 shows the troubled situation.

The goals of family intervention would include strengthening the parental subsystem by weakening the coalition/alliance of mother and son,

FIGURE 3.3. **Mapping Key or Legend**

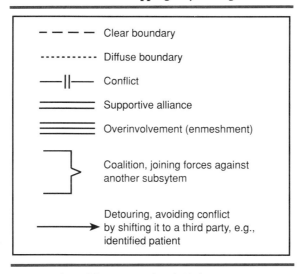

Source: Adapted from Minuchin (1974).

FIGURE 3.4. **Map of Dysfunctional Family Structure**

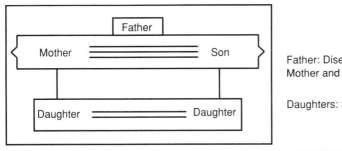

Father: Disengaged
Mother and son: Enmeshed coalition/alliance
Daughters: Sibling subsystem

and reinforcing the parental role of father. If this approach proved success-ful, the son would become part of the sibling subsystem where he belongs. Figure 3.5 shows changes in the family after successful family intervention.

Family positions and relationships may be altered by clarifying and reinforcing natural boundaries and subsystems and by encouraging the in-clusion of left-out family members. Minuchin finds that family members in a therapeutic interview reveal alliances and disengagement through their

FIGURE 3.5. **Map of Family Structure after Intervention**

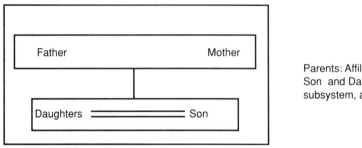

Parents: Affiliated subsystem:
Son and Daughters: Sibling
subsystem, affiliated

Parents: Affiliated subsystem
Son and daughters: Sibling subsystem, affiliated

seating arrangements. This spatial distribution occurs spontaneously in early family sessions if members are permitted to seat themselves. In subsequent meetings the practitioner has opportunities to manipulate space by moving family members or rearranging furniture. In the family just described, the practitioner might modify preferred arrangements by choosing a seat so that parents are placed together on one side and the three children on the other. Without words, the practitioner indicates that the parents represent a leadership subsystem that does not include any of the children.

FAMILY ROLES

Family roles are perhaps more difficult to assess than family positions. Every family has rules and expectations that regulate role enactment, thus allowing the family to function. Patterns formed by durable, repeated family interactions determine how and by whom family roles are enacted. Formal or ascribed role enactment consists of activities widely assigned to a specific role. For instance, the ascribed role of nurturer or caretaker is commonly assigned to mother; the role of provider is still assigned more to father than to mother. Working women expect husbands to share the nurturing and caretaking functions of the family, just as women share the role of provider. There is, of course, more shared role enactment in some families than in others, and the voluntary features of role sharing may be hard to assess. Achieved role enactment includes informal patterns in a particular family not often found elsewhere. A son in one household may, for instance, assume the authority and responsibilities of an absent father. This then becomes his achieved role. Role distribution and role differentiation are two important concepts in role theory. Role distribution assigns different roles to family members. If mother takes on the obligations of family manager, she is expected to act in ways that promote family efficiency. If father is the family jokester, his messages are taken less seriously than those of practical mom. Role differentiation does not designate certain persons for certain roles, but does stipulate what activities accompany different roles, and what a role enacter may or may not do. In some families role enactment poses few problems. In other families conflict and discontent surround role enactment. Conditions related to role enactment color the entire fabric of family life. Some of these conditions are described briefly as follows.

- *Role conflict:* This refers to disagreement among family members regarding the way roles should be enacted and by whom.
- *Role incompetence:* This leads to dissatisfaction about the way roles are enacted. Adequate role enactment does not guarantee satisfaction. A wife whose role enactment is adequate may resent the lesser enactment of her husband. He, on the other hand, may resent the superior enactment of his wife. Role adequacy or role competence leads to marital satisfaction only if it gratifies both partners.
- *Role consensus:* Sometimes called role consonance, role consensus refers to agreement regarding family role enactment, role distribution, role differentiation, and role competence.
- *Role dissonance:* This refers to disagreement or lack of consensus regarding family role enactment, role distribution, role differentiation, and role competence.
- *Role complementarity:* This deals with role enactment in which the actions of one person reinforce the actions of another. Even when role complementarity gratifies both persons, their role enactment is unidimensional and may inhibit emotional development.
- *Role symmetry:* This is role enactment in which persons vie for the same patterns of role development. If both seek dominance, conflict results. If both seek to be dependent, leadership and direction are lacking.

ROLE THEORY TERMS

Definition of Roles

Roles are sets of expected, predictable behaviors we enact when dealing with other people.

Characteristics of Role Enactment

- All of us must assume a variety of roles depending on circumstances.
- The roles we enact are greatly influenced by what went on in our original families.
- Role enactment requires the consent and cooperation of those around us; therefore, roles are *interdependent.*

Types of Role Enactment

- *Ascribed/formal:* Family members enact roles appropriate to their actual position.
- *Achieved/informal:* Family members enact roles inappropriate to their actual position.

Negative Consequences of Achieved Role Enactment

Examples:

- Daughter becomes daddy's sweetheart.
- Son becomes mother's little man.
- Husband becomes father to his wife as well as to the children.
- Wife becomes her husband's mother as well as the children's mother.

Effects:

- Individual life tasks are not accomplished in sequence.
- Development of members may be premature (child enacts parental role).
- Development of members may be arrested (parent enacts childish role).
- *Family system becomes distorted and confused.*

Variation in Family Role Enactment

- *Complementary roles:* Usually produce stability but at the price of individual development.
- *Symmetrical roles:* Usually produce family conflict and instability.
- *Flexible roles:* Role enactment adapts to individual and family needs.

Examples of Complementary Roles

- Wife is cautious and frugal; husband is impulsive and extravagant.
- Wife is managerial and dominant; husband is docile and passive.

Examples of Symmetrical Roles

- Both husband and wife struggle to be dominant and assertive.
- Both husband and wife wish to be dependent and nurtured.

Family Structure and Role Enactment

- Family starts out with a subsystem composed of husband and wife.
- As children are born they form a sibling subsystem.
- Large families may have more than one sibling subsystem.
- *No child belongs in the parental subsystem.*

TABLE 3.1. Abbreviated Chart of Family Role Enactment						
	Mother		Father		Children	
Positive features: Role consensus Role competence						
Negative features: Role dissonance Role conflict						
Questionable features: Role complementarity Role symmetry						

Note: Use a plus sign (+) to denote functional role enactment; use a minus sign (−) to denote dysfunctional role enactment.

The true nature of family role enactment is not immediately discernible, and observations must be made over time in order to be valid. A practitioner trying to assess family role enactment may find it helpful to apply some of the concepts just described by means of a family chart, as shown in Table 3.1. In this way some of the significant aspects of family role enactment become accessible.

DIFFERENTIATION OF SELF SCALE

Bowen (1971) defines *differentiation of self* as the extent to which individuals separate emotionally from their families of origin. Self-differentiation also refers to the level of individuation existing between members of the nuclear family. In refining the concept, Bowen adds that self-differentiation distinguishes between thought and feeling, and that persons who cannot separate cognitive processes from emotional processes are not apt to function well (Bowen, 1976). The terms *solid self* and *pseudoself* are applied to contrasting poles on the differentiation of self scale. The solid self consists of internalized values and beliefs that slowly evolve. These fixed principles may be modified by learning and experience but not by coercion or external persuasion. Persons who function near the solid self polarity can differentiate themselves from others, engage in goal-directed activity, and seek intimacy without enmeshment or fusion. Persons operating near the pseudoself polarity are excessively concerned with love and approval, even at the price of their own development. They constantly look to others for acceptance and are unhappy without it. At the same time, they hold others responsible for their happiness and blame others when their needs are not met. They rarely distinguish between what they can do for themselves and what they ask others to do for them. Theirs is a world of strong emotions and heavy demands. In contrast, persons near the polarity of solid self usually separate thoughts from feelings. Their sense of self is based on reality, not on what others do or say. They do not shrink from emotional closeness per se but strive for balance in the emotional domain. They are more autonomous and do not consider other people responsible for their emotional well-being. In general, they have more energy for goal-directed activity and therefore function well.

The concept of differentiation of self is subtle and requires subjective appraisal on the part of the health care professional. Some attempts have been made to develop a differentiation of self scale that quantifies behavior, but such work has not been validated to any extent (see Figure 3.6). An

FIGURE 3.6. **Differentiation of Self Scale**

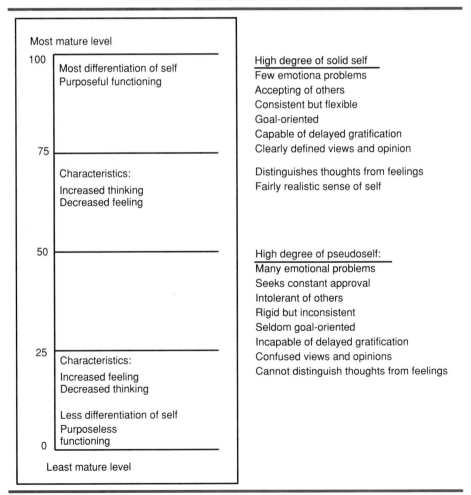

Source: Adapted from Bowen (1971, 1976) and Kerr and Bowen (1988).

impressionistic tool does give the practitioner a method of comparing behaviors of family members, if the deficient aspects of the scale are kept in
mind.

FAMILY CHRONOLOGY

A family chronology, or family history, is an extremely useful assessment
tool. The chronology is a sequential record of family events occurring since

FIGURE 3.7. **Family Chronology Diagram: The Grant Family**

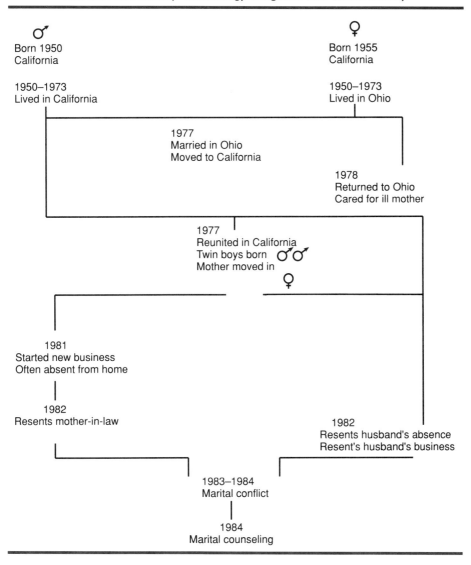

FIGURE 3.8. **Family Chronology, Narrative Format: The Grant Family**

1950–1973 Richard Grant was born and raised in California. He has two older sisters. His father is a practicing lawyer and his mother manages a dress shop.

1955–1973 Rosemary Cooper was born and raised in Cleveland, Ohio. After high school she attended a business college, where she earned an associate degree. Her father died the year Rosemary found her first job. Rosemary is an only child.

1973–1975 Richard graduated from college and began working for an insurance company. He attended a sales conference in Cleveland, where Rosemary was working as a secretary. The couple met when Rosemary was assigned to help Richard finish a report.

1975–1977 Rosemary and Richard corresponded and saw each other as much as possible. They were married in June 1977 and moved to California.

1978 Rosemary's mother had a stroke and she returned to Cleveland to look after her mother. The stay lasted eight months, and although he visited occasionally Richard became increasingly unhappy with the separation.

1979 Rosemary became pregnant and agreed to return to California if her mother could come live with her. Twin boys were born in November 1979. The first year after the birth was hectic, but the couple managed well by sharing parenting tasks.

1981 Richard left the insurance company to go into business for himself. The move was financially successful, but Richard was absent from home much of the time.

1982–1983 Rosemary and her mother, who still lived with the couple, formed a coalition that excluded Richard. Rosemary often felt torn between her mother and her husband, who did not get along well with each other. She felt lonely at times, was impatient with her sons, and resented Richard's absences from home. Richard was proud of the way he had provided for his family, was devoted to his sons, was resentful of his mother-in-law's presence, and worried about Rosemary, who did not seem like the bright, confident young woman he had married.

1984 At Richard's insistence, the couple went to a marriage counselor to try, in Richard's words, to "revitalize the marriage."

the family unit was established. The family chronology may deal only with the nuclear family or may be extended to include the whole family network. Gathering facts about the family not only enlightens the health care professional but is informative for the family members. The chronology includes the names of the members, their ages, dates of marriages, divorces, separations, and illnesses or accidents. Information about education, occupation, and life changes are also significant. The format of the chronology is less important than the information that is revealed (Cain, 1980).

Some health care professionals prefer to diagram the family chronology by means of commonly used symbols and a key (Figure 3.7). Others choose to utilize a narrative format (Figure 3.8). There are advantages to both methods. Diagrams allow other practitioners to absorb considerable information at a glance. Because there is no official way to chart the chronology, however, the use of symbols may be subject to misinterpretation. The narrative format takes longer to read but is less open to misinterpretation. Moreover, the narrative chronology can be shared with the family. Compiling the chronology emphasizes the centrality of family life as it relates to the past as well as the present. Family members gain a sense of proportion about current problems as they recall previous crises that were surmounted. This is a cognitive exercise for family members that helps reopen communication channels.

The focus of the chronology depends on the presenting problem and the clinical needs of members. Sometimes the chronology deals mostly with psychosocial events and issues. At other times the focus is on physical or biological experiences such as illness or disability. Since the family chronology is usually concerned with what has happened to the contemporary family, it is frequently used in conjunction with a genogram that collects data across two or more generations.

FAMILY GENOGRAMS

A family chronology reveals the centrality or significance of family life. A family genogram (Figure 3.9) reveals the continuity of family life across generations. The genogram is essentially a family tree showing various branches. Like most of the tools described here, the genogram is a subjective instrument based on observed or factual data. Many health care professionals compile a family history based on data gathered in early sessions and subsequently begin a genogram. Because families are preoccupied with current issues, they tend to be more responsive if the practitioner asks about family composition at present. From this beginning, the practitioner can go on to ask about earlier generations. Usually the genogram data are explored in early family sessions but may be revised or augmented as new information is learned. The genogram is concerned with current and historical information, and is often used with the more detailed family chronology.

In these days of complicated family arrangements resulting from marriage, divorce, and remarriage, the genogram can give the practitioner an accurate picture of family configurations. Details are gathered that help practitioners make inferences about family similarities and differences. Genograms begin in the present with at least two different strains or branches, each attributed to one member of the marital dyad. The two branches increase geometrically to four, and eight, and sixteen as earlier generations are traced. Comparing aspects of these different branches shows how they differ from one another and how these differences have affected the life experiences of various members. If branches of the wife's family are dissimilar from those of the husband, these differences may contribute to tension and conflict.

FIGURE 3.9. Family Genogram

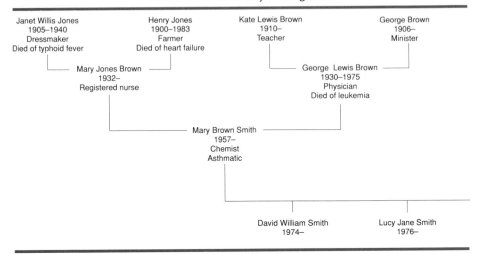

Genograms owe much to the work of Bowen (1971, 1976; Kerr & Bowen, 1988), who maintains that family events repeat themselves across generational boundaries, and that gender and birth order affect personality development and family life. These points are undeniable, but genograms in themselves do not show the depth of emotional relationships or the nature of family transactions. Their value lies in the historical record they provide.

Demographic data constitute the first level of a genogram. This includes dates of births and deaths, and longevity of family members. Often place of residence, educational level, and occupation are included. The second level of the genogram consists of information about major life transitions, separations, divorces, accidents, and illnesses. There is usually a pivotal individual or individuals in a genogram, and the data gathered are facts likely to have significant impact. McGoldrick and Gerson (1986) describe genogram construction as a net cast in ever widening circles, and ask practitioners to take the following steps:

- Move from the central figure or problem to broader considerations.
- Move from members of the current household to the extended family.
- Add information about previous generations to data about the current generation.
- Include any facts that have probable impact on the central figure or problem.

One practitioner constructing a genogram might be interested primarily in psychosocial factors and discount extraneous details. Another practitioner might be concerned with biological factors such as the existence of

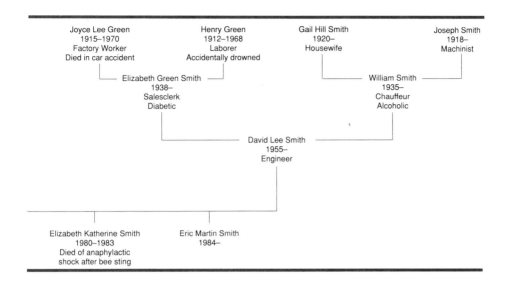

FIGURE 3.10. Sample Genogram of Four Generations

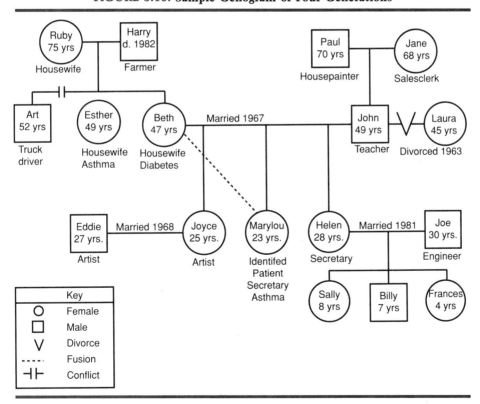

Source: Adapted from Simon (1985).

familial illnesses. If such illnesses are genetic in origin, the genogram is an excellent teaching device. Prevalence of certain conditions among members of succeeding generations indicates to contemporary families the risks they and their children may face. Even when genetic counseling is unnecessary, the presence of heart disease, diabetes, or hypertension in a family is easily noted in a genogram and can be used to encourage preventive measures.

The family genogram is a device used to trace families across several generations (Figure 3.10). Demographic data regarding family health, longevity, occupations, marriages, and divorces can be shown on a genogram, and information is available at a glance.

FAMILY SOCIOGRAMS

The sociogram was first used by Jacob Moreno, an innovator in the field of group work (Phipps, 1986). It is a sociometric tool that may be used in different ways. Members of a group may be asked to choose the person in the group who is admired most or least, who has most or least power, or who is the most or least active. By using a sociogram, the group leader can use directional arrows to show positive or negative feelings between members. Used in this way, the sociogram generates data about status, dominance, affection, and other emotional forces existing between members.

The sociogram may be employed to show the direction and frequency of messages transmitted between family members. After a family meeting has ended, the health care professional can diagram the spatial positions of members, who spoke to whom and how often, and who failed to speak to certain family members. This tool may be used for assessment and to evaluate progress. If a sociogram is prepared after each family session, the practitioner can see changes occurring as intervention proceeds. The sociogram may be developed by a participant observer sitting with the family and the practitioner, by an unseen observer behind a two-way mirror, or by the practitioner immediately after the meeting ends. Figure 3.11 shows an example of a sociogram.

Although sociograms help the practitioner to recall the direction and frequency of family communication, they have limitations. Unless the sessions are videotaped and later analyzed or there is an observer present to make notes, total accuracy cannot be guaranteed. In addition to providing quantitative data, sociograms can be used qualitatively if the following questions are considered by the practitioner.

- Are messages transmitted directly from sender to recipient or mediated through a third person who acts as a switchboard or interpreter?
- What subjects are not discussed by the family even when introduced by family members?
- What issues absorb the attention of the family even when other matters seem to be more urgent?

FIGURE 3.11. Family Sociogram

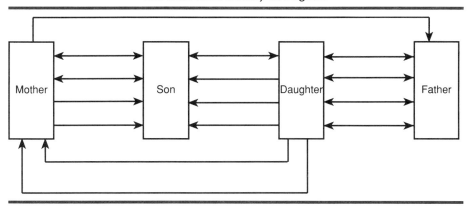

Note: In this sample sociogram, each arrow represents communication from one person to another. The daughter, for example, communicated four times more frequently to the son than the son to the daughter.

FAMILY INTERACTION ANALYSIS

A relatively complicated tool for examining what goes on in a family is Bales Interaction Process Analysis (IPA) (Table 3.2; Zastowny & DeFrank, 1986). This is a standardized measure developed by Bales (1950), which looks at twelve categories of communication. Three categories are concerned with positive communication behavior within a family or group; three are concerned with negative communication behavior, three with problem-solving communication, and three with information-seeking communication. The degree to which families engage in the four categories of communication depends somewhat on the nature of the family problem but is greatly influenced by the family's accustomed communication methods. In a family where a member has been given a medical diagnosis, the family will use information-seeking forms of communication. An identified patient with a psychiatric problem may cause the family to blame or find fault with one or more members. Thus, the problematic issue may affect communication as well as the family's habitual patterns of behavior.

The Bales Interaction Process Analysis takes practice on the part of the observer. So much goes on at a family meeting that a single scorer may easily be overwhelmed. A solution to this is to use more than one scorer, perhaps making each scorer responsible for only two family members' communication. Another solution is to videotape the meeting so that the communication process may be analyzed at a more leisurely pace. Naturally, the family must give written permission for the taping after being told its purpose.

There are limits to the value of the IPA. Reliability cannot be ensured unless more than one person scores the interaction and compares the re-

TABLE 3.2. Interaction Process Analysis

Family socioemotional behavior:

A. *Positive communication:*
1. *Shows support:* Acknowledges status of others, offers help, uses humor in nonthreatening ways.
2. *Offers tension release:* Laughs, acknowledges, shows satisfaction, gratifies.
3. *Shows agreement:* Expresses acceptance and/or understanding, complies.

B. *Negative communication:*
4. *Shows disagreement:* Expresses rejection, witholds help, uses humor harshly, threatens the status of others.
5. *Exhibits tension or aggravates tension:* Looks for help, withdraws from interaction, shows dissatisfaction.
6. *Displays antagonism:* Behaves aggressively, defends self, blames others, issues challenges.

Family task behavior:

C. *Problem-solving communication:*
7. *Offers suggestions:* Gives advice and direction without questioning the autonomy of others.
8. *Offers opinions:* Engages in analysis and evaluation, shares feelings and desires.
9. *Offers information:* Repeats, clarifies, confirms, and summarizes content; orients others when appropriate.

D. *Questioning communication:*
10. *Asks for information:* Seeks clarification, confirmation, and summarization.
11. *Asks for opinions:* Seeks analysis and evaluation, searches for expression of feelings by other members.
12. *Asks for suggestions:* Seeks direction and guidance; looks for alternative actions and solutions.

spective ratings each has given to the same transaction. Each scorer makes a judgment as to which categories are correct for each family response (see Figure 3.12) and scorers may disagree. Some limitations of the IPA stem from the fact that actual content of communication is ignored, and the scorer can only surmise the intent, purpose, and motivation of family members. No mention is made of the meaning of messages sent by members communicating with one another. Thus, the IPA tool simply categorizes family communication according to predetermined guidelines. It does, however, introduce some element of objectivity and helps the practitioner analyze the theme of a session, as well as the responses of individual members.

FIGURE 3.12. Interaction Process Analysis (IPA) Scoring

Member	Category (Positive)						Category (Negative)					
	A-1	A-2	A-3	B-4	B-5	B-6	C-7	C-8	C-9	D-10	D-11	D-12
Mother												
Father												
Daughter												
Son												
Grandma												

Source: Adapted from Bales (1950) and Zastowny and DeFrank (1986).

FAMILY PROCESS ANALYSIS

The interaction process analytic tool helps practitioners identify the tone and theme of family interaction, and reveals the interactional styles of individual family members. A theoretical model entitled *Levels of Marital Conflict* is offered by Leas (1985). This model assists practitioners as they examine family dissension patterns. After noting the conflict level at which a family operates, the practitioner can endeavor to reduce dysfunctional conflict and promote problem-solving behavior. Originally intended for management consultants, the model has been adapted for use with couples and family units (Weingarten, 1986). The principle underlying this model is that family conflict is not always detrimental, provided it is handled in positive ways. There are five levels of conflict behavior, all of them characterized by clusters of behavior, each of which is less constructive than the preceding cluster. The behavior levels are (1) problem solving, (2) disagreeing, (3) competing, (4) fighting or fleeing, and (5) waging war (see Tables 3.3 and 3.4).

Level One Behavior

This is the most effective level, and families who adopt problem-solving behavior function well even when they face serious problems. Not every family functions at this level at all times or in all situations. Sometimes the gravity of a problem may overwhelm a family for a while. However, Weingarten and Leas (1987) note that some families never regress to unproductive behavior, while other families never use problem-solving tactics

TABLE 3.3. Levels of Conflict

Behavior Level	Major Objective	Emotional Climate	Interaction Style	Clients' View of Practitioner
Level 1 – Problem solving	Solve or resolve the problem	Hope and optimism	Open, direct, focused communication; little or no distortion of content; recognition of common interests	Advisor and objective facilitator; resource person and expert
Level 2 – Disagreeing and arguing	Protect oneself. Compromise if necessary.	Uncertainty and vigilance	Vague, unfocused communication; cautious and calculated discussion	Mediator, enabler, intermediary
Level 3 – Competing and contending	Win or lose the competition.	Frustration and resentment; fear of losing	Distorted communication; personal attacks and manipulation	Arbiter, referee, judge
Level 4 – Fighting and/or fleeing	Injure the other person. Ignore the other person.	Hostility, antagonism, alienation	Stubborn unwillingness to change self or opinions; distorted perceptions; mixed messages; refusal to take responsibility for self or situation	Ally or enemy
Level 5 – Waging all-out war	Eliminate the other person by any means possible.	Revenge and destructiveness; retaliation and vindictiveness	Extreme volatility; no recollection or understanding of issues; self-righteous, compulsive, driven behavior	Rescuer or destroyer

Source: Adapted from Weingarten and Leas (1987).

TABLE 3.4. Therapeutic Guidelines Based on Conflict Levels

Behavior Level	Behavior Pattern	Therapeutic Guidelines
1. Problem solving	Effective interaction is used in dealing with tasks and decisions, even in difficult situations.	Support customary adaptive interaction of the family.
2. Disagreeing	Saving face and not being hurt are more important than solving problems; outside advice may be sought; members disagree but are not wholly antagonistic.	Offer support and protection to entire family; avoid becoming part of a family triangle; insist that members be clear, specific, and focused on problems.
3. Competing	Anger and resentment surface; self-protection is less important than getting even.	Outline communication rules; explore separate goals and experiences of members; use a cognitive approach; construct a genogram to defuse anger and promote sharing of information among members.
4. Fighting/fleeing	Goals and basic issues are forgotten in attempts to hurt other members either through confrontation or withdrawal.	Conflict has produced an impasse. Set rules for communicating; search for issues where a degree of agreement is possible.
5. Waging war	Injury and revenge are a way of life; spouse and child abuse may be present; victim and victimizer are locked in a life-threatening struggle.	At this level, reconciliation is not an immediate goal; suggest a period of separation to control family violence; utilize legal and protective services.

Source: Adapted from Weingarten and Leas (1987).

regardless of their circumstances. In other words, the behavioral level of a family tends to be persistent despite temporary modifications.

Level Two Behavior

Families functioning at this level find it hard to reach a consensus. Self-protection, saving face, and avoiding risk are more important than dealing with issues directly. Families using this behavioral level are not actually antagonistic toward each other, but seem deficient in trust. This causes them to feel uncertain, anxious, and vulnerable. Because they do not trust each other, they are inclined to seek advice and help from others. If appropriate help is available, these families often begin to resolve their problems.

Level Three Behavior

Here there is considerable anger and resentment in the family. Issues are confused and distorted; family members are disheartened and feel that they may never solve their problems. Instead of dealing with real issues, family members simply collect grievances. Support for one family member is interpreted as attack on another. Family members are unwilling to bestow praise or approval on fellow members. Competition and blaming characterize most family behaviors.

Level Four Behavior

At this level, winning becomes less important than hurting others. Usually a marital partner is the target of fight/flight actions, but sometimes it is a child or children. When marital partners are involved, they do not try to work out their difficulties but want only to injure each other. If such couples divorce, they are caught up in bitter disputes about property and child custody. If they stay married, they maintain great distances from each other by being unavailable, by not talking, and by concealing their actions and whereabouts. Failing this, they continue to ridicule, disparage, and humiliate each other.

Flight behavior may be more destructive than fight behavior, for fighting participants are at least involved. Flight actions decrease involvement and replace indignation with indifference. Participants need assistance to understand that flight can be as threatening to family members as fight, and offers no greater potential for solving problems.

Level Five Behavior

At this level, revenge and destruction have become a way of life for the family. This is the kind of behavior engaged in by the husband and wife in the 1989 film *The War of the Roses*, where sanity and survival yield to murderous impulses. Families that abuse or mistreat weaker members clearly operate at this level. Here, victims receive no mercy, and the role of victim may be shared among several members. A state of war makes all family members volatile and unpredictable. Flight behaviors are infrequent, partly because victims feel they have no where to go. It is possible that after years of being abused a victim may finally rebel and kill an abusing parent or spouse after years of passive acceptance.

Couples and families operating at this level rarely seek help except through court referrals or protective service agencies. Until the potential for change can be assessed, it may be necessary to see warring spouses separately. Their relationship is sufficiently pathological to require a cooling off period of indeterminate length. Programs for battered women and children have proliferated in recent years and provide a haven for victims. The best programs are those that encourage self-control and taking charge of one's life. Control is a crucial issue for the perpetrators of violence and for their victims. People who have little control over themselves or their lives are prone to violence or to accept the role of victim. A sense of control and autonomy reduces tendencies to abuse others and, conversely, to tolerate abuse of oneself.

Levels of conflict behavior constitute an admirable family and marital assessment tool. Recognizing the level at which a couple or family function gives direction to planning and intervention. A warning must be issued to generalist health care professionals who want to give family-focused care and find themselves working with families that operate at levels three, four, or five. At these dysfunctional levels, generalist practitioners should request consultation or supervision from more experienced colleagues. Levels three, four, and five indicate considerable family pathology; knowing one's own limitations and securing backup expertise are essential in working with families that are seriously dysfunctional.

The comprehensive nature of family assessment means that the practitioner must employ effective and sensitive interviewing techniques, as well as carefully selected assessment tools. Data collection continues as long as the family is in contact with the practitioner and the health care system. A nonjudgmental attitude, sensitivity, and timing are important in all family work. Developing trust and rapport is always a goal of early meetings. Timing of interventions is facilitated by analyzing family progress during the therapeutic process.

FAMILY PROGRESS ANALYSIS

Families who seek professional help for a physical, social, or psychological problem have already made a hard choice in entering the health care system. They are upset and worried; they are afraid of what might be revealed about their family. They are unsure of many things, but they usually have some ideas about the nature of the problem and the kind of help they want. A good opening, then, is for the practitioner to explore the family's perception of the problem as family intervention commences.

Introductory Sessions

An introductory session or sessions is a time for getting acquainted with family members who are present and for finding out about members who are not present for one reason or another. As the practitioner observes members' interactions with each other and tries to reduce their anxiety, it helps to ask who initiated the referral. Was a recommendation made by another health care professional, by a friend or relative, or by a family member. If the family acts as if there is an identified patient, this should be acknowledged.

However, the practitioner explains that the family is the focus, rather than any individual. This can be done by insisting that every family member is equally important and contributes to family operations. The practitioner should state the purpose of the meeting and share information about his or her professional role. While trying to establish a calm, reassuring climate, the practitioner should bring up contractual matters such as where and when the family will meet. If the family can tolerate exploration at a first meeting, the practitioner might ask what the family hopes to accomplish as a result of the sessions. As a rule, some but not all members will respond to this question.

During the introductory stage the practitioner will select tools to organize data in a coherent way. The family map, the chronology, and the sociogram are especially helpful in early sessions. When family members disagree about facts or give inaccurate information, their inconsistency may not be deliberate but merely indicate anxiety or embarrassment. Inaccuracy and distortion can be reduced by avoiding emotionally charged words, and by not evincing shock or disapproval. Instead of asking what the problem is, the practitioner might say, "What has been happening in the family that brings you here?" Throughout the course of family sessions it is permissible and even desirable to refer to what was discussed at a previous meeting. Very often important disclosures are made at the end of a session and cannot be dealt with fully. Referring back to unresolved issues provides continuity and shows the family that what members say is important.

There is no real consensus among practitioners as to whether every member must be present at every session. This decision is a matter to be settled jointly by the practitioner and those family members who are present. If a practitioner will continue only when every member attends, absent or reluctant members are given undue control. Sometimes a reluctant member will participate later on, especially if the family appears to benefit from the sessions.

Working Sessions

As families continue to meet with the health care professional, they become better able to trust and to take risks. Even so, hazards persist. Attrition rates are high, since many families are frightened by the prospect of change and terminate prematurely. For families who continue to meet, trust and rapport must be maintained. Interpretations and confrontations must be carefully worded and should be in the form of suggestions or reflective comments rather than challenges. Examples of such techniques are: "How have things changed at home since we've been meeting?" "You may be right, but there is another way of looking at what happened." "I wonder if you were really as hurt as you say. Is it possible that you were angry as well as hurt?"

During the working phase, family members become more open, and their dysfunctional interactional patterns become more overt. Feelings of bitterness may be expressed, and even experienced clinicians become uneasy. At the first sign of great acrimony, the practitioner can insist on ground rules for behavior during the sessions. Ground rules establish behavioral norms to which members are expected to conform. Not interrupting, speaking only for oneself, and listening to each other are some of the ground rules that might be enforced during sessions. Ideally, the family and the practitioner should collaborate in establishing these rules.

Termination Sessions

Many families terminate sessions without the authorization of the health care professional. Even the most adept professional cannot change the family. The family is given an opportunity to deal with problems and to make internal changes, but only the family can take advantage of the opportunity. A great disparity may exist between what the family is willing to change and what the practitioner hopes to change. If there is a gulf between the family's and the practitioner's goals, agreement must be negotiated. More often it is the practitioner who must compromise.

In the introductory sessions specific goals were formulated. Goals give family and practitioner a sense of purpose and direction. Without specific goals, neither the family nor the practitioner has standards for evaluating progress. Termination should not find the family unprepared. If an agreement has been reached that the family will participate in twelve sessions, this should be referred to as termination approaches. Summarization of the family's progress and references to goals achieved are constructive ways of preparing members for termination.

CLINICAL VIGNETTE: FAMILY CONFLICT DUE TO DIVERSE VALUES

Flora and Jay grew up in the same neighborhood and attended the same schools and church. Flora was the oldest of eight children; her father was a truck driver and the undisputed boss of the family. Flora's mother worked in a fast food restaurant. When her mother was at work, Flora was expected to look after the younger children and soothe the uneven temper of her father when he was at home. The household was noisy, crowded, and disorganized in spite of Flora's efforts to maintain order.

Flora was an attractive girl, quiet, unassuming, and busy with school and her tasks at home. While in high school, she began dating Jay, whose home life was as orderly as Flora's was disorderly. Jay's mother was a schoolteacher before marrying, and Jay was her only child. His father was a plumber who earned a good living; Jay's mother did not work outside the home but was active in community affairs. She was a meticulous housekeeper who spent a great deal of her time with Jay. Even in grade school Jay showed academic promise, which his parents tried to cultivate. They had high ambitions for Jay and were disappointed when he began dating Flora, particularly when she left high school before graduating. During her senior year her father was ill for a time and could not work. As a result, the family could not pay its debts.

The money earned by Flora's mother was not enough to feed and clothe a large family, so Flora dropped out of school to work with her mother as a waitress. When her father recovered, Flora tried to return to school but became discouraged when she realized how far behind she was. Flora attended her high school prom with Jay and accompanied his parents to graduation, where she watched her former classmates receive their diplomas. The friendship between Jay and Flora continued while he was in college in spite of the objections of his mother, who thought that he should look for a college girl instead of wasting his time with "that dumb little waitress around the corner." Jay usually listened to his mother, but showed no signs of giving up Flora. They were married shortly after he finished college. At that point Jay had a fellowship for graduate work and was self-supporting. The years in graduate school were rewarding for Jay, but less so for Flora. Because all their friends were struggling to make ends meet, their lack of money did not bother Flora. What bothered her was her inability to feel comfortable with the wives of other graduate students. It was easier after her son was born, for then she had more in common with some of the other wives who had children.

In this marriage the husband and wife came from working-class families, but Jay's family was upwardly oriented whereas Flora's was not. There was more stability and affluence in Jay's family. As an only child, he received a great deal of parental attention, especially from his mother, who had many middle-class values. By means of higher education, Jay had clearly moved into the middle class and identified with middle-class attitudes toward career and family. Flora now lived in a middle-class neighborhood but retained the lower-class values that made her more comfortable. Five years after the birth of her son, Flora found herself in a suburban home with four bedrooms, landscaping, and no close friends. She was close to her mother and sisters, whom she visited several times a week, taking her son with her to the old neighborhood. These visits were the only times when Flora felt relaxed and comfortable.

Although Flora attended company functions with Jay, these were stressful events that often left her with a throbbing headache. The headaches were relieved only when she lay down in a darkened room while Jay or a baby sitter cared for her son. At Jay's insistence, Flora visited an internist who told her she suffered from migraine headaches. She also saw a gynecologist because of her concern that she was unable to become pregnant. Neither the internist nor the gynecologist found a physiological basis for the headaches or her infertility. Jay became impatient as Flora's headaches increased in frequency. She was often unable to attend company functions.

Their sex life, which had been gratifying to them both, began to deteriorate. Jay worried about the welfare of their little boy when Flora was "out of it," as he described her headaches. Noting the strain in the couple's relationship, the internist suggested a psychiatric referral for Flora.

After an assessment of Flora and several conjoint interviews with the couple, marital counseling was suggested. It was concluded that Flora's problems originated in her feelings of inferiority, her loneliness as a corporate wife, her husband's immersion in his career, and her inability to ask him for emotional support. Jay was devoted to Flora and willingly involved himself in marital counseling. Counseling sessions helped him appreciate the stress that social and economic advancement had brought to Flora. This understanding of his wife's feelings made him more supportive of her efforts to fit into his world. Learning of her need to see her family of origin, he was more willing to see them often. His increased interest was reassuring to Flora and made her more willing to find a place for herself in the environment he had chosen. Flora progressed enough to accept a recommendation that she join a group for mothers of preschoolers that dealt with personal and parenting issues. Communication between the couple was enhanced by marital counseling and their own high motivation. Figure 3.13 shows the family map for this family, Table 3.5 shows their family chronology, Figure 3.14 shows the differentiation of self scale for Flora and Jay, Figure 3.15 shows the family genogram, and Table 3.6 shows the family conflict level.

SUMMARY

A number of assessment tools have been developed to aid in assessing families and planning therapeutic intervention. This chapter describes various tools, shows how they might be used, and discusses their advantages

FIGURE 3.13. Clinical Vignette: Family Map of Jay and Flora Ott

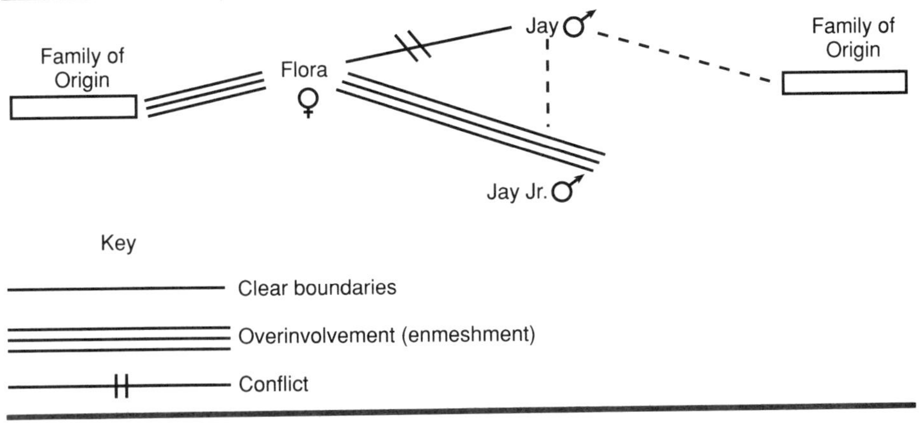

Key

——————— Clear boundaries

=========== Overinvolvement (enmeshment)

———H——— Conflict

TABLE 3.5. Clinical Vignette: Family Chronology of Jay and Flora Ott

1975	Jay and Flora met while both were in high school.
1977	Jay graduated from high school; Flora did not.
1980	Jay graduated from college.
1982	Flora and Jay married.
1983	Jay finished graduate school; Jay awarded an MBA.
1984	Jay Jr. born.
19851988	Flora's health problems began.
1989	Jay and Flora moved to suburban home.
	Marital dissatisfaction developed.
	Sexual problems arose.
	Jay and Flora sought marital counseling.

TABLE 3.6. Clinical Vignette: Family Conflict Level

Jay and Flora Ott operate at level two. Occasionally regress to level three.

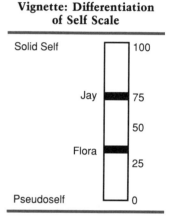

FIGURE 3.14. Clinical Vignette: Differentiation of Self Scale

and limitations. The assessment tools are derived from a number of conceptual frameworks. The following mechanisms used to organize family data appear in the chapter: family maps, family role enactment, differentiation of self scale, family chronology, family genogram, family sociogram, family interaction analysis, family process analysis, and family levels of conflict.

Attrition rates are high in family work, but the health care professional who times interventions to coincide with a family's capacity for change is more likely to forestall premature termination. Even the most experienced professional cannot modify family interaction unless the family is willing. Specific goals are necessary in working with troubled families; goals give practitioners and family members a way to evaluate progress. When there is disagreement between a family and a practitioner regarding goals, mutual accommodation and compromise help resolve the impasse.

Some practitioners insist that every family member attend the therapeutic sessions; others are willing to meet with those family members who

FIGURE 3.15. Clinical Vignette: Family Genograms, Jay Ott and Flora Daly

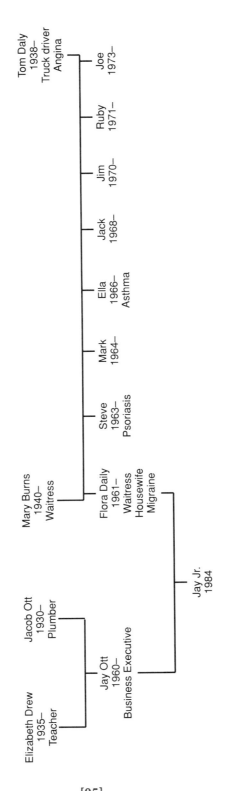

wish to attend. Still others choose to meet with family subgroups even when the entire family is willing to participate. Since family needs vary and clinical considerations prevail, flexibility in this regard is the best course of action.

REFERENCES

Bales, R. F. (1950). *Interaction Process Analysis: A Method for the Study of Small Groups*. Cambridge, MA: Addison-Wesley.

Bowen, M. (1971). "The Use of Family Theory in Clinical Practice." In J. Haley (Ed.), *Changing Families*. New York: Grune and Stratton.

Bowen, M. (1976). "Theory in the Practice of Psychotherapy." In P. Guerin (Ed.), *Family Therapy*. New York: Gardner.

Cain, A. (1980). "Assessment of Family Structure." In J. R. Miller and E. H. Janosik (Eds.), *Family-Focused Care*. New York: McGraw-Hill.

Kerr, M. E., & Bowen, M. (1988). *Family Evaluation: An Approach Based on Bowen Theory*. New York: Norton.

Leas, S. (1985). *Moving Your Church through Conflict*. Washington, DC: Alban.

McGoldrick, M., & Gerson, R. (1986). *Genograms in Family Assessment*. New York: Norton.

Minuchin, S. (1974). *Families and Family Therapy*. Cambridge, MA: Harvard University Press.

Phipps, L. B. (1986). "Group Work: History and Overview." In E. H. Janosik & L. B. Phipps (Eds.), *Life Cycle Group Work in Nursing*. Boston/Monterey, CA: Jones and Bartlett.

Simon, R. (1985). "Family Therapy." In H. I. Kaplan & B. J. Sadock (Eds.), *Comprehensive Textbook of Psychiatry*, 4th ed. Baltimore, MD: Williams and Wilkins.

Weingarten, H. (1986). "Strategic Planning for Divorce Mediation." *Social Work*, 31(3): 194–200.

Weingarten, H., & Leas, S. (1987). "Levels of Conflict: A Guide to Assessment and Intervention in Troubled Marriages." *American Journal of Orthopsychiatry*, 57(3): 407–416.

Zastowny, T. R., & DeFrank, R. S. (1986). "Empirical Investigation: Research Strategy." In E. H. Janosik & L. B. Phipps (Eds.), *Life Cycle Group Work in Nursing*. Boston/Monterey, CA: Jones and Bartlett.

PART

TWO

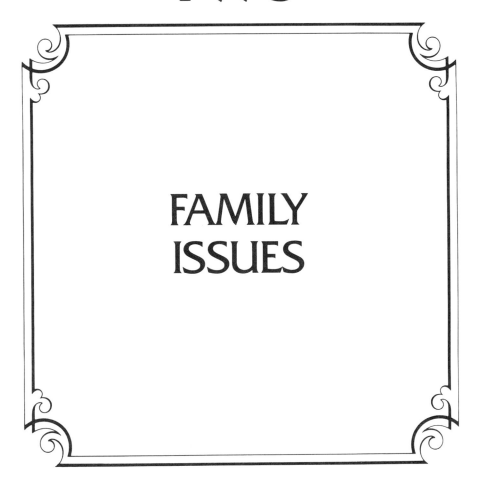

FAMILY
ISSUES

CHAPTER FOUR

Internal Family Issues:
Ethnicity, Race, and Class

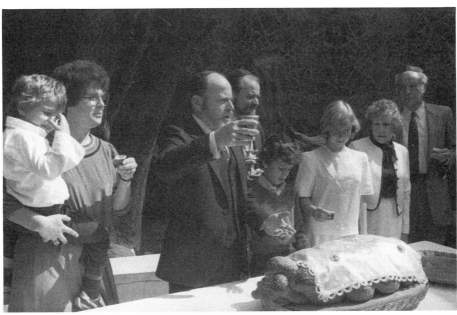

© Frank Siteman MCMLXXXV

The life history of the individual is first and foremost an accommodation to the patterns and standards traditionally handed down in his community. From the moment of his birth, the custom into which he is born shapes his experience and behavior. By the time he can talk . . . and by the time he is grown and able to take part in its activities, its habits are his habits, its beliefs his beliefs, its responsibility his responsibility.

Ruth Benedict

The United States is a heterogeneous country made up of many families and groups of families who arrived at different historical moments, for different reasons, and from places all over the world. Over the last few decades many of the minority groups in the United States have sought a greater share of economic and political power. What was once a self-effacing acceptance of minority status has given way to militancy and pride in the group heritage. The climate of minority assertiveness places new demands on the health care professional. Because families are less defensive about their national origin and their values, caregivers must be more knowledgeable about minority group experience before and after the momentous arrival in the United States. Daniel Moynihan (1965, 1986) noted that the past and present of an ethnic group are one. An unexamined past, therefore, omits much that is needed to understand minority group experience. Failure by caregivers to consider the historical memory of minority groups is a threat to effective care.

During the 1960s, cultural and ethnic consciousness was invoked in black communities to reduce racial stigma and enhance the self-image of black Americans. In a relatively short time, ethnic awareness spread to other groups — Asians, Puerto Ricans, Mexican Americans, and American Indians. These groups, which had not previously shown much ethnic awareness, formed a loose-knit coalition bent on asserting a special identity. Cultural and ethnic awareness also intensified among minority groups of European descent — Irish, Italians, and Poles, among others. Until then, the tendency of most minority groups in the United States had been to strive for integration. The ethnic awakening did not actively discourage integration and assimilation, but it affirmed the right of minorities to retain a shared identity while accepting the benefits of a pluralistic, democratic society.

Steinberg (1981) assigns a negative side to pluralism, alleging that American pluralism had its beginnings in conquest, slavery, and the exploitation of newly arrived groups:

Conquest first in the case of native Americans who were systemat-
ically uprooted, decimated, and finally banished to reservation
wastelands; and second in the case of Mexican Americans in the
Southwest who were conquered and annexed by an expansionist
nation. Slavery, in the case of the millions of Africans who were
abducted from their homelands and forced into perpetual servitude
on another continent. (p. 5)

These harsh words are cited here to emphasize the bitterness and pain that
often accompanied the immigrant experience. An important point is that all
families leaving a homeland, however ungiving, for a strange country suffer
severe culture shock. An early immigrant in an autobiographical account
vividly expresses the confusion of immigrants "cut adrift suddenly from
their ancient moorings, they were floundering in a sort of moral void. Good
manners and good conduct, reverence, and religion had all gone by the
boards, and the reason was that these things were not American" (Ravage,
1917, p. 79).

Leaving one's native land for another country sets in motion a long
process of bewildering change. Depending on differences between the new
land and the one left behind, accommodation is easier for some immigrant
groups than for others. It is important for health professionals to learn the
circumstances surrounding the arrival of these families in the new world,
the reception they received, and the cultural baggage in the form of race,
religion, and traditions that accompanied them. Only through such knowledge can caregivers recognize and deal with internal family issues. Except
for American Indians, every minority group in the United States originated
elsewhere. Even though they carried little in the way of material goods,
immigrant families brought customs that were rich and meaningful for
them.

Every family, regardless of its origin, engages in practices that reflect
shared ideas about what is important and worth preserving. Aspects of
family relationships such as courting, choosing a mate, rearing children, or
caring for the elderly are determined to a large extent by family ideas of
propriety. Ideas about what is appropriate develop slowly over generations
and do not vanish quickly when transplanted from one geographic location
to another. Indeed, the experience of migration or immigration may reinforce the family's attitudes, at least for a time. For example, an Irish family
living in the United States may be more loyal to tradition than an Irish
family living in Dublin, merely to safeguard that which is meaningful but
seems in danger of being lost.

There is a tendency for persons who are not members of a minority
ethnic group to make superficial judgments about the group. In dealing with
individuals or families who are part of an ethnic minority, one must realize
that there is great diversity among people who at first glance appear similar.
Asia, for example, is a huge land mass encompassing ancient nations,

agrarian and industrial, who resemble each other only slightly. It is offensive to Chinese, Japanese, Korean, and Vietnamese people to be seen as a monolithic population segment. The same is true of Hispanic people, who may have come from Cuba, Puerto Rico, or Mexico and whose experiences are quite diverse. Indigenous black Americans and West Indian immigrants may share an African heritage, but their group experience differs greatly. In order to emphasize the differences between ethnic groups that resemble each other superficially, four population segments comprising more than one ethnic group are presented in this chapter. The purpose is to promote sensitivity and reduce misinformation about ethnic groups. Ethnicity and minority status are only two of the variables affecting immigrant families. The preimmigrant experience is crucial, as are the variables of race, language, and religion; the length of time an immigrant group has been in this country and the way the group is perceived by outsiders are other significant variables. Throughout its history the United States regarded newcomers with suspicion, even when their energy and skills were needed. This was especially true if they were not white, were not Protestant, or were from non-English-speaking countries. In 1751 Benjamin Franklin asked "Why should Pennsylvania, founded by the English, become a colony of aliens, who will shortly be so numerous as to Germanize us, instead of our Anglifying them?" Thomas Jefferson in 1782 wrote that the importation of foreigners would "bring with them the principles of the government they leave, imbibed in their early youth; or if able to throw them off, it will be in exchange for an unbounded licentiousness, passing, as usual, from one extreme to another" (Grant, 1928).

When the thirteen colonies won their independence, the population was homogeneous. The original settlers did not consider themselves immigrants but founders and colonizers. The native Indian population numbered less than one million people scattered across a huge continent. Of the white population, 80 percent spoke English; 61 percent claimed English descent, and 90 percent were Protestants. The population distribution of the young republic is shown in Table 4.1.

For many years the growing, expansionist nation accepted immigration as a necessity, but imposed restrictions as needs lessened and the political

TABLE 4.1. United States Population
Distribution at the Time
of the American Revolution

English origin	61%	German origin	9%
Scottish origin	17%	Dutch origin	3%
Irish origin	2%	Swedish origin	1%

Source: Adapted from Steinberg (1981).

climate changed. In this chapter, selective restrictions are described in terms of the minority groups affected by them. Four broad categories of ethnic minorities are presented; within the categories are subdivisions chosen because they show distinctions and differences. No single chapter can adequately discuss all groups making up the polyglot population of the United States. It is possible, however, to select representative groups and draw comparisons. The purpose here is to explore the historical experience of the group, develop hypotheses about group values, and sensitize the health care professional to nuances of the group cultures. Every minority group in this country has a history to unfold, and the following groups are indicative of the population diversity of the United States. Contrasting subgroups within the broad categories allows distinctions to be made. The generalizations made in this chapter are not applicable to every family, and a warning is issued that the chapter offers guidelines, not blueprints, for understanding minority families.

   I. American families of European origin:
      The Irish American family
      The Italian American family
  II. American families of Asian origin:
      The Chinese American family
      The Japanese American family
 III. American families of African origin:
      The Indigenous Black American family
      The West Indian American family
 IV. American families of Hispanic origin:
      The Puerto Rican family
      The Mexican American family

AMERICAN FAMILIES OF EUROPEAN ORIGIN: THE IRISH AMERICAN FAMILY

Historical Background

Minority ethnic groups entered the United States in one of three ways. Some, like the Mexican Americans and the American Indians, were subdued by an aggressive nation seeking territory. Some, like the indigenous American blacks, were kidnapped and brought here in chains. Others came willingly, enduring long, unpleasant journeys in the hope of finding a better life. The Irish immigrants were among the last group. They had the advantage of speaking English, but in other respects they differed from the English and Scottish families already arrived. Even though the Irish were among the first wave of immigrants, they seem to retain more cultural allegiance than some other groups. Greeley (1972, 1977, 1981) attributes this to the following circumstances: (1) They did not have to learn a new language; (2) they developed a parochial school system that respected Irish values, religious and secular; (3) they had already learned to oppose cultural domination in their centuries of dealing with Great Britain.

In 1126 A.D. an English pope, Adrian IV, handed Ireland over to the English king, Henry II. This began a long cycle of rebellion, repression, famine, and misery, as England invoked various measures to control the troublesome Irish. In the early years of occupation, an Irish parliament operated under the control of England. Then Oliver Cromwell and succeeding English kings confiscated Irish lands and awarded ownership to Englishmen. With English landlords in control of the Irish parliament in Dublin, Penal Laws were passed that excluded the Catholic population from education, political expression, and religious freedom. In the nineteenth century the Penal Laws were gradually revoked, and land reform gave the Irish peasantry some rights of ownership by the late nineteenth century. For many years poverty and exploitation were the daily experience of the Irish in their own land.

Irish agriculture was varied and productive, but most of the harvest was shipped from Ireland to England. As a result, the potato was the mainstay of the Irish diet, and failure of the potato crop meant disaster. The Great Potato Famine, which lasted from 1847 to 1850, decimated the population and caused thousands of starving Irish men and women to emigrate. There had been periodic failures of the potato crop before this, but the Great Famine caused more than a million Irish to emigrate within twenty years. Ireland has given a higher proportion of its people to the United States than has any other country (Bernardo, 1981). Those Irish who immigrated before 1850 were mostly farmers and craftsmen from Protestant North Ireland, whose ties to Great Britain were strong. After 1850 Irish immigrants were usually from the rural Catholic South. Although they had been farmers, these immigrants landed in American cities and congregated in Irish neighborhoods. Like the immigrant groups that came later, they accepted physically demanding, poorly paid jobs building railroads, bridges, and canals.

In the homeland, any farms owned by the Irish were small and relatively unprofitable, since large tracts were usually owned by English absentee landlords. In order to improve living conditions by stabilizing the size of their precious farms and by controlling population growth, the Irish adopted the "stem" family structure. Under this system the farm was managed by the parents until they grew too old. At that point the undivided farm was turned over to a selected son (or daughter), who might or might not be the oldest. In the stem family arrangement, only the chosen heir could afford to marry. Parents remained on the farm for their lifetime and were cared for by the heir and his wife.

Having no land of their own, unchosen siblings did not marry. Regardless of their age, these landless, unwed brothers and sisters did not enjoy full adult status. More often than not, they continued to work on the family farm, where they were referred to as "boys" and "girls." Although the stem family served a purpose, it deprived many of their natural rights and privileges. A significant result was that few Irish immigrated as intact families. With marriage at home beyond reach, unmarried women without dowries came to find jobs or husbands in America. Unlike other ethnic groups, the number of female Irish immigrants exceeded that of males. This, along with the custom of late marriages, further reduced their prospects. Many young, unmarried Irish women accepted work as domestic servants, where they were in great demand.

In the absence of a unified nation, Irish identity was based on allegiance to the Roman Catholic Church and aversion to England. In America, Irish affiliation with the Church was viewed with alarm by the Anglo-American majority. As was their custom, the Irish drew strength from their religion, and the Church responded by establishing parishes where a church, parochial school, and convent were conveniently located. For the Irish immigrant, the parish was a more important dimension than the neighborhood. Social norms were defined and upheld by the local parish and its administrators.

In their economically and politically deprived homeland, sexual repression was almost a necessity. One consequence of years of sexual repression is fear of the consequences of physical affection and emotional intimacy. In this, as in many other areas, the Irish are contradictory and puzzling. Despite their verbosity they are uncomfortable in expressing deep feelings, and often hide behind a joke and a laugh. Perhaps because of their long distrust of England and fear of retaliation, they are seldom direct and tend to prefer ambiguity to openness.

Poverty and the influence of the Church not only encouraged sexual repression among the Irish but led to preoccupation with sin, evil, and guilt. Such preoccupation relates to the concept of original sin, which persuades believers that evil-doing is part of the human condition, and that suffering is the price that everyone must pay. Because of internalized guilt, the Irish tend to assume they have caused their own troubles. They suffer in silence, believing that pain is a road to sanctity. Not only is suffering deserved, but it is considered inevitable. This leads to pessimism and wariness in everyday matters. The Irish saying "Sing before breakfast, cry before dark" expresses the idea that if things are going well, they are apt to change soon. Rotunno and McGoldrick (1982) cite a prevailing belief among the Irish that the tragedies that befell the Kennedy family were due to their excessive privilege and success.

The Church in Ireland exerted great influence on its followers, and the influence continued in America through the parochial school system and the unquestioned authority of priests. Modifications introduced by the Vatican and the financial problems of parochial schools have moderated the authority of the Church. As debate about contraception and abortion continues, Irish Americans have begun to explore their options, and their effort to accommodate to Church rules is an issue for many. In dealing with any Catholic family, especially an Irish American one, it is advisable to explore their attitudes toward the Church so that therapeutic tactics are considerate of family beliefs (Greeley, 1981).

Relationships between men and women in the Irish family are also full of contradiction and ambiguity. It is probably significant that there is no Irish equivalent of either the Latin lover or the *pater familias*. Indeed, Irish women seem to dominate family life. Their harsh experiences in Ireland have tended to make Irish Americans pragmatic. They hope that their children will make good marriages, preferably to a Catholic who is hard-working and has some money laid aside. Irish reluctance to engage openly in tenderness or expressiveness may pose problems for Irish Americans who marry persons of Italian or Hispanic origin. What the Irish construe as self-control may seem cold and distant to others. Differences between Irish and Italian religious patterns have been explained as reflections of national attitudes about women. Celibacy was considered by the Irish to be a desirable state, and sexuality within marriage was advocated only for procreation, although many couples have abandoned these views. In Italy the Madonna is worshiped as a tender, nurturing maternal figure, whereas in Ireland the Virgin Mother is venerated but from afar. Biddle (1976) wrote that for the Irish the Virgin Mother was a deity with power in her own right, to whom one could appeal directly in time of need. For Italians, the Madonna functioned as a mediator whose power lay in the love her Son had for her. The implication here is that the Irish mother is extremely powerful in the family, and is subordinate only because she chooses to be.

In the immigrant Irish family, daughters are considered worthy of attention and education, but indulgence is often shown to sons (Blessing, 1980). Children are disciplined, but not always consistently. Affection is not lacking, but it is not often expressed except through teasing and frequent admonishment. More is expected of girls than of boys in the way of behavior and manners. Allowances are made for the behavior of sons, just as they are for the husband and father. Most Irishmen consider their wives to be morally superior to themselves, and the women are inclined to agree even though they make a pretense of deferring to the husband's authority. The attitude of girls toward their brothers, and later toward a husband, is copied from the mother's manipulative, ambiguous interactions with the father.

When experiencing physical pain, the Irish are apt to be vague and inaccurate in describing symptoms. They rarely seek treatment unless the pain is severe or they cannot work. Although they believe that life brings pain, they seldom exaggerate discomfort. This means that their complaints, physical or psychological, should not be minimized by the health care professional (Zborowski, 1969; Novak, 1972).

The psychiatric disability that plagues the Irish, in America and in their homeland, is alcoholism. As early as 1840 an Irish priest wrote that "not only were our countrymen remarkable for their intemperate use of intoxicating liquors, but intemperance had already entered into and formed part of the national character" (Bales, 1946). Irish alcoholism has been attributed to three factors: (1) belief that drinking was manly and drunkenness the weakness of a good man, (2) belief that the drinker is not responsible for acts committed when under the influence, and (3) belief in alcohol as a universal panacea that dulls pain, cures colds and fevers, enlivens celebration, and smooths the sharp outlines of reality (Bales, 1962).

Therapeutic Guidelines

The contradictions that characterize Irish behavior and Irish temperament may cause problems for the health care professional, but there are some useful guidelines. Their strong sense of privacy and propriety makes it hard for members of this group to talk of personal matters. They are more likely to respond to specific, goal-directed interventions than to self-disclosure or emotional catharsis. Tasks assigned at home protect family privacy, and the authority of the health care professional makes it likely that the tasks will be attempted. The Irish family tends to be outwardly compliant, accords the health care professional due respect, but prefers to keep some distance. Although humor is appreciated, crude language and even mild swearing usually meet with disapproval.

Disengagement is more common in Irish American families than enmeshment. The Irish have great respect for personal and family boundaries. They may wish to renew or revive relationships, but be unable to acknowledge this either out of reticence or from fear of destroying boundaries. If emotional issues can be reframed or relabeled in commonsense, down-to-earth language, they appear less threatening and can be handled. For example, a young couple estranged from the husband's family who wish to mend fences are more likely to respond to a specific plan for contacting the parents than to open-ended discussion of feelings about the situation. With their propensity for repression and denial, and their feelings of personal responsibility, the Irish are more interested in finding a remedy than in dealing with the emotional causes of disengagement or estrangement.

The working-class Irish family has deviated least from its past. Always practical, many have found careers in government service as policemen or civil servants. Though loyal, they are confused by their changing church. Middle-class Irish are more diversified and more integrated into American life. They are more accepting of changes in the church and may not heed restrictions against contraception, divorce, and even abortion. Many American values are congenial to the Irish. The hard-working Irish father and the mother who works both inside and outside the home fit neatly into American life. Ambivalence and contradiction are still discernible in family relationships. The man is the ostensible head of the household, but his wife is often the family executive. Boys may be favored by their mothers, but girls are treated in ways that enhance their capabilities. The Irish American family represents a minority group whose complexities are understandable in light of their historical experience.

THE ITALIAN AMERICAN FAMILY

Historical Background

The family, nuclear and extended, is the most important institution in Italian life. To casual observers, all Italian families, regardless of local origin, share common attributes. In reality, most Italian immigrants to the United States came from southern Italy, and differ in life-style, habits, and cuisine from their northern neighbors. Early immigrants from Italy came from the prosperous, industrialized north; after 1900 the majority came from the impoverished, agrarian south. Between 1880 and 1920 about 4 million Italians entered America.

Throughout the Middle Ages and the Renaissance, Italy was a divided land plagued by invaders, shifting alliances, and natural disasters such as flood and earthquake. When Italy was unified in the 1860s, unification was not followed by land reform. This embittered the peasant population and intensified ill will between southern Italy and the north where wealthy landowners lived. Their turbulent national history made Italians distrustful of anyone who was not part of the family or well known to family members. Peasants were exploited by landowners, by the state, and by other vested interests. In Ireland the Church was banned by England and was perceived by the Irish as a protector of native values. In Italy the Church was considered an ally of the rich and powerful, rather than the protector of the poor. For Italians, then, continuity and safety could be found only within the family. It was the family that deserved one's deepest loyalty. Protecting the family and upholding family honor remain for Italians the surest means of protecting one's own interests (Rotunno & McGoldrick, 1982).

The immigrants from southern Italy were people whose rough, unpolished ways embarrassed their countrymen who had arrived earlier and begun to prosper. Because they had been exploited by the upper classes at home, Italians defined themselves by their family and village connections. Upon arrival Italian immigrants joined countrymen from their own or nearby villages and clustered in enclaves housing others from the same region. Within the enclaves family was the sustaining force and the means of judging individuals. Outsiders were acceptable only if this served the needs of the family. The family included *cognates* (blood relatives), *affines* (in-laws), *comparaggio* (godparents), and *paisano* (fellow villagers). Honor and dishonor were attributed to all persons in the same family. Family loyalty extended outward in concentric circles, as shown in Figure 4.1. The rest of the world was regarded with indifference or hostility. *Amoral famil-*

FIGURE 4.1. Concentric Relationships
of Italian Families

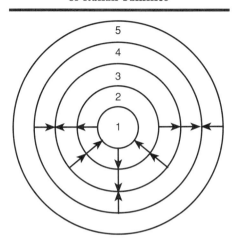

Key

1: Immediate family (including godparents)
2. Extended family related by blood
3: Extended family related by marriage
4: Trusted friends, associates, neighbors
5: Strangers and outsiders

Source: Adapted from Glazer and Moynihan
(1970) and Miller and Janosik (1980).

ism is the term coined to describe this absence of trust or concern for those outside the family (Glazer & Moynihan, 1970).

Unlike the Irish, whose values coincided with those of America, Italians, who valued group affiliation over individualism, sometimes found adjustment difficult. Once settled in a neighborhood, the Italian immigrant was more or less reluctant to move or travel. Italian Americans enjoyed spending a lifetime in the same place; even now, married sons and daughters often choose to live only a few houses away from their parents. The same tendency to reject geographic mobility extended to social mobility. Rising in the world was not a primary goal for Italian immigrants. Because they disliked working for outsiders, many Italians formed small businesses that were family-operated and family-centered. Education received less priority than was the case in other ethnic groups. Even among Italian Americans today, worldly success that does not separate the individual from the family is the success that is truly welcome. Jewish parents rejoice in the success of their children, but Italian parents are happy only if they are included in it (Glazer & Moynihan, 1970; Rotunno & McGoldrick, 1982).

Italian families fear that education and success might strengthen outside influences at the expense of family bonds.

In Italian marriages the father is considered the authority figure and apparent decision maker. Nevertheless, the mother is not subordinate, for her role is central to the family. Positions of husband and wife are equivalent in subtle ways, and the wife's skill as mother and homemaker are highly regarded. It is sometimes said of Italian families that the father is the head of the house but the mother is the heart of the home. Male and female relationships are strictly defined, although definitions have blurred as second- and third-generation Italians enter the middle class. A high value is placed on all family members regardless of age and gender, but cross-sex relationships are handled cautiously. Men tend to turn to other men for help and advice, while women customarily seek help from female relatives and friends. Casual, platonic relationships between men and women of the same age are the exception, not the rule.

Italian fondness for dramatization and histrionic behavior has been explained as a coping mechanism that helps them deal with the vicissitudes of life. By expressing emotion freely, Italians manage to reduce their sense of being passive victims. Dramatizing life's joys and sorrows helps the Italian to "get on in the world and obtain what he wants, solves many problems, lubricates the wheels of society, protects him from the envy of his neighbors and the arrogance of the mighty" (Barzini, 1964, p. 104). A more mundane explanation is that expressive Italian behavior reduces anxiety by releasing emotions that can be shared and appreciated by others. It is also possible that emotional reenactment of events and sensations reduces their impact through repetition. It is true that emotional expressiveness is more permissible in women than in men. This is not because expressiveness is devalued but because men are expected to control their feelings before outsiders.

The Italian way of life is expansive in that joy, grief, pain, and suffering are seldom solitary experiences. An interesting description of Italian reactions to pain and illness is offered by Novak (1972, p. 44):

> The Italian has no worries about disease or being ill—these are future things. The only thing that worries him is the present pain which prevents enjoyment. . . . He couldn't care less about analysis, diagnosis, mechanics. The Italian hates "the knife" and "the needle." He likes personal things. His parents took such personal interest in him that he sees the world almost wholly in personal terms.

Interestingly, although Italians may respond intensely to pain, they also respond strongly to measures designed to relieve pain, perhaps because they are eager for relief.

The importance of alcohol in the Italian family is secondary to the emphasis on food, especially food prepared in mama's customary fashion. In

Italy alcoholism is rare, partly because drinking was part of a social occasion but not the reason for it. Men and women drank together, usually in the home. Children were allowed to drink watered wine on occasion, and attitudes about drinking were matter-of-fact. Alcohol was not used to transform reality but to enjoy life as it was. Wine was the preferred beverage rather than the distilled liquors that the Irish consume. Second- and third-generation Italians have adopted some of the drinking habits of Americans, such as the cocktail party at which little food is served. However, they remain an ethnic group whose problems with alcohol are minimal. In this they resemble Jewish Americans, whose drinking habits continue to provide safeguards against overindulgence (Nelli, 1980).

Therapeutic Guidelines

Attempts of Italian Americans to solve problems within the family help explain their low rates of psychiatric hospitalization and utilization of mental health facilities (Vecoli, 1978). In the Italian language there are two words for walls; one describes internal and the other describes external walls. This indicates the difference in the way internal and external living is seen, and the significance that is placed on family boundaries (Rotunno & McGoldrick, 1982). As a result, one problem faced by health care professionals is that of being accepted by the Italian American family. Initially the caregiver may be distrusted, but this is cultural, not personal. The Irish family in its interactions with the health care system uses distance and reticence as coping maneuvers. Outwardly compliant, they may offer silent resistance to change. In contrast, the Italian family may use guile and charm to conceal their suspicion. Because they look first for help from family members, the problems of Italian families may be serious before they apply for professional assistance. Once in treatment they give colorful accounts of their problem, and their communication style, characterized by elaboration and exaggeration, may overwhelm a caregiver from another culture. Italians are likely to be very concerned about their physical and psychological state, and Ragucci (1981) noted tendencies toward elaborate descriptions of symptoms. In Zbarowski's classic study (1969), Italians were concerned primarily with prompt relief of discomfort and equated freedom from pain with alleviation of the illness.

Although they appear to be articulate and open, divulging family secrets is difficult for members of this group. Urging them to disclose secrets is counterproductive, and caregivers must constantly evaluate the family's readiness to trust. The respect for secrets in Italian families is explained by their desire to avoid revelations that might damage relationships within the family or impair family honor with outsiders. One elderly Italian woman who had had a backstreet abortion years ago shared the secret only with her mother and a sister. For years the knowledge was held between the three, and was told to the woman's grown daughter only as a warning of the consequences of premarital sex. The information never became general family knowledge, and was jealously guarded for many years. To be effective in helping these families, one must move from being an outsider to being an advisor who is devoted to family interests. Enmeshment between members is a fact of life and should be interpreted as cultural rather than pathological.

Once the family accepts the health care professional, a major goal is to help family members extricate themselves from enmeshment without violating family traditions. As children become adolescents and young adults, they may become impatient with family closeness. This is very threatening for parents, and conflict results that threatens family balance. Here a caregiver might use reframing and relabeling tactics by complimenting parents on having raised such stalwart, self-reliant children. At the same time, troubled parents need reassurance that family love and influence are not limited in quantity, and that permitting children to grow up is the best way of preserving family integrity. Reminding parents that they once broke with tradition by coming to a new country may reinforce feelings of connectedness between parents and children. A self-assertive son or daughter may be more acceptable if seen as a "chip off the old block" or "her mother's daughter." The caregiver must maintain a neutral stance between supporting individuation and family values. Emotional disengagement is difficult for these family-oriented people to tolerate. Boundary maintenance may be explained as one way of making family life more satisfying for everyone. What is essential is to help members to move in the direction of self-differentiation, if they are so inclined, without arousing feelings of betrayal in other family members. Health care professionals from other ethnic groups should know that Italian families are among the most stable in the United States. They have a low divorce rate, care for their elderly, and deal constantly with conflicting messages they receive in American life.

Cultural dissonance is frequently experienced by Italian American families. Parents are torn between American values and those of the old country. Children are torn between American values and those of their traditionally minded parents. For example, staying close to home and questioning upward mobility are not highly regarded in the present-day United States. There is ongoing conflict about personal growth versus family stability. Second- and third-generation Italian women tend to become dissatisfied with their status as home-oriented wives and mothers. And bright adolescents are encouraged by their teachers to become all that they can be, even if this means moving outside the limited realm of the family.

The health care professional involved with Italian American families needs to screen their volubility in search of valid data. Expectations of the family for rapid solutions to problems must be confronted. Emotionality and tension may rise and fall in these families, but involvement and caring are constant. This means that many family strengths are available; these can be mobilized and channeled into problem-solving modes that are acceptable. When emotionality runs high, the caregiver should remain neutral and temperate. With Irish families, connections should be made between events and the feelings evoked by them; with Italian families connections should be made between feelings and the events that precipitated them. Remember that the vitality and interactional style of this minority group are propelled by memories of a difficult past. They are characterized by their commitment to family continuity and gradual acceptance of American values.

Stereotypes are hazardous because:

- Within each racial and ethnic group, there are subgroups that resemble and differ from one another in various ways.

- Within each racial and ethnic group are families who adjust to mainstream culture in different ways and at different rates.

- Within each family, regardless of racial or ethnic origin, are members who adjust to mainstream values in different ways and at different rates, depending on the importance they place on stability versus progress.

FIGURE 4.2. **Traditional Irish American Family**

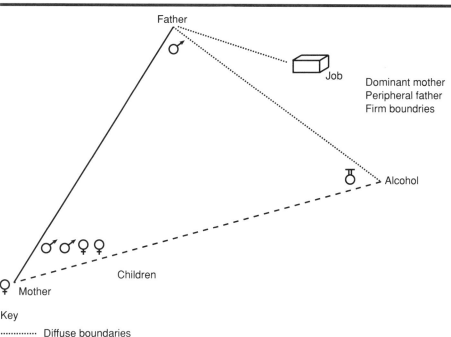

Father

Job

Dominant mother
Peripheral father
Firm boundries

Alcohol

Children

Mother

Key

··········· Diffuse boundaries
– – – – Clear boundaries
——— Rigid boundaries

The examples in Figures 4.2 through 4.7 show ways of mapping representative ethnic minority families. The maps are intended to suggest possible family structures and therefore will not apply to all ethnic families.

FIGURE 4.3. Traditional Italian American Family

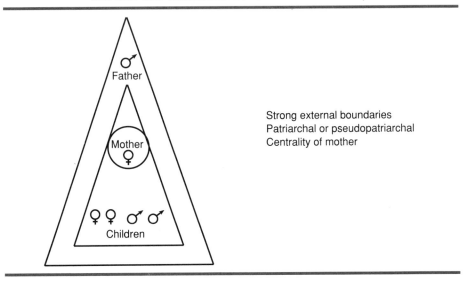

Strong external boundaries
Patriarchal or pseudopatriarchal
Centrality of mother

FIGURE 4.4. Traditional Chinese American Family

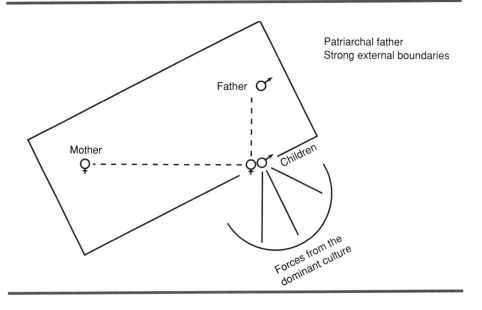

Patriarchal father
Strong external boundaries

FIGURE 4.5. Indigenous Black American Family

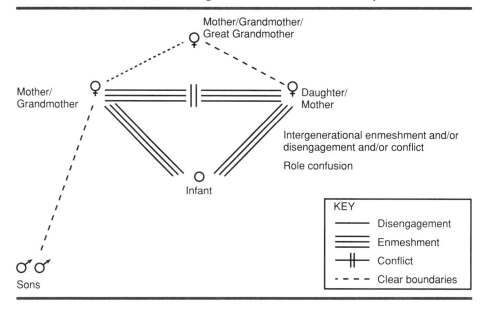

Mother/Grandmother/
Great Grandmother

Mother/
Grandmother

Daughter/
Mother

Intergenerational enmeshment and/or
disengagement and/or conflict

Role confusion

Infant

Sons

KEY
——————— Disengagement
═══════ Enmeshment
—‖— Conflict
- - - - Clear boundaries

FIGURE 4.6. Traditional Puerto Rican Family

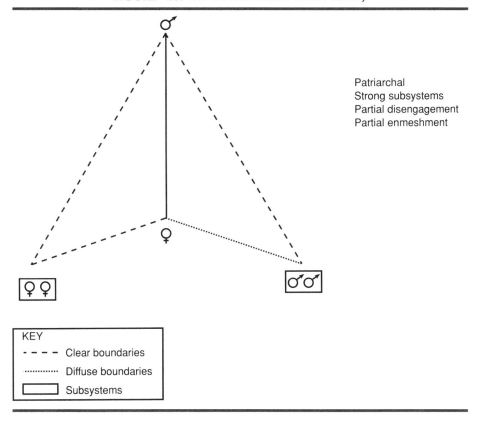

Patriarchal
Strong subsystems
Partial disengagement
Partial enmeshment

KEY
- - - - Clear boundaries
.... Diffuse boundaries
☐ Subsystems

FIGURE 4.7. Traditional Mexican American Family

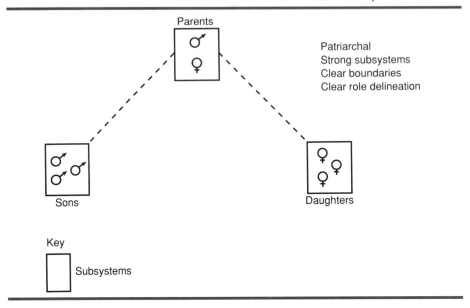

AMERICAN FAMILIES OF ASIAN ORIGIN: THE CHINESE AMERICAN FAMILY

Historical Background

Problems of immigrant families are compounded when racial differences intrude. Racial prejudice in turn is compounded when economic issues enter the picture. The phrase "yellow peril" was used early in this century by the influential publisher William Randolph Hearst, whose warnings of inundation by Asian immigrants fell on attentive ears. Bias feeds upon ignorance, and Asia was, and still is, a mysterious continent to most Americans. Caucasians tend to consider all Asians alike in appearance and heritage, but as Tsui and Schultz (1985) suggest, Asians are a heterogeneous group that includes Chinese, Japanese, Vietnamese, and Koreans, among others. Even though each group has unique characteristics, they share enough characteristics to warrant some generalizations. Most Asians believe in deference to authority, restrained and appropriate verbal and behavioral expression, strong family organization, and prescribed family and personal responsibilities. Most Asian families are patriarchal and non-democratic, with explicit role expectations. In their family life, upheld by years of tradition, dissension and confrontation are avoided at all costs (Tsui & Schultz, 1988).

Besides national differences based on their historical experience, variations result from the arrival time of different groups. Asian immigration, especially Chinese, was heavy in the nineteenth century when canals and railroads were being built and labor was needed. It decreased drastically early in the twentieth century when severe limits were imposed. This was a time of American isolationism during which European immigration was also limited, but quotas set for Asians were lower than for other groups. The Exclusion Act of 1882 prohibited immigration of the families of Chinese workers already in the United States, so that for many years Chinese communities here were overwhelmingly male. Later, when immigration quotas were liberalized, family life was normalized to some extent. In 1980 about 60 percent of all Chinese Americans were first-generation immigrants, mostly women and children who had suffered separation from family members who preceded them to the United States.

The diversity of the Asian population in the United States increased after the Korean and Vietnamese military actions. In recent years a great number of Asian refugees and immigrants have arrived on American shores. Many of these later arrivals are not laborers but members of the mercantile or professional ranks. They undoubtedly have problems related to cultural adjustment, language, and status, but they are likely to be less conservative and more sophisticated than Asian immigrants of a hundred years ago. Thus, time of entry affects social class, which in turn affects the adjustment process of the immigrant. A Chinese immigrant from rural China will have more difficulty adapting to American life than a college student from Beijing. Many elderly Chinese Americans who have lived for years in a Chinese ghetto are less accepting of American customs than a newly arrived youngster attending an American school. Some elderly residents of the "Chinatowns" in American cities have been frozen in time, so to speak, and cling to familiar customs as long as they live.

For most Asian groups, the family is the crucial organizing structure. During dangerous times the Chinese family proved adaptable and resourceful despite relentless political events. Before and after World War II, a strong nationalist party, headed by Generalissimo Chiang Kai Chek, ruled China. The nationalist movements and its leaders retreated to the island of Formosa, now Taiwan, when the Communist party led by Mao Tse Tung took power. Each wave of Chinese immigration brought people who came for different reasons. Early immigrants came in hopes of finding a better life, but others were sojourners who worked here for a time, saved their wages, and returned to their families in China. Some were emigres or refugees who feared for their lives as one uncompromising political party succeeded another. To most Chinese immigrants, family continued to be important; separation from the extended family made the nuclear family more precious.

The Chinese family, like most Asian families, is more authoritarian than democratic. Husband, wife, sons, and daughters learn how and when to interact with each other. It is expected that father will work hard and be respected. Sons are greatly cherished; daughters are expected to be caring and obedient. Mothers are loving and may mediate between father and children, but they also insist on strict role performance. To outsiders it seems that the family is merely an appendage to father, but the purpose of life is not to satisfy the father. Instead, it is the family that gives all members a reason for their existence. The purpose of all members is to bring honor to the family, and this is a purpose that guides the father also. The power vested in the father is accompanied by great responsibility. The primary responsibility of the father is to leave the family as honorable and vigorous as he found it.

Industry, responsibility, and achievement are virtues that help Chinese Americans succeed in the dominant culture. A crucial difference is that parents in these families do not value independence and autonomy in their children. Competence and expertise are desirable because these bring material benefits to the family. However, these qualities must be controlled in order to avoid threats to family continuity. The child who brings greatest joy to parents is highly disciplined, capable, and ambitious but is still dependent on parents for approval and counsel. One Asian college student confided to a professor the conflict she experienced on returning home and transforming herself from an articulate, outgoing college student into a docile, submissive daughter.

A symbiotic relationship exists between father and sons; this is intensified by the veneration given to all family ancestors. Because family life is cyclical, sons realize that someday they will enact the role of husband and father. For as long as one's parents live, one must behave in a filial way. As parents grow old, the obligation of adult children is to recreate for parents the comfort and indulgence that are the right of small children.

Daughters face problems related to their place in the family. Many daughters are well loved but know they occupy places of inferiority. When they leave home for college or business, they readily abandon their acceptance of inferior status. Their behavior often puzzles parents accustomed to clearly defined role performance.

Upon arrival in the United States, Chinese immigrants tend to live in native communities that are major centers of transaction, social, economic, personal, and political. For the residents these neighborhoods have the character of a village or of an extended family. In their attempt to survive in a strange country, Chinese Americans are likely to turn to their own kind for help. Many Chinese immigrants have already endured deprivation and even persecution in their homeland. United for a time by a nationalist leader, the country moved to a communist system that introduced some reforms but was very coercive, especially on middle- and upper-class citizens. As always, the needs of this immigrant group change after arrival. The immediate need is for work and a place to live. After survival needs are met, the impact of new ways may lead to intergenerational conflict, role confusion, and mourning for family members who were left behind.

Therapeutic Guidelines

Chinese Americans find it easier to express somatic complaints than psychological ones. Some organs, such as the heart, liver, or kidneys, seem to have a symbolic meaning, and complaints of Chinese Americans often focus on these organs. Since there may be an organic basis for the complaints, physical as well as psychological assessment is needed. Shame and shaming are mechanisms used to reinforce appropriate role enactment. Living up to one's obligations is the best way to avoid *tiu lien* or loss of face following a shameful experience. Suppression of one's negative feelings is stressed, especially if they are directed toward parents or those to whom one is obligated. Shon and Ja (1982) quote Confucius, who said, "In serving his parents, a son may gently remonstrate with them. When he sees that they are not inclined to listen to him, he should resume an attitude of reverence and not abandon his effort to serve them. He may feel worried but he does not complain" (p. 214).

The ever-present threat of shame and the need to suppress negative feelings are potential sources of psychological distress. A parent whose children do not meet filial obligations, a son or daughter frustrated by family rigidity or insensitivity, faces the dilemma of adhering to old habits in a land where they are no longer considered necessary. Free and open expression of feelings is not the Chinese way. Such variables as age, gender, social status, and family role determine the nature of an interaction. Who speaks first, who bows lowest, who is most deferential are all determined by the identity of the participants and the nature of the situation. This means that the health care professional operates in circumstances that seem ambiguous to the Chinese American, even though they have been carefully explained. Ambiguity causes the Chinese American to be fearful of being shamed and losing face. To avoid this, the Chinese American is inclined to be watchful and vigilant, looking for cues and maintaining silence as much as possible. These precautions place an added burden on the health care professional.

Suicide is not uncommon in the Chinese culture, but the voluntary death of a family member brings grief to the family. The suicide rate of men exceeds that of women by four to one. Chinese men usually commit suicide by ingesting barbiturates; for women hanging is the most frequent method. This is a contrast to suicide methods used in Western societies, where women tend to overdose on pills and men use violent methods such as shooting or hanging themselves. Suicide in Chinese men is usually caused by loneliness or physical debility; women are driven to suicide by chronic conflict with their husband or their parents. Unfortunately, the discouraging of free expression among Chinese Americans causes many to find a solution for interpersonal problems in suicide.

In working with Chinese American families the health care professional should accept and uphold hierarchical family structure by such simple means as addressing father first. To decrease uncertainty, the health care professional should share information about himself or herself without going into detail. The family hierarchy must be acknowledged and never challenged directly. To do otherwise would shame the family. A father would suffer loss of face if contradicted by his wife or a daughter or even by a son. The oblique, indirect communication style of the family may be difficult for a health care professional who is eager to move things along. "Make haste slowly" is a good axiom to bear in mind when working with members of this strong, complex, intricate family system.

Talking about one's problems seems strange to Chinese Americans who believe that physical and mental health depend on harmony, moderation, and discipline. Because the role of physician is better understood than the role of counselor, the Chinese American is more comfortable if the care provider acts somewhat like a physician. By making a diagnosis of sorts and assigning specific tasks to be accomplished, the care provider acts as the authority in charge. Even so, there is a high attrition rate among this group unless problems are physical. If they are to continue to meet as a family, the counselor's role must be explained and time given to discuss the family's expectations of what will follow.

An egalitarian relationship should be avoided because these families are accustomed to vertical relationships and respect expertise. The health care professional should appear confident and dignified. Diffidence or modesty on the part of the caregiver may be interpreted as incompetence. Nondirectiveness and neutrality on the part of the caregiver may be construed as indifference. This can be modified by offering expressions of concern for the family's well-being. With their history of forced separation from family members, they may look for parental affection from the caregiver. Dependency may result, but can be discouraged by introducing collateral caregivers while maintaining connection with the original care provider. When rapport is established with the health care professional, the relationship may become precious to the family. Although tendencies to keep in touch must be monitored, the trust that persists will facilitate reentry to the health system in time of need.

Because of close ties with extended family members, decisions concerning who attends family sessions demand careful judgment. Occasionally a family group may resist being involved because of embarrassment, which is a euphemism for shame or losing face. Parents are frequently reluctant to disclose their reactions before the children; children may hesitate to confront parents in the presence of an outsider. The health care professional may choose to meet first with the identified client and member(s) of his or her choice. Once their trust has been won, other members or subgroups may be invited. At some point older family members such as grandparents who wield power may be invited to meet. Initial sessions may need to be devoted to learning just who does what in the family. Exploration regarding role performance should be factual rather than abstract, and thus less threatening to family members.

THE JAPANESE AMERICAN FAMILY

Historical Background

Like Chinese Americans, the Japanese do not believe that marriage of two people establishes a new family. Instead, it merely perpetuates the family of the husband. The woman leaves her parental home to become part of her husband's family. The status of the bride is low, especially before she becomes a mother. She is subordinate to her parents-in-law, her husband, and her husband's older siblings. A girl should obey her father, a woman her husband, and a widow her oldest son. Actually, this pattern may exist only on the surface and is altered by events and by the personalities of those involved. The strongest attachments are those between mother and children. After the disability or death of the father, the oldest son is the head of the family, but he is often so respectful of his mother that she actually rules the family.

The position of the oldest son is one of privilege in Asian families, and the Japanese family is no exception. Sons are more valued than daughters, who are fated to become part of another family. Along with privilege, the oldest son has obligations. He is expected to set a good example; younger siblings defer and are guided by the oldest son before and after the death of the father. The independent, self-made man does not exist in the Japanese mind. What one becomes is due to the combined efforts of the family. The greatest obligation is to one's parents, and it can never be fully paid. No matter how bitterly parents and children disagree, one's parents are entitled to reverence and obedience.

Shaming tactics are used by Japanese parents to eradicate unacceptable behavior. Shaming is painful because it demonstrates that approval has been withdrawn and personal security endangered. The Japanese word *amae* denotes an embracing, universal kind of love, and it links the ideas of shame and obligation. Obligation does not only mean paying what is owed. It is also a voluntary way of expressing *amae* or love. When a Japanese does not fulfill obligations, he feels shame and loses the sense of security he once enjoyed. He feels exposed and diminished in the eyes of others. Thus, the pressure to meet one's obligations, and the fear of shame if obligations are not met, are powerful motivators for this minority group.

The Japanese American family has a dubious claim to distinction. They are the only minority group who have been subject to incarceration because of their racial heritage. On February 19, 1942, ten weeks after the attack on Pearl Harbor, an executive order was signed giving the secretary of war power to exclude citizens and aliens from designated areas when their presence might endanger the security of the United States. A short while later, all U.S. citizens of Japanese descent were banned from working or traveling on the West Coast (U.S. Commission, 1982). Prejudice against Japanese Americans had long been present in California, where most Japanese Americans lived. Immigration from Japan had been restricted in 1908 and fully prohibited in 1924. Issei (the immigrant generation of Japanese) were banned from citizenship, even though their children (Nisei, first-generation Japanese born in the United States) were citizens because they were American-born. Internment of Japanese Americans was justified by the rationale that "racial affinities are not severed by immigration. The Japanese race is an enemy race and while many second and third generation Japanese born on United States soil, possessed of United States citizenship, have become Americanized, the racial strains are undiluted" (U.S. Commission, 1982).

A civilian bureau, the War Relocation Agency, was established to oversee relocation and internment of Japanese Americans then living on the West Coast. Conditions in the internment camps permitted survival but not much more. Family life was disrupted; fathers who had been household heads found their authority eroded. Some camps were better than others, but educational and medical facilities were minimal. More painful than loss of home and possessions was shame at having been brought so low by their adopted land.

The response of Nisei to the wartime experience differed markedly from that of Issei. Issei tended to believe that they were deficient in some way and hesitated to call relocation and internment unfair. The Nisei, who considered themselves natural-born Americans, felt that their constitutional rights had been breached. They had learned that it was not enough to be a citizen if your ancestry was Japanese. They found different modes of dealing with the experience. Among the most frequent reactions were the following:

- Denying the importance of the experience and trying to forget it
- Losing faith in America and trusting only people of Japanese ancestry
- Dedicating their lives to economic prosperity to overcome feelings of inferiority
- Identifying with the aggressor by becoming very American and avoiding any association with Japanese culture or people

"Before internment" and "after internment" are markers used by many Japanese Americans in describing the experience of their people. As stated in the commission report (1982), "Even after four decades, it is the mournful reference point from which these Americans describe changes in their communities, their personal lives, their aspirations. It is the central experience which has shaped the way they see themselves, how they see America, and how they have raised their children."

Therapeutic Guidelines

The behavior of Japanese Americans is partly a by-product of the institutionalized prejudice that was inflicted upon them. The sense of injustice still held by the group may contribute to their will to succeed and their efforts to master situations. Comas-Dias and Minrath (1985) suggest that therapeutic work can progress only if "reality is acknowledged from the start of treatment, and the manifest and symbolic meaning of sociocultural factors carefully explained and worked through." Perhaps the most important consideration in working with these families is the issue of power. The power of the family must be reinforced, not imperiled, by a care provider who acts all-powerful. Premature requests for personal disclosure may be seen as intimidation and invasion of family boundaries. The family may hesitate to challenge the health care provider directly but may engage in avoidance behavior. Smiles and polite nods as well as tangential dialogue may be employed to avoid genuine involvement. If the health care professional shows interest in the chronological experience of the family, members may become willing to move from general to specific events. Discriminatory laws on citizenship, marriage, and property may need to be acknowledged before the family can describe current needs (Takiki, 1989). Many Japanese Americans struggle with issues of superiority versus inferiority and passivity versus assertiveness. They need assurances that they are respected by the care provider before they confer respect.

Japanese Americans, like other Asians, are reluctant to go outside the family for help except as a last resort. Pressure, sometimes excessive, is placed on young people for academic achievement. Students who cannot meet parental expectations may recognize their own limitations before the parents do. Some youngsters react by withdrawing from family life or by challenging the father's authority. This has the usual effect of making father more insistent on compliance. The result is disruption of family life and alienation between father and children. A Japanese American wife may find work outside the home for economic reasons. This can undermine father's hierarchical position and create a different set of problems for parents.

Role theory can be used to advantage with these families because it depersonalizes issues. The health care professional can point to a new environment in which the family now functions. Instead of trying to change family members, the care provider can suggest ways of being and acting compatible with society that do not attack family organization. Redefining some aspects of role performance helps family members adopt new behaviors while retaining some that are meaningful. A cognitive approach is acceptable in most instances because emotions tend to be suppressed rather than expressed. As problems are disclosed, the family may discount or minimize their importance. This kind of denial, like most denial, is a protective mechanism arising from fear of being stigmatized or losing face.

A frontal assault on the family's defenses or interdependence will probably lead to premature termination. The health care professional needs to be sensitive to indirect, implied messages, and tolerant of evasion and circumstantiality. And it must be acknowledged that even the most experienced care provider may have difficulty dealing with the guardedness that Japanese Americans bring to encounters in a society that has sometimes been hostile to them.

THE INDIGENOUS BLACK AMERICAN FAMILY

Historical Background

Most immigrants came to this country voluntarily, but the ancestors of indigenous black families came unwillingly, shackled, herded into the miserable holds of disease-infested ships. Forcibly torn from their families, they began years of servitude with no hope of returning to familiar tribal life. Wideman (1989) describes the journey of an African as follows: "Curled in the black hold of the ship, he wonders why his life on solid green earth had to end, why the gods had chosen this new habitation for him, floating, chained to other captives, no air, no light, the wooden walls shuddering, battered, as if some madman is determined to destroy even this last pitiful refuge. . ." (p. 130).

Invariably, the journey into slavery terminated the strong family and tribal bonds that permeated the lives of Africans before they came to this country (Nobles, 1980; Franklin, 1969). During the years of enslavement, their recollections of family and tribal life in Africa were discouraged by slave owners and lasted only a few generations.

The slave owner was intent only on making slavery profitable; if slaves were treated humanely, it was because they were valuable property. Attitudes of owners toward family and marriage among slaves were erratic and guided by the profit motive. Slaves had no rights and were not permitted the comfort of formal marriage. Breeding activities, especially between slaves on the same plantation, were allowed because slave children were valuable merchandise. A semblance of family life was permitted because domesticity was thought to make slaves more docile. Some blacks shared a cottage with a mate and children, but changes in the life of the owner often disrupted these quasi-marital arrangements and cruelly separated families.

Even though family life was controlled by the owner, enslaved blacks valued their mates and children. Because they could not marry, they developed their own rituals to make family meaningful. Some of their rituals resembled old tribal ceremonies; as memories of Africa faded, new rituals were devised. Some slaves, when permitted to choose a mate, adopted a marriage ceremony called "jumping over the broom." Although it probably seemed ludicrous to whites, this simple ceremony had poignant overtones. It was meaningful to the participants, and the symbolic use of a broom may have been due to its availability. After all, not many slaves could afford a wedding ring (Miller & Janosik, 1980).

The recurrent theme in the lives of enslaved blacks was loss—loss of freedom, loss of identity, and loss of family members to the auction block. Regardless of the importance of family life to blacks, they were not empowered to begin or end relationships. It was the white owner who sanctioned partnerships, controlled access to females, and defined family life. After the Emancipation Proclamation, blacks struggled to maintain intact families. Many freed men and women continued to live and work on Southern plantations, hoping that lost loved ones would return (Hines & Boyd-Franklin, 1982).

A study of family records after 1960 indicated that the black family was nuclear in form and headed by an adult male. Although this pattern was prevalent in the South, migration to Northern cities contributed to the fragmentation of black families. In 1900 three-quarters of black families lived in the rural South; by 1950 less than one-fifth did (Lewis, 1965). Moving to urban centers changed the form if not the substance of black family life. One change was the erosion of the large kinship group, because many family members remained in the South. Economic progress was made during World War II, but the return of veterans created a labor surplus that even the pent-up demand for consumer goods could not absorb. Three factors have contributed to the heavy unemployment of black men: racial prejudice, lack of seniority, and exclusionary policies of many unions.

Unemployment was less of a problem for black women. Domestic work in white households was always available because it was not sought by many others. Underpaid and overworked, black women were able to contribute to the support of their families. Entering the homes of affluent whites, the women often became trusted confidantes. They learned how the system worked and used this knowledge on behalf of their own families. A consequence of the intermittent employment of black men and the constant employment of black women was the evolving of a managerial role for women, even when the husband was present in the home.

A great strength of black families is their willingness to delegate and distribute roles. Role flexibility enables grandmothers to raise grandchildren and foster children when the need arises. It has contributed to the competence of black women and the esteem they enjoy within the family. The other side of this role flexibility is the undermining of the black man, who often feels powerless both inside and outside the family. His response to this feeling of powerlessness may take various forms. He may withdraw from family life and look for gratification elsewhere. Another consequence of role flexibility is the parental child who foregoes childhood to become the caretaker of siblings (Pinderhughes, 1982).

Many black families have increased their incomes over the last twenty years. In 1968 black families in which both parents worked earned an income 73 percent as high as white families in the same category. By 1981 black families were earning 84 percent of white families' earnings. This is shown graphically in Figures 4.8 and 4.9. However, female-headed households are the most rapidly rising segment of all black families, and their economic losses more than offset the gains made by two-parent black families. Black children are particularly subjected to conditions of poverty, being about three times more likely to live at poverty levels than whites. Again, this may be attributed to the fact that so many black children do not live in more affluent households with two wage earners. Almost half of adult black males are unemployed, and this is related to the rise in households headed by women. As men lose their jobs, the burden of providing for children falls on women, many of whom resort to welfare. In many states, two-parent families are not eligible for welfare, and this contributes to the creation of households where the father is absent, voluntarily or forcibly (Joe, 1983).

Over the last twenty years black Americans have surpassed whites in making educational progress. Between 1960 and 1981 black males achieved

FIGURE 4.8. Family Income: Median Income, in Thousands of 1981 Dollars, Adjusted for Inflation

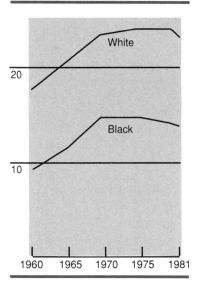

Source: U.S. Census Bureau.

FIGURE 4.9. Single Mothers: Families Headed by Women with Children under 18, as a Percentage of All Families of Each Race with Children under 18

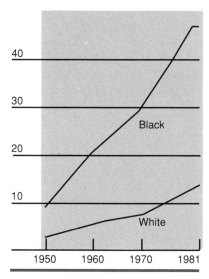

Source: U.S. Census Bureau.

a 4.4-year gain in schooling, whereas white males achieved an average gain of 1.9 years. The illiteracy rates for blacks dropped rapidly, until there is now little difference between blacks and whites in reading ability. School dropout rates have fallen for blacks, and college enrollment of this group has risen greatly. However, the financial rewards for education are different for the two groups. Of blacks with four or more years of college, 47 percent earned between $20,000 and $40,000 annually. This record was equaled by whites who had only a high school education (Herbers, 1983, 1985) (see Figure 4.10).

In the last two decades the unemployment ratio of blacks to whites has remained constant at two to one. From 1972, when affirmative action was implemented, until the present, blacks increased their share of administrative, professional, and technical jobs in fields that were once closed to them. Even so, the U.S. Census Bureau, using its most current data, estimates that between 45 and 50 percent of black men are unemployed (see Figure 4.11).

Indigenous black Americans have been described as bicultural (Pinderhughes, 1982). Because color prevented them from moving easily in white society, they lived apart from other groups and developed their own rich culture. Many black Americans are ambivalent and distrustful toward

FIGURE 4.10. Years in School:
Median Years in School of
Those over 25 Years Old

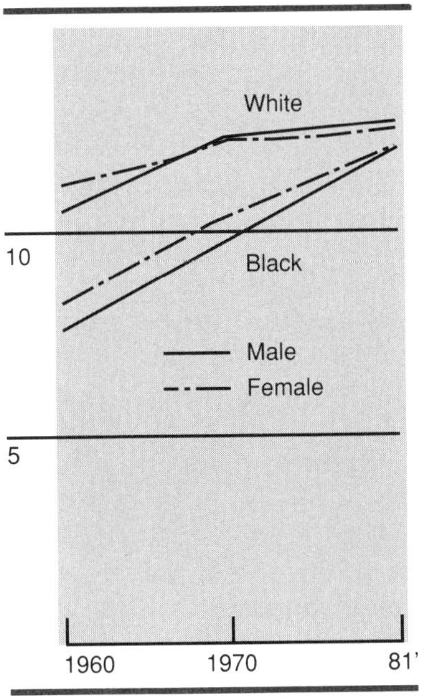

Source: U.S. Census Bureau.

FIGURE 4.11. **Employment in the United States**

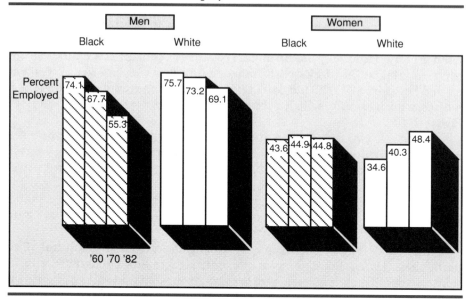

Source: U.S. Census Bureau.

white society. Their racial awareness and heightened pride in being black is one method of dealing with these feelings. Reaching into their African past helps blacks handle biculturalism and their identity crisis. Given their history in America, it is hard for them to know who and what they are. Many humiliating stereotypes have been inflicted on black Americans. There is the stereotype of the inarticulate noble savage who can sing, dance, play, and outrun most whites. There is the stereotype of the broken home where mother and children live in poverty, visited occasionally by a propagative, "love them and leave them" man. And there is the stereotype of the outlaw, prone to violence, drug-addicted, AIDS-wracked, and always dangerous.

What must be recognized is that no group bears a heavier cultural burden than American blacks, who must handle the tensions of white society along with their own anxiety. Every day they face discrimination and uncertainty about what is expected of them. The social critic Max Lerner (1957) wrote that achievement only brings more problems. It is the black moving up in the world who is most prone to self-doubt and guilt. Many feel that they are neither one thing nor another. Genuine equality in white society seems just beyond reach, and affinity with other blacks is lost. Blacks have their own class distinctions, and there is an expanding middle class that is trapped between an inferior status it rejects and equality that remains elusive.

In a controversial report, Daniel Moynihan (1965) presented two messages. One message was that blacks should receive preferential treatment to compensate for past injustice. The second message concerned the relationship between poverty, unemployment, and family disorganization. In 1986, Moynihan added the phenomena of the single-parent family and teenage mothers as contributors to the problems of black families. His solution to these problems is more government subsidy, national standardization of benefits, encouragement of adoption, and more programs that protect teenagers from pregnancy and abortion. In a critique of Moynihan's proposals, Minuchin (1986) asks for measures that would strengthen the black family. His suggestions include day care, preschool and parenting programs, and greater involvement of black churches. Moynihan looks to more government intervention; Minuchin looks to more family and community involvement. Martin and Martin (1986) state that mutual aid was a tradition among blacks even in slavery times. Depending on the extended family and on each other lessened only in the last sixty years, as blacks learned to look outside their communities to government agencies for help.

Slavery encouraged a mother-centered family with tenuous bonds to father. Political and economic conditions since that time have perpetuated that pattern. Attachments to extended family and community continue but have been altered by migration and pressures of inner-city life. Boyd-Franklin (1987) states that many black women are pessimistic about male–female relationships because of what they learned in family life. Some have been told by female relatives that black men are unreliable and exploit women. Others believe that black men are not faithful, and that if they enter a relationship, they will have to share the man with other women. Some relationship problems in black families are attributable to the heavy responsibilities of men and women. Demands from employers, children, and extended family members are unending. Privacy and time alone are difficult to find.

In most cultures the mother is central in a child's life; this is especially true in families where mother is a single parent. The importance of black women as breadwinners and household heads influences the socialization of children in unusual ways. In most white households children see that father is the primary provider even when mother has a career of her own. There is less of this role modeling in black households. Limited employment prospects for males cause preferential treatment for girls, especially in regard to education. Behaviors that are unrewarded tend to be extinguished. Lack of incentive may be one reason that many black men lose interest in advancement, responsibility, and delayed gratification, since few rewards are in sight. Very few black women would reject a satisfying marriage leading to an intact family. Far from insisting on a matriarchal family, most women, regardless of race or origin, prefer to share family life and family obligations with a lasting partner (Gutman, 1967).

Therapeutic Guidelines

Helping a black family requires an ecological perspective that examines the relation of the family to external systems such as school, church, housing, welfare, and perhaps the criminal justice system. Therefore, extensive knowledge of community resources is helpful in guiding families through the labyrinth of many agencies. It is not advisable to perform tasks that rightly belong to the family, but coordination and encouragement are certainly warranted. The concern that many black families have that they will be casually dismissed or simply told what to do has basis in fact. Every family member must be treated with respect. The use of first names is questionable except with the very young. Addressing older members as "Mr." or "Mrs." reinforces their status and role in the family and indirectly strengthens the boundaries between individuals and subsystems.

The centrality of the mother in the black family may lead to conditions of enmeshment, and the mother may be overly powerful in family life. Enmeshment may be manifested in the actions of a parental child or in the actions of a child who is not free to separate from mother. The mother's centrality minimizes the involvement of the father, as children respond primarily to the moods and demands of mother. Teaching the family about the developmental tasks of young people and about appropriate role enactment helps modify dysfunctional interactions. Because many black families feel that they live in a hostile world, suggestions for change may be more acceptable if they are called survival tactics. Because having choices increases the families' sense of power, a discussion of possible options is often fruitful.

An ecological approach emphasizes the support to be found in community groups beyond the nuclear and extended family. Church groups, scout troops, Big Sister and Big Brother organizations all have the potential to reduce distrust between the family and society. At the same time the family may need to express resentment engendered by years of discrimination. If the health care professional is not black, care must be taken not to challenge or undermine the right of families to their own values and belief systems. This is especially true where religion is concerned. Church affiliation is important to black families, many of whom belong to strict denominations whose rules are resented by young family members. Here it is important not to become the ally of any faction. When conflict is related to an adolescent's rejection of religious beliefs or to troubles a child is having in school, the care provider may act as an intermediary between parents and child, clarifying the issues and helping the participants explain their views directly to each other (Hines & Boyd-Franklin, 1982).

Whether they come for help voluntarily or at the request of an official agency, black families are most likely to respond to time-limited, goal-oriented problem-solving methods that do not make family members defensive. Black families may feel overwhelmed at times and may need reassurance that they do have the power to improve family life. The work of the health care professional should be explained as part of a process of growth or empowerment in which the family determines what it would like to change, and begins to move toward achieving change.

THE WEST INDIAN AMERICAN FAMILY

Historical Background

The West Indies are a group of islands in the Caribbean Sea, some of which are independent and some of which are administered by Great Britain, the Netherlands, France, or the United States. The black population, which constitutes a majority on most of the islands, are descendants of African slaves who were brought to the islands in the sixteenth century. The white population of the islands, a decided minority, are descendants of European explorers and colonists. Must of the population is of mixed blood and is considered neither white nor black but mulatto. Slavery undoubtedly was difficult for West Indian blacks, but emancipation occurred earlier in the islands than in the United States. With emancipation, land ownership and upward mobility were open to blacks. During the eighteenth century there was little immigration from the islands to the United States, but numbers increased after 1940 (Ueda, 1980). Usually one family member came first, and other members were sent for later. Because it was easier for West Indian women to find work, more women immigrated than men. Frequently several families shared a house or apartment, with each family occupying one bedroom. Conditions were crowded, but the West Indians had the companionship of other people from the islands.

The cold winters in American cities pose a problem for these immigrants, and the sheer size of the cities intimidates arrivals from the small islands. The racial discrimination endemic in the United States constitutes another problem, because color distinctions in the islands are more subtle. Gradations of color are on a continuum, with light-skinned islanders enjoying higher status than those with dark skins. The custom in the United States of labeling people as "black" or "white" is unfamiliar to West Indians. Many of them are proud of their island culture and their link to the nation that colonized it. Most of them have been indoctrinated with the work ethic and are willing to defer immediate gratification for eventual prosperity.

Marriage is highly regarded by islanders and gives status to the principals. Usually couples marry only after they have attained some financial security. However, unions apart from formal marriage are also common. There are purposive unions in which a couple live together, have children, and eventually marry. There is also nonpurposive union, in which a couple lives together, may or may not have children, but do not intend to marry (Brice, 1982).

It is considered more important for women to be good housekeepers and mothers than seductive sexual partners. Child-rearing practices are loving but strict. Spankings, scoldings, and warnings are frequent; children are expected to behave themselves and respect their elders. Girls are taught to be obedient and sensible. Their activities are supervised by parents who are watchful and protective of daughters. Boys are given more freedom but are expected to work hard and move up in the world. Child lending is a common occurrence; school-age children are sent to live with relatives for various reasons; for example, a working mother may not be able to care properly for a child or a childless woman may need companionship. Islanders may be either Catholic or Protestant, depending on the dominant religion of the colonizing country.

Therapeutic Guidelines

Traditions of stoicism and self-reliance make West Indian people reluctant to accept help from outsiders. Their respect for authority causes them to follow through on referrals from school personnel or family physicians. Once referred, they tend to continue in treatment until progress is made. Folk wisdom and folk medicine are prominent in the lives of islanders. They may simultaneously follow the advice of a folk healer and of a conventional health care professional. They are not inclined to challenge care providers, but they are more comfortable with those who are mature in age and demeanor. An educational approach that includes teaching and explaining is likely to be effective.

The West Indian family is often multigenerational, and it may be helpful to ask about events that took place many years ago. Sometimes it is beneficial to work with and through grandparents if problems surround a child. Therapeutic sessions should be time-limited, specific, and goal-directed for these work-oriented families. The families tend to be enmeshed, but their devotion to one another is there to be mobilized for solving problems. If families have sufficient intellectual ability, the concepts of Bowen may prove compatible. Although emotionally bound together, these families are accustomed to planning and forethought, and give grave consideration to suggestions from care providers. Working with West Indian families can be very rewarding because of the adaptive resources of the strong family system.

AMERICAN FAMILIES OF HISPANIC ORIGIN: THE PUERTO RICAN FAMILY

Historical Background

The Puerto Rican family traces its lineage to three ancestral strains. The first inhabitants of the island were an Indian people, most of whom died of hunger or overwork after the Spanish explorers arrived. Although the Indian way of life did not survive, its influence persists to some extent. More pervasive, however, is the Spanish influence introduced by Christopher Columbus, who discovered the island in 1493. The Spanish brought their language, customs, and religion to Puerto Rico. Other aspects of Spanish influence are the patriarchal family structure, the Roman Catholic belief in saints and a hereafter, and a double standard that permits sexual freedom for males but not for females. A third racial strain was introduced in 1511, when African slaves were imported by the Spaniards to work in the sugar cane fields. The Africans contributed to the cuisine and music of the island. They also relied on medicine men and folk medicine, and added these beliefs to the cultural blend.

In 1898 Puerto Rico was ceded to the United States by Spain. A U.S. commissioner was appointed to head a civil government. The commissioner represented Puerto Rico in the House of Representatives but had no vote. The United States retained the power to veto any law passed on the island. English was declared the official language in the public schools. In 1917 a bill of rights increased island participation in its own government. Citizenship was granted and Spanish was reinstituted as the language of instruction in the public schools, with English as the second language.

Puerto Rico is now a commonwealth of the United States, but its people cannot vote in U.S. elections. They do, however, have free access to the United States and must be considered migrants, not immigrants. Because passports and visas are not required, to-and-fro migration from the island to the mainland continues. Free access "reinforces many links to the island, although it also reflects repeated ruptures and renewal of ties, dismantling and reconstruction of familial and communal networks in old and new settings" (Rodriguez et al., 1980, p. 2). Puerto Ricans came to the United States in search of work, education, and opportunity. Garcia-Preto (1982) believes that the motivation is often some family problem such as illness or marital dissatisfaction.

An interesting effect of the Spanish heritage is the importance of lineage. This is shown in the Puerto Rican custom of using a given name first, the father's surname second, and the family name of the mother in third place. Many follow the Roman Catholic faith, but Protestant missions on the island have attracted some converts. Most marriages are formalized by religious and legal ceremonies, but some are consensually made. As stipulated by Roman law, which prevails on the island, consensual unions are not legally binding. Although the children of these unions are not legitimate, they seldom suffer shame or discrimination. They are known as "natural" children.

Relatives may live in separate households or be separated by migration, but kinship bonds are very strong. Traffic between the mainland and the island preserves the extended family network, although this is less true of the middle class. In middle-class Puerto Rican families, competition and upward mobility have weakened traditions of group dependence, but the extended family continues to be influential. The prevalence of consensual unions has given rise to numerous families in which "his" children, "her" children, and "their" children live together.

In the Spanish tradition, family structure is likely to be patriarchal, but an absentee father is not uncommon. Within the family the man seems to have considerable authority over wife and children, although many women engage in role redefinition after coming to the mainland. As is true of many newcomer groups, the women seem to find jobs more easily than the men. This reduces the emotional and economic dependency of the women. Conflict often follows as the husband tries to oppose new role enactment, while wives welcome it. Although the men tend toward authoritarianism, Puerto Rican women are inclined to be more assertive and outspoken than their counterparts in Mexican American families. Undoubtedly there is a limit to female assertiveness based on the tolerance of the Puerto Rican male.

Puerto Ricans place great value on honor, dignity, and respect, or *respeto*, which may be defined as a high regard for authority, order, and self-worth. It is reciprocal in that if one behaves appropriately, one is entitled to the respect of others. Failure to respect the Puerto Rican male insults not only the man but his entire family as well. The machismo associated with being male is linked to *respeto*. *Machismo* is a term fraught with meaning. It implies certain power within the family, and authority over wife and children. It also implies a swaggering possessiveness toward wife or sweetheart, and greater sexual freedom for men than for women, who are expected to be modest and faithful and to suppress their sexual feelings, with the result that many regard sexuality as a duty rather than a pleasure.

Child rearing is the responsibility of the mother, although the father often acts as disciplinarian. Children are expected to be obedient and helpful. Scoldings and spankings are commonplace; praise and recognition are withheld for fear of spoiling children or causing them to lose respect for the parents. The influence of the wife increases as she grows older. The Puerto Rican mother usually has close ties to her sons and may act as intermediary between her husband and her sons. Like her husband, she fiercely guards the virtue and reputation of her daughters.

The absence of an extended family is a problem for Puerto Ricans on the mainland. Islanders usually marry young and have large families. Without help from the extended family, the wife often feels overwhelmed by her duties. The extended family helps control dissension by upholding traditional values. Moving children from one nuclear family to another within the extended family is a frequent occurrence. This may be done to relieve a mother with many children, either by reducing the size of her brood or by providing an older child who can help her. Although the practice may be worrisome to the health care professional, it is culturally acceptable and represents no problem to the participants. Transferring children within the extended family may also be done to remove a child from peer group influences that the parents distrust.

Therapeutic Guidelines

Many Puerto Ricans believe in *spiritism*. Spiritism is a mystical believe that powerful, invisible spirits surround us, and spiritists are individuals with special ability to communicate with this unseen world. When under stress, Puerto Ricans develop somatic complaints. Their first recourse is to visit a physician, but if their symptoms are not relieved, they will consult a spiritist. Spiritists often include family members in meetings called re-unions, where the spirit world is invoked. Malignant spirits are asked to help, not harm, the sufferer. Benign spirits are asked to do more. In a sense, the group of neighbors and family members become a therapeutic force. The problems of the sufferer are discussed, evaluated, and explained within the belief system of the group. Garrison (1977) states that spiritism merely represents a healing cult compatible with Catholicism, and functions as a mental health resource in the Puerto Rican culture. Belief in spiritism and in folk medicine causes Puerto Ricans to question conventional treatment methods, and to prefer treatment from a native folk healer called a *curandero* or *curandera*. Many Puerto Ricans subscribe to the hot–cold etiology of health and illness, which was part of Spanish and Portuguese medicine over three hundred years ago. All ailments are classified as either hot or cold; foods and medicine may be hot, cold, or cool. Cold diseases must be countered by hot substances and vice versa. Thermal temperatures play a part but are not the whole picture. For example, a respiratory infection is a cold ailment whether or not a fever is present. Therefore, it may not be treated with fruit juices, which are also cold. Cool foods should not be eaten during menstruation or after childbirth. Because cool foods include fruits and vegetables that are rich in vitamins and minerals, this belief presents problems for the health care professional. Vitamin and iron supplements are considered hot and will be refused by pregnant Puerto Rican women who fear that these substances will cause the child to be born with inflamed skin. Knowing something about the hot–cold theory will enable an innovative care provider to suggest needed substances in forms that neutralize hot-cold incompatibilities (Harwood, 1971).

As noted previously, family consensus on role enactment is threatened by life on the mainland. The result is confrontation between husband and wife or between parents and children. The response of parents may be to withdraw from their unfamiliar surroundings. The task of learning a new language seems easier for children than for parents. Children then become interpreters, and parents suffer a loss of dignity and authority. Polarization occurs in the family as children welcome change and parents oppose it. Feeling beleaguered, the parents become stricter and resort to punishment that further alienates the children. What the parents want is to protect their children, especially daughters, from becoming part of a more permissive society. Often their fears of violence, crime, drug addiction, and sexual freedom are justified, but their methods are counterproductive. Rebellion by the children may be used to persuade parents that coercion is not working. Physical and psychological change may be introduced by assuring all family members that their turmoil will decrease if they talk and listen to one another. Working to establish family consensus is imperative, whether the issue is birth control for the wife, improved nutrition for the family, or negotiated curfews for the adolescent children. What the health care professional models is mediation and compromise to encourage all members to adapt gradually to their new environment. Garcia-Preto (1982) warns the care provider to participate actively in family sessions but not to deal immediately with crucial issues. The Puerto Rican family is most responsive to a warm, almost personal relationship with the care provider, rather than a distant one. Exploring the nature of the family's problems, what has been done to solve them, what sources of support are available, and what they would like to change allows for a comprehensive assessment while allaying the family's fears. Discussing migration and ties to the island clarifies problems that are cultural and environmental in origin. In instances where the husband is absent from the home or uninvolved with the family, the wife can be encouraged to turn to the extended family for help. If no extended family members are available, access to community support through welfare, child care, or church groups should be arranged for the wife. The authoritarian structure of Puerto Rican families means that many concerns of the wife and children go unheard and unheeded. Providing a forum where needs can be safely expressed and problems analyzed is a primary objective, after which compromise and the art of negotiation can be modeled.

THE MEXICAN AMERICAN FAMILY

Historical Background

The history of Mexico is one of violence and exploitation. Like Puerto Rico, Mexico was colonized by Spanish explorers who arrived in the sixteenth century and overcame the Indian population. The Spaniards took possession of the Indians' treasure and taught Roman Catholicism to the native population, who combined the religion of the Spaniards with their own beliefs. Most Mexicans are *mestizos* of mixed Indian and Spanish descent. In 1821 Mexico obtained independence from Spain and, for a time, encouraged European immigration. After 1821 Anglos or non-Mexicans came in large numbers to the part of Mexico now called Texas. By 1834 Anglos outnumbered Mexicans by a ratio of six to one. Less than ten years later Texas was annexed by the United States, an event that led to the Mexican War. This war lasted two years, intensified bitterness between Anglos and Mexicans, and fostered an image of Mexican Americans as inferior.

Immigration of Mexicans grew rapidly at the turn of the century, when labor was needed, but was discouraged during periods of economic depression. Even so, Mexican Americans make up one of the largest minority groups in the United States. Most of them congregate in the Southwest, near the Mexican border; a sizable number are illegal aliens who crossed the Rio Grande in order to work on American farms. Recent legislation extended amnesty to illegal aliens who met stipulated terms regarding residence in the United States, but many Mexican Americans did not apply for amnesty either because they could not meet the requirements or because they distrusted government promises.

Mexican Americans tend to work hard at low-paying jobs. Many are migratory farm workers whose problems are aggravated by language deficiencies, minimal education, fear of deportation, and unwillingness to seek help through official channels. After World War II, younger Mexican Americans became resentful of social injustices suffered by their people. The restless political climate that pervaded the 1960s saw the emergence of Chicano activists who tried to improve conditions. Traditionally, Mexican Americans were an accepting, fatalistic group, but new attitudes of self-help have begun to appear.

There are several similarities between Puerto Rican and Mexican American families in addition to their shared Spanish and Indian heritage. Both groups subscribe to a family-centered way of life known as *familism*. A hierarchical family structure, male-dominated and based on age and gender, is characteristic of the two groups. For the Mexican American male, as for the Puerto Rican, machismo is a complicated and paradoxical idea. Machismo may be expressed through sexuality and infidelity but also may be expressed in honor, courage, and devotion to the family. The motherhood of the Mexican American woman expresses and fulfills the machismo of her husband. It also defines and fulfills her own selfhood. In the Mexican American family, role enactment is complementary for children as well as for parents. All children are instilled with such values as hard work, discipline, and respect for others. Girls, whose virtue must be safeguarded, are given less freedom and more responsibility than their brothers. Tasks necessary in the household are delegated according to the age, ability, and gender of the children. Although families tend to be patriarchal, the parental dyad made up of husband and wife runs the family, with children performing their assigned chores. Clear boundaries are upheld between parents and children. Sibling subsystems are also important; order is maintained through subordination of female to male and younger to older family members. Interdependence characterizes the Mexican American family and extends beyond the nuclear form across generations into the extended family network. In general, nuclear families live in separate households but close to extended family groups. Thus, nuclear boundaries remain despite proximity, affiliation, and interdependence.

After marriage a Mexican American woman is unlikely to enter the labor force, except on a temporary basis. Alvirez and Bean (1976) believe this is related to the following causes: (1) large numbers of small children in the family because of a high birth rate, (2) traditions that encourage wives and mothers to remain at home, and (3) educational disadvantages that limit employment opportunities for women. Many Mexican Americans in the Southwest live in the *barrio*, which offers some security but reinforces old values and opposes change. Within the barrio Spanish is the primary language. This means that as children attending school become bilingual, their parents do not. When parents must use their children as interpreters, they suffer role reversal and loss of authority. The barrio may be a comfortable refuge for a time, but family dissension is almost inevitable. Prosperity and the aspirations of some members cause families to leave the barrio for mixed neighborhoods with better housing and more varied opportunities. Any Mexican American family leaving the barrio confronts ongoing conflict between tradition and progress.

Therapeutic Guidelines

The health care professional working with a Mexican American family must respect the constraints imposed by tradition. Stoicism and resignation have contributed to a lack of interest in preventive health measures. If Mexican Americans are not in great pain and can accomplish their daily tasks, they consider themselves to be healthy. Their fatalism persuades them that misfortune in this life will be corrected in the next, if only they display courage and endurance. Disease or illness may be the result of sinfulness or misbehavior for which one deserves punishment. *Mal Ojo*, the evil eye, may destroy a person who has erred or been guilty of excessive pride. Therefore, no one should be praised too much lest the evil eye fall upon him. Minor illnesses are ignored as much as possible. Even when a family member is very ill, there is reluctance to seek help or enter a hospital. Often the extended family gathers round the sick person, trying various home remedies. Precautions against communicable disease may not be followed simply because of the belief that relatives and common household objects cannot transmit infection. Mexican Americans are reluctant to challenge authority figures directly, but manage to circumvent measures that are unacceptable to them. Any disability that can be treated within the family is not greatly feared, but if separation from the family occurs, the situation is seen as dangerous and frightening (Cirredondo et al., 1982).

Mexican American families are responsive to child-centered approaches that deal with family interaction in a problem-solving manner. Because family life is so important to this group, they are usually willing to attend family meetings. Inhibitions about criticizing family members can be reduced by care providers who are skilled in reframing and relabeling techniques. A father whose authoritarianism is resented by his teenaged children may, for example, be described as caring too much rather than disciplining too fiercely. Children torn between respect for parents and the allure of the dominant culture can be directed to a middle ground where parents feel less threatened and therefore more reasonable. The use of analogies, anecdotes, and metaphors by the care provider is more acceptable than direct confrontation or requests for early disclosure. Marital disharmony is difficult for Mexican Americans to reveal. However, recognizing the commitment of parents to children, and the loyalty of all members to the family unit, allays mistrust and helps forge an alliance with the care provider. Since most of the family's problems have a cultural basis, the care provider may choose to act as an intermediary who interprets new behavior patterns and reinterprets traditional behavior patterns to children. In this way, shifts and imbalances caused by change become less ominous.

BUILDING COMMUNICATION BRIDGES

The use of translators is an important issue when dealing with clients who are not fluent or comfortable in the caregiver's language. The basic question is whether to use a translator at all and, if one is used, what characteristics are important in the translator. Some Spanish-speaking clients reported more satisfaction when a professional translator was present during psychiatric interviews. However, caregivers in the same study were less satisfied when a professional translator was present and reported that clients who were interviewed in the presence of a translator seemed less "appreciative" and were less likely to return for subsequent visits. The disparity between the reactions of clients and those of caregivers suggests that the clients felt more at ease with a translator present, whereas caregivers found the presence of a third party intrusive and unproductive. The reactions of the caregivers were supported in part by higher attrition rates following the presence of a translator (Grosjean, 1982; Westermeyer, 1987).

Translators who are inexperienced or not psychologically well informed may be reluctant to ask questions about sex, violence, suicide, or finances unless they have been prepared in advance for the content areas that will be explored. If a professional translator is not available, the caregiver may try to facilitate communication and/or decrease the clients' anxiety by asking a friend or relative to be present. This sometimes works well but often does not. Unfortunately these "translators" are rarely objective. As a result, they tend either to minimize or to exaggerate the family's problem, depending on what they consider relevant. They may selectively omit data or distort what the family members are actually saying. Sometimes it is necessary to depend on a professional translator or a family friend or relative, but in all cases it is essential to discuss with the translator what is expected of him or her. Advance preparation helps translators avoid making their own interpretations and places them in their appropriate auxiliary role.

Even when a translator is considered unnecessary, an uncomfortable family may feel more at ease if an ethnic companion is permitted to be present in early interviews. A good way to increase the family's comfort is to begin by asking how the members feel about the encounter and what their expectations are. Clarification of what is said and what is meant must be undertaken repeatedly during the interview to ensure that client and caregiver understand each other's viewpoints.

Direct, probing questions should be used with great care and sensitivity so that clients do not become defensive. By asking open-ended questions and expressing empathy for the client, the caregiver will facilitate progress. Cultural taboos against self-disclosure vary from group to group, and the caregiver should expect some reluctance to share embarrassing information until trust has developed. Care providers first should ask questions in ways that allow the client some choices in replying. Questions that permit the client to avoid premature revelations without being compelled to tell lies help develop a therapeutic relationship that eventually causes the client to share more information. Naturally, there are some situations in which a client may be a source of harm to himself or others. In these cases, the indirect, time-consuming approach is not appropriate. Frequently, however, the person who is working in a transcultural situation will be more effective if time is taken to work within racial and ethnic guidelines.

Confrontation is another communication technique that may be seen by the client as a form of criticism or accusation, and therefore should be employed carefully, if at all. A better technique for caregivers is not to confront but to point out apparent contradictions or discrepancies and ask for clarification. An example might be to comment, "You said your husband was a good provider who works hard for the family even though he often misses work and is hard on the children. Tell me more about that so I can understand how things are for you and your family." When family and care provider come from different ethnic or racial backgrounds, additional time must be made available for their interactions, especially in the first stages of the therapeutic relationship when each may be puzzled by aspects of the other. In order to maintain a reassuring, unhurried atmosphere, it is wise to allow from 50 to 100 percent more time than would ordinarily be arranged. Any language deficiency introduces complicating factors into the health care picture. Many ethnic families have members for whom English is not a primary but a secondary language. As a result, communication becomes more challenging for everyone involved. Some clients may be able to report factual details in their second language but unable to deal with emotions, abstractions, or subtle distinctions in that language. The stress of the clinical encounter, especially if the client is depressed or anxious, or has a thought disorder, will further impair the ability to communicate. Westermeyer (1987) reported that some clients seem to be more confused and disorganized when using a second language because their knowledge of the acquired language is less extensive than their knowledge of their original tongue. Conversely, it has been noted that other clients exhibit less confusion and disorganization when using a second language. In these instances, less knowledge of the language is thought to lend them greater control of disturbing thoughts and ideas. Because it is difficult to predict what the repercussions will be when selecting the language to use in interviewing such clients, it might be advisable to validate information by communicating with the family in both the primary and secondary language on separate occasions.

Health care is facilitated by professionals who have:

- Knowledge of the historical experience, recent and long-term, of ethnic groups composing the community
- Demographic data that include family size, socioeconomic status, and future expectations characteristic of diverse ethnic groups
- Recognition of folk beliefs and cultural attitudes toward health and illness
- Awareness of the nature of problems encountered by ethnic group members when they enter the health care system, including fear and distrust of new methods, language barriers, and discrimination by caregivers

---

SUMMARY

The description of minority families presented in this chapter is by no means exhaustive. The intent is to explore salient characteristics of selected minority groups in a manner that sensitizes care providers to the ethnic experience and encourages them to use greater understanding and knowledge. Culture and ethnicity include ideas about health, illness, and family life that persist across generations and survive even the upheaval of coming to a new country. All ethnic groups confront repeated challenges as they transfer their families from familiar to unfamiliar surroundings. An important consideration in working with members of any ethnic minority is to look at all customs and values in relative terms, seeing none as altogether good or bad. Change is inevitable in family life, whether it is resisted or welcomed. An important function of health care professionals is to help families monitor the rate of change that is acceptable to various members, and reach a consensus.

When families and the health care professional represent groups that have little in common, additional time is needed to establish trust. Knowledge of the historical experience of the group to which the family belongs can be very helpful to the care provider, and to the family as well. Unless the care provider is aware of group history, of the immigration experience, and of group norms, the accuracy of any assessment is questionable. Similarities and differences based on group experience exist among families often categorized under a single adjective such as European, Asian, black, or Hispanic. Every minority group category contains families that exhibit remarkable diversity. At the same time, some generalizations are possible if they are constantly subjected to scrutiny and qualification. As health care professionals become more knowledgeable about cultural influences, and more sensitive to the values of ethnic minority families, perhaps these families will be more receptive to efforts on their behalf. Respect for cultural norms must be supplemented with knowledge of how norms evolved and why they persist. Only then can the health care professional intervene in ways that are compatible with a family's belief system.

There is a duality in the adaptational task of immigrant families (Aroian, 1990). One aspect of the immigrant task is dealing with grief over losses caused by departure from the homeland. The second is meeting resettlement demands associated with adjustment to unfamiliar language, occupation, customs, and status. Adjustment is an ongoing process complicated by experiencing grief linked to the past while simultaneously meeting resettlement demands oriented to the future. Immigrant families, whatever their country of origin, need to learn that old attachments need not be altogether discarded but may have to be reshaped in order to conform to new requirements. Health care professionals can help immigrant families to find a balance between valuing what was lost and building anew. In many ways, the duality of the immigrant task, the energy and compromise it requires, can be the focus of family intervention.

REFERENCES

Alvirez, D., & Bean, F. D. (1976). "The Mexican American Family." In C. H. Mendel & R. W. Habenstein (Eds.), *Ethnic Families in America.* New York: Elsevier.

Aroian, K. J. (1990). "A Model of Psychological Adaptation to Migration and Resettlement." *Nursing Research*, 39(1): 5–9.

Bales, R. F. (1946). "Cultural Differences in Rates of Alcoholism." *Journal for the Study of Alcohol*, 6(March): 400–449.

Bales, R. F. (1962). "Attitudes toward Drinking in the Irish Culture." In D. Pittman & C. Snyder (Eds.), *Society, Culture and Drinking Patterns.* New York: Wiley.

Barzini, L. (1964). *The Italians.* New York: Atheneum.

Bernardo, S. (1981). *The Ethnic Almanac.* New York: Doubleday.

Biddle, E. A. (1976). "The American Irish Catholic Family." In C. H. Mendel & R. W. Habenstein (Eds.), *Ethnic Families in America.* New York: Elsevier.

Blessing, P. J. (1980). "Irish." In S. Thernstrom (Ed.), *Harvard Encyclopedia of American Ethnic Groups.* Cambridge, MA: Harvard University Press.

Boyd-Franklin, N. (1987). "Group Therapy for Black Women." *American Journal of Orthopsychiatry*, 57(3): 394–401.

Brice, J. (1982). "West Indian Families." In M. McGoldrick, J. K. Pearce, & J. Giordano (Eds.), *Ethnicity and Family Therapy.* New York: Guilford Press.

Cirredondo, R., Weddige, R. L., Justice, C. L., & Fitz, J. (1982). "Alcoholism in Mexican Americans." *Hospital and Community Psychiatry*, 38(2): 180–183.

Comas-Dias, L., & Minrath, M. (1985). "Psychotherapy with Ethnic Minority Borderline Patients." *Psychotherapy*, 2(2): 421–426.

Franklin, J. (1969). *From Slavery to Freedom: A History of Negro Americans*, 3rd ed. New York: Vintage Books.

Garcia-Preto, N. (1982). "Puerto Rican Families." In M. McGoldrick, J. K. Pearce, & J. Giordano (Eds.), *Ethnicity and Family Therapy*. New York: Guilford Press.

Garrison, V. (1977). "Spiritism in Harlem, Adjunct to Religion." *New York Times*, November 6.

Glazer, N., & Moynihan, D. (1970). *Beyond the Melting Pot*. Cambridge, MA: Harvard University Press.

Grant, M. (1928). *The Founders of the Republic on Immigration, Naturalization, and Aliens*. New York: Scribner's.

Greeley, A. M. (1972). *That Most Distressful Nation: The Taming of the American Irish*. Chicago: Quadrangle.

Greeley, A. M. (1977). *The American Catholic*. New York: Basic Books.

Greeley, A. M. (1981). *The Irish Americans*. New York: Harper & Row.

Grosjean, F. (1982). *Life in Two Languages: An Introduction to Bilingualism*. Cambridge, MA: Harvard University Press.

Gutman, H. (1967). *The Negro Family*. New York: Pantheon.

Harwood, A. (1971). "The Hot–Cold Theory of Disease." *Journal of American Medical Association*, 216(7): 1153–1158.

Herbers, J. (1983). "Income Gap Between Races Widens." *New York Times*, July 18.

Herbers, J. (1985). "New Class of Children Is Poorer." *New York Times*, October 20.

Hines, P. M., & Boyd-Franklin, N. (1982). "Black Families." In M. McGoldrick, J. K. Pearce, & J. Giordano (Eds.), *Ethnicity and Family Therapy*. New York: Guilford Press.

Joe, T. (1983). *A Dream Deferred: The Economic Status of Black Americans*. Washington, DC: Center for Study of Social Policy.

Lerner, M. (1957). *America as a Civilization*. New York: Simon and Schuster.

Lewis, O. (1965). *La Vida: A Puerto Rican Family in the Culture of Poverty*. New York: Random House.

Martin, J. M., & Martin, E. P. (1986). *The Helping Tradition in the Black Family and Community*. Silver Springs, MD: National Association of Social Workers.

Miller, J. R., & Janosik, E. H. (1980). *Family-Focused Care*. New York: McGraw-Hill.

Minuchin, S. (1986). "Beyond Benign Neglect." *Readings: A Journal of Reviews and Commentary in Mental Health*, 194(December): 4–5.

Moynihan, D. (1965). *The Negro Family: The Case for National Action*. Washington, DC: U.S. Department of Labor.

Moynihan, D. (1986). *Family and Nation*. New York: Harcourt Brace Jovanovich.

Nelli, H. S. (1980). "Italians." In S. Thernstrom (Ed.), *Harvard Encyclopedia of American Ethnic Groups*. Cambridge, MA: Harvard University Press.

Nobles, W. (1980). "African Philosophy: Foundations for Black Psychology." In R. Jones (Ed.), *Black Psychology*. New York: Harper & Row.

Novak, M. (1972). *The Rise of the Unmeltable Ethnics*. New York: Macmillan.

Pinderhughes, E. (1982). "Afro-American Families and the Victim System." In M. McGoldrick, J. K. Pearce, & J. Giordano (Eds.), *Ethnicity and Family Therapy*. New York: Guilford Press.

Ragucci, A. T. (1981). "Italian Americans." In A. Harwood (Ed.), *Ethnicity and Medical Care*. Cambridge, MA: Harvard University Press.

Ravage, M. (1917). *An American in the Making*. New York: Harper.

Rodriguez, C. E., Sanchez-Korrol, V., & Alers, J. O. (1980). "The Puerto Rican Struggle." *Essays on Survival*. New York: Puerto Rican Migration Research Consortium.

Rotunno, M., & McGoldrick, M. (1982). "Italian Families." In M. McGoldrick, J. K. Pearce, & J. Giordano (Eds.), *Ethnicity and Family Therapy*. New York: Guilford Press.

Shon, S. P., & Ja, D. Y. (1982). "Asian Families." In M. McGoldrick, J. K. Pearce, & J. Giordano (Eds.), *Ethnicity and Family Therapy*. New York: Guilford Press.

Steinberg, S. (1981). *The Ethnic Myth: Race, Ethnicity, and Class in America*. New York: Atheneum.

Takiki, R. (1989). *Strangers from a Distant Shore*. Boston: Little, Brown.

Tsui, P., & Schultz, G. (1985). "Failure of Rapport: Why Psychotherapeutic Engagement Fails in the Treatment of Asian Clients." *American Journal of Orthopsychiatry*, 55(3): 561–565.

Tsui, P., & Schultz, G. (1988). "Ethnic Factors in Group Process: Cultural Dynamics in Multi-Ethnic Therapy Groups." *American Journal of Orthopsychiatry*, 58(1): 136–142.

Ueda, R. (1980). "West Indians." In S. Thernstrom (Ed.), *Harvard Encyclopedia of American Ethnic Groups*. Cambridge, MA: Harvard University Press.

United States Commission on Wartime Relocation and Internment of Civilians. (1982). Washington, DC: U.S. Government Printing Office.

Vecoli, R. T. (1978). "The Coming of Age of Italian Americans, 1945–1974." *Ethnicity*, 1591(January 1978): 119–147.

Westermeyer, J. (1987). "Clinical Considerations in Crosscultural Diagnosis." *Hospital and Community Psychiatry*, 38(2): 160–164.

Wideman, J. E. (1989). *Fever: Twelve Stories*. New York: Henry Holt.

Zborowski, M. (1969). *People in Pain*. San Francisco: Jossey-Bass.

CHAPTER FIVE

External Family Issues: Mobility, Unemployment, and Natural Disasters

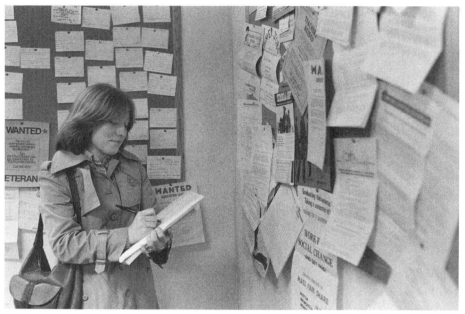

© Frank Siteman MCMLXXX

*Some terrors are beyond human endurance.
A man who was not afraid of anything,
even of waves and earthquakes, would be
mad or insensible.*

Aristotle

[145]

This chapter reviews pertinent external issues that have an impact on family life: mobility, unemployment, and natural disasters. It looks at American mobility in historical perspective and documents immigration laws in the United States from the late 1800s to the present. It discusses five stages of the migration experience for families and examines problems for refugee families. The next section deals with the impact of unemployment on family relationships and describes how the marital alliance and parental roles are affected by the prolonged unemployment of the family breadwinner. It looks specifically at the psychological impact of unemployment.

The third part of the chapter defines natural and environmental disasters and their impact on the family. It describes phases of families' reactions to disasters and identifies the families' emotional responses that need to be understood. Briefly mentioned is the ultimate disaster of war and how it brings havoc and destruction to families, communities, and whole nations. Following this section is a description of issues for families of Holocaust survivors.

Therapeutic guidelines for the health care professional are offered with each of the three sections in this chapter. A clinical example of a refugee family's difficulties is also presented.

MOBILITY AND ITS IMPACT ON THE FAMILY

American Mobility in Historical Perspective

From colonial times, Americans have been a migratory people. With the exception of the Native Americans, all of us moved here from somewhere else, and even Native Americans moved freely on the continent according to their needs. Thus, a yearning to be "on the move" is a uniquely American characteristic. In the United States prior to the twentieth century, mobility meant freedom and the ability to own land, to succeed, and to govern one's own destiny. The whole family had to work hard together to maintain its freedom in the wilderness. In the mid-1800s new territories were explored; the railroads opened up the continent, which meant new markets and new ways of transporting goods. The technological revolution, including the invention of the automobile, came at about the time the frontier disappeared. Migrants must move to another part of the country to find seasonal work, suffering many disadvantages. For the most part, migrant workers are underprivileged ethnic minorities who endure impoverished conditions much like that suffered by eighteenth- and nineteenth-century European peasants. The experiences of migration and immigration are similar, but migrants must adjust over and over. Immigrants must endure massive culture shock which may last for years, but lacks the repetitiveness of migratory life, which may cause permanent displacement.

Immigration to the United States

For many decades, immigrants coming to the United States via New York City arrived at Ellis Island and were accepted or rejected there. It is estimated that almost 20 percent of those seeking entry were denied access to the United States. Ellis Island is now restored as a museum and was opened to the public in September 1990. This project—the most costly restoration in U.S. history—was funded by private donations. Public interest and support attest to the significance of the immigrant experience for thousands of Americans. In 1891 Congress established federal control over immigration, and in 1892 immigration supervision began there. Of the 12 million people who came through New York Harbor between 1892 and 1954, 900,000 came through Ellis Island in 1907. They were persuaded to leave southern and eastern Europe by poverty, anti-Semitism, and overpopulation. The main building at Ellis Island opened in 1910. A hospital had already opened in 1902; persons with physical illness or disease were detained there. There were also large kitchen facilities and a laundry. Meals were provided by concessionaires, and typical American food was represented. Feeding the great hordes of diverse people was difficult. Chinese requested rice, Italians wanted wine, Scandinavians preferred dried fish, Jews herring. Laws restricting immigrants were passed in the 1920s, and eventually persons wishing to immigrate were required to be inspected by U.S. consulate officials abroad (Hall, 1990).

The passage of the 1976 and 1978 amendments to the Immigration Act and the Refugee Act of 1980 opened worldwide immigration on a first-come, first-served basis. Hundreds of thousands of people enter the United States yearly—now mostly from Central America, South America, and Asia. Many of these people have suffered violence, torture, and extreme oppression (Hartman, 1990).

Hall (1990) states that people still come for opportunity—to escape oppression and to provide a better life for themselves and their children. The entry into the United States today is a streamlined process in contrast to the early days of Ellis Island. Prescreened and approved by U.S. embassy or consulate officials in their home country, once here, immigrants are given a forgery-proof permanent alien registration card (called the "green card"), which is proof of legal entry and is also a work permit. This green card entitles the bearer to permanent residence; and, if he or she so wishes, the immigrant can apply for citizenship after five years. From 1924 until 1965 Europeans were favored; in 1924, Congress, in the Johnson-Reed Act, set quotas based on the percentage of a nationality in the United States population. Eventually this was thought to be discriminatory, and in 1965 the Hart-Cellar Act gave applicants from *all* countries a chance to apply for permanent residence. Under special rules passed in 1988, spouses, parents, and young unmarried children of U.S. citizens came without any limit. In 1986 Congress passed a law that penalized employers who knowingly hired workers without the green card—or those who entered the country illegally. The 1986 immigration bill also offered amnesty to any illegal entrants who could prove U.S. residence prior to 1982.

There are those who decry the changing composition of America's population, but recent demographic studies suggest that today immigrants contribute more in income, sales, and Social Security taxes than they get back in social services. In the meantime, debate over immigration laws continues in Congress. Some say that the preference given to families handicaps others without such ties who may have advanced degrees, needed skills, or money to invest. Thousands of people still clamor to be admitted to the United States. "Unchanged is the vision of millions abroad that America is the land of promise" (Hall, 1990, p. 105).

World Status of Refugees in 1989

From other sources comes tragic and disheartening information ("The New Refugees," 1989). Today there are 15 million refugees in the world who have been uprooted from their homelands by war, famine, political repression, and economic hardship. Only 1 percent of the world's homeless resettle each year; most will spend the rest of their lives near starvation in poorly constructed refugee camps, located from Malawi and Pakistan to Honduras and Thailand. Many elderly Palestinians, no longer hopeful, expect to end their days in a refugee camp near Beirut. A recent influx to the United States of Laotians and Cambodians has brought specific problems. Often lacking in skills and education, they have trouble finding jobs, and many remain indefinitely on welfare. Coming from male-dominated societies, the men have trouble working for female employers or managers, because they consider this to be a loss of status. Many of the adults are illiterate and have great difficulty learning to speak and write the English language even in a rudimentary way.

On a more positive note, the United States is one of the few societies that believes that "people from different races, cultures, and ethnic backgrounds can be assimilated as citizens and as equals to those who preceded them" (Fallows, 1989, p. 47). Fallows spells out two truths about the United States' long experience with immigrants and refugees: (1) There is widespread disdain for the immigrant groups most recently arrived, and (2) there is tacit acknowledgment of the success of newer immigrant and refugee groups once they have had time to establish themselves. In the 1980 census, the four ethnic groups with the highest average incomes were mainly composed of Asian immigrants.

Some refugees and immigrants come from a culture in which geographic mobility is customary, and they can rely on certain learned skills to help them cope. Conversely, some of these families come from a very sedentary culture in which pulling up their roots means near disaster. Yet, great numbers of people manage to leave their familiar surroundings, break ties with people and places, and transplant their homes and goods, their goals and dreams, and even their ghosts (Sluzki, 1979).

The Five Stages of Migration for Families

Sluzki presents five stages of the migration process and discusses preventive and therapeutic implications. The five stages are described as follows:

I. *Preparatory stage:*
   A. The family makes a commitment to migrate, makes application for visas, writes official letters required.
   B. The family members express negative motivations (to escape political or religious oppression/persecution) or positive motivations ("to make a better life," etc.).
   C. The family experiences ups and downs in its emotional responses to the move.
   D. The family members examine their motivations for the move more closely. Whose idea was it? Is the move pushed by one, dragging the others behind? Is the move to a better climate motivated by a chronically ill child? Who is rescued? Who will experience the greatest loss?
   E. In this stage there is the frequent assumption that if the family's motivations are mainly positive, then there is no need to mourn. (Feeling sorry or sad is not allowed.) Those family members who *do* express feelings of mourning and loss may be scapegoated by the others. In some instances, where leave-taking is difficult, those members who do *not* mourn are seen as disloyal to the previous family life.
   F. Family members begin to negotiate new family rules about roles and functions to be assumed after the move.
II. *The act of migration:*
   A. The amount of *time* involved in the migration has a significant influence on the family's response and adjustment. The move may

be a four-hour plane ride, a more prolonged process involving long stays in refugee camps, or a period of residence in another country different from the one the family left and different from the one to which the family will migrate.

B. The bonds established with other persons with whom the family shares the migration experience may be as strong as those ties left in the country of origin. For example, the Jews who shared the Holocaust, or the Vietnamese boat people who were together for weeks at sea, establish emotional ties that may last a lifetime.

C. Some families move very cautiously—send family members ahead to the new country to find places to live and employment. Some families plan to move only temporarily and will return if things do not work out. Other families, especially in the case of war or political upheaval, are forced to move suddenly, with no time to plan ahead or prepare themselves for the changes.

III. *Period of overcompensation:*

A. Migratory stress and reaction to it is usually delayed; families are so preoccupied with logistics that they are not fully aware of the emotional impact of what has happened to them.

B. Intellectually and emotionally, the family's primary focus is on survival—how to get basic needs met—food, clothing, shelter, medical attention, how to be safe from harm. In strange cities, getting a bus to work or school or walking to a grocery store can be a momentous ordeal. Getting medical care for a child who becomes ill can also be a frightening task, especially if supportive family members have been left behind, and the migrating family does not yet have language facility.

IV. *Period of decompensation or crisis:*

A. Adjustment to a new way of life is hard for everyone in the family. With the occurrence of family conflict and ongoing adjustment problems, stress reaches its peak. Often, crisis enters the family through the changed behavior of children. In most instances, children learn the new language more quickly than the parents and are assimilated more readily into the culture. This is especially true of school-aged children who are exposed to spoken English every day and have the opportunity to relate to other children and adults from the new country. Usually, there is a clash of values, especially around adolescent behavior and parental authority, particularly about some aspects of sexuality. It is at these times that the family may come to the attention of a mental health clinic or a family service agency for professional help. This may be after numerous confrontations with school authorities and the police.

Other family problems develop if the wife finds employment before the husband, which may be a direct challenge to previously held traditional structure and roles. Many family values and rules will prove to be adaptive in both cultures. Some patterns of behavior are retained even though they are alien to the mainstream culture, because they are crucial to the family's identity. The nature and severity of the family's crisis in the new country depends on the family's own style, its strengths, and the presence of supports in the new environment.

V. *Transgenerational impact:*

    A. Any long-term delay in the family's adaptation to the new culture becomes apparent when a second generation is born and raised in the newly adopted country.

    B. The generational clash between the old culture and the new is more accurately felt in those families that have been isolated by choice or by circumstance, such as living in a barrio or other segregated community in the new country.

Therapeutic Guidelines: Migration/Immigration

Emotional distress experienced around the migration process is to be expected and does not necessarily indicate pathology or the presence of psychiatric illness. Leaving one's native land, relinquishing all that was held close, and moving to a new country with its unfamiliar language and customs is indeed a complex and momentous task. The health care professional should be aware of his or her own beliefs concerning family roles, especially those having to do with husband–wife and parent–child relationships. American middle-class beliefs that emphasize the autonomy of the individual, independence from family ties, and egalitarian roles between men and women contradict some Asian and European cultural beliefs. In some cultures, mutual dependency is equated with loyalty, and encouraging independent strivings from the family of origin may be construed as an attack on family values (Sluzki, 1979).

In assessing the impact of such a move on a family, it is important to know where they were in regard to certain life cycle issues. Is this a family with young children? Were older family members from the extended family included in the move? The adjustment of the traditional older generation may be more difficult and, therefore, slower to occur. Is the mother in the family still in her childbearing years? If so, there may be two subgroups of children — those born in the old country and those in the new. It is also important to evaluate the sibling relationships with regard to the timing of the move. For example, if the family prospers and children born in the new country have more advantages, what impact will this have on the sibling relationships (McGoldrick & Gerson, 1985)?

If the migration of the family is a planned one, it is wise to encourage family members to learn some of the language of the new country prior to leaving the old one. Some "survival" words and phrases that will enable people to meet their basic needs are crucial: how to buy food, find a place to live, find medical services, and call the police when needed, to name a few.

Some guidance about social behaviors can be crucial, such as how to meet and greet people. Do people shake hands, for example? What behaviors, such as eating from a common bowl, are considered unacceptable? Once in the new land, learning the language more comprehensively, both speaking and writing it, is very desirable. Some public school systems provide free instruction in English as a second language. Some urban areas have an organization known as Literacy Volunteers of America (LVA), that uses trained volunteers to teach English as a second language.

From the psychological viewpoint, it is helpful for families to anticipate some of the emotional responses they may experience. For example, in the new country they will probably experience sadness and feelings of not belonging. They should be given permission to have these natural feelings of loss and to express their grief, even if the family has primarily positive motivations for moving. People who flee a country to escape persecution and oppression will also grieve, in addition to suffering the consequences of a sudden involuntary uprooting. Many refugees must leave behind extended family members whose lives may be endangered by their very departure. In some circumstances, many of these extended family members may never be heard from again. The grief of some families is compounded by feelings of guilt. Like disaster survivors, they question why and how they escaped. Whenever possible, families should be encouraged to keep in touch with people back home. This mitigates their feelings of guilt and reduces uncertainty regarding the fate of persons left behind. At the same time, they should be encouraged to establish links with people of their own culture in the new country. Their own countrymen, already here for a while, can be a valuable resource in sharing experiences and relating how they coped with their move. The immigrating family can derive comfort from any memorabilia brought from home—photographs and treasured objects. Above all, the immigrating or refugee family needs a supportive, caring network in the new country.

FAMILIES AND UNEMPLOYMENT

Unemployment is a devastating experience not only for the person who is jobless but also for the family. For the unemployed person, self-esteem is eroded and confidence is threatened. Unemployment, especially of the primary wage earner, creates havoc in the life of the family and has a major impact on the family's social and economic functioning. Regardless of its duration, unemployment has some emotional consequences. When unemployment is prolonged, it has far-reaching effects from which some families never recover.

The Elizabethan Poor Laws, established in England in 1601, required each parish to impose a tax for the purpose of furnishing employment to able-bodied jobless persons. These laws created a system in which all impoverished unemployed persons were assumed to be poor and jobless by choice. Additionally, these poor laws provided too little sustenance for health and decency. In some respects public attitudes toward the unemployed poor have not changed much. The more fortunate public either blames unemployed people for not finding work or criticizes social and economic programs that do not offer a quick solution.

In 1986 the unemployment rate in the United States was between 6 and 7 percent, and this seemed to cause little concern except among the unemployed themselves (Macarov, 1988). Joblessness seems to worry politicians and the public only when national unemployment rates reach 8 or 9 percent. Because unemployed persons are usually family members, the number of persons directly affected by unemployment rates is two or three times greater than the official rate. Since ethnic minorities, women, young people, and the elderly are disproportionately victimized by joblessness, unemployment among these groups may be twice that of the general population (Briar, 1983).

Despite the advantages of modern technology, progress in this area has reduced the need for unskilled and semiskilled labor. In the United States, technological changes in agriculture have reduced the agrarian proportion of the work force from 90 to 3 percent. Employment in industry accounts for less than 20 percent of all jobs, and it is predicted that this figure will be lowered to between 3 to 5 percent by the year 2000. In the long term, technology has caused unemployment to rise, despite an overall reduction in work hours. If the role of human labor in society becomes less important, as seems likely, there need to be radical changes in public value systems. The work ethic as a major criterion of human worth may need to be replaced by other standards and attributes (Macarov, 1988).

Families become trapped when they cannot afford to move to look for work. For many, chronic unemployment becomes the norm; having a job becomes a sporadic and uncertain occurrence. As industries change or relocate, workers become superfluous. Decent-paying jobs under acceptable conditions and offering a measure of security then become only a dream. Self-sustaining citizens complain that some families are welfare recipients for generations, and call for restrictions. Rein (1982) makes it clear that for employment to be attractive to welfare clients, jobs must pay more than the minimum wage, be stable, and provide adequate fringe benefits. All too often the jobs available to most welfare clients do not have these characteristics.

Psychological Impact of Unemployment

In the crisis brought about by unemployment, the hard-earned possessions of a lifetime — car, home, savings — may be lost, sometimes to the extent of bankruptcy. Many people feel that they have no control over their lives or their future. In such situations suicide sometimes seems the only recourse.

Briar (1983) reports research data showing that in England and the United States sharp increases in unemployment are followed by increases in deaths, suicides, homicides, and stress-related health problems. Research findings also show that joblessness leads to hypertension, depression, domestic violence, child abuse, and various mental health problems.

In exploratory research on unemployment among low-income women, Donovan et al. (1987) notes five areas the subjects considered crucial in coping with joblessness: (1) loss of income, (2) loss of fulfillment and self-esteem, (3) strain on the family, (4) loss of social support from the workplace, and (5) loss of structure and purpose. Strained family relationships are most likely to occur when unemployment brings about shifts in the members' roles. A husband's unexpected job loss makes a working wife the primary breadwinner and changes the balance of dependency between the partners. According to Donovan et al., loss of social interaction for these low-income women made them feel lonely and depressed. Often they had formed close friendships within their group of co-workers, and these disrupted associations added to their sense of deprivation.

For both men and women, feelings of worth and self-esteem are linked to employment. For many, personal identity and selfhood are interwoven with their job or profession. When the wife does not work outside the home, the husband is clearly designated as the provider and head of the household. In these traditional families, loss of employment fiercely attacks the husband's feelings of status and competence. It often forces the wife into a job market for which she may be poorly prepared and may be reluctant to enter. The impact of a parent's unemployment is felt by the children as well. They not only have to cope with living on a reduced scale, but also must adjust to living with parents who are preoccupied with personal problems and reality issues concerning survival.

The widespread unemployment and economic depression following the stock market crash of 1929 in the United States brought unprecedented pressures on family life that were not limited to any one social or ethnic group. In 1933 the Federal Emergency Relief Act (FERA) was enacted, accepting federal responsibility for unemployment relief in the emergency. Almost sixty years have elapsed since then. Today the availability of public funds fails to solve the unemployment problems of our complex technological society, where permanent unemployment is becoming part of the national scene in some regions.

Therapeutic Guidelines: Unemployment

Health care professionals are obligated to find ways to help unemployed persons in a manner that removes the stigma of being jobless and avoids any suggestion of prejudice or discrimination. Jobless people should not be blamed for their situation. Usually they experience enough anxiety and depression about not finding work that their ability to present themselves as good job risks is already impaired. There is urgent need for advocacy, retraining programs, social action campaigns, and self-help groups to aid unemployed persons and their families. A referral to a mental health clinic is indicated when there are signs of emotional disturbance in the wage earner and of turmoil in the family.

NATURAL AND ENVIRONMENTAL DISASTERS

A *disaster* has been described as "an extreme social crisis situation in which individuals and social systems become dysfunctional and disorganized, sustain personal, collective, and public hardships, and also become a community of sufferers" (Siporin, 1976, p. 216). Because disasters are more severe than previous events, alterations of individual, family, and community behaviors occur. Ambiguity concerning the outcome of disaster causes anxiety, which is exacerbated when customary behaviors prove inadequate. The unexpectedness of a disaster and the inexperience of the inhabitants in coping with disaster can drastically alter the outcomes. People who live where landslides are common, for example, become practiced in preventive and restorative measures. The same is true of inhabitants of arid regions, where a brush fire can become a conflagration of terrifying proportions. Relatively isolated communities often suffer undue hardship because of their inaccessibility to rescue workers. An example of unexpectedness, unpreparedness, and relative inaccessibility may be found in the accounts of a severe earthquake that occurred in the northeastern part of the United States and Canada, where such events are rare. When a severe earthquake did occur in this region, the tremors annihilated three farming communities and caused damage from Portland, Maine, to Halifax, Nova Scotia. All along the coastline, small communities lost contact with the outside world for forty hours. Houses were flattened, and water, gas, and electric lines were severed. A forty-eight-car Canadian Pacific train plunged into a river, creating more havoc when sixteen railroad cars loaded with propane gas exploded with the fiery intensity of an atomic explosion. Additional injuries were suffered when flying debris landed on a busy highway, igniting buildings and vehicles in the suburbs of Fredericton, New Brunswick, which was located at the center of the earthquake.

Natural and environmental disasters can take many forms, and their impact is influenced by a number of uncontrolled variables. Table 5.1 depicts representational forms of community disasters and the global range of their occurrence.

Each year thousands of lives are lost because of disasters in both underdeveloped and highly developed societies. Two disasters of equal magnitude will have significantly different consequences depending on population density in the affected areas and the support systems available to stricken

TABLE 5.1. Location, Type, and Fatalities for Representative Disasters, 1963–1991

Date	Location	Type	Fatalities
1963	U.S.S. Thresher	Submarine lost	129 lives
1964	Alaska	Earthquake	117 lives
1970	Bay of Bengal, East Pakistan	Tidal wave	200,000 lives
1974	Zagreb, Yugoslavia	Train wreck	153 lives
1977	Canary Islands	Airplane crash	582 lives
1979	Chicago, Illinois	Airplane crash (DC-10)	272 lives
1980	St. Petersburg, Florida	Ship and bridge collision	36 lives
1981	Las Vegas, Nevada	Hotel fires:	
		Hilton Hotel	8 lives
		MGM Grand Hotel	84 lives
1988	San Francisco, California, area	Earthquake	?? lives
1991	Philippines	Volcano	341 lives

Source: Adapted from Janosik (1986). Information prior to 1981 from the *Information Please Almanac* (New York: Simon and Schuster, 1981).

communities. Highly industrialized societies with dense populations and complex technology are prone to greater impact but have more resources to alleviate suffering and disruption (Berren, 1980). Another classification of disasters considers the expected or unexpected nature of the disaster. Disasters that have occurred before, or that give warning signals, allow for a degree of preparedness. People living in a valley that is periodically flooded are better prepared to cope with flood control, just as people living in the vicinity of a volcano have learned evacuation procedures based on careful estimates of potential danger. Whenever the onset of disaster is gradual rather than precipitous, those who are threatened have time for anticipatory planning. Other factors that warrant consideration are the duration of impact of disaster and the broad distribution of consequences throughout the population. When disasters are sudden, unprecedented, and nondiscriminatory in their effects, there is greater likelihood of severe community disruption. Regardless of classification, disasters disturb community equilibrium and create conditions of crisis for families, as well as for whole communities.

Disaster conditions disrupt patterns of role performance established over the years. Under ordinary circumstances, role performance is distributed among family, job, and social responsibilities. In times of disaster, additional demands are made at all three levels of role performance. When individuals must choose between meeting the responsibilities of one role at the expense of other roles, the result is ambivalence and role conflict. Disasters impose internal strains on family role enactment because members are not sure what is expected of them or what the future will bring. When central family members, such as parents, cannot meet their own role expectations in protecting and caring for the family, the result is role strain accompanied by feelings of personal inadequacy. Most people experiencing disasters exhibit behavior that is adaptive and functional, and many families have the ability to adopt new patterns of role enactment when necessary. Personal and family losses are handled better when borne in the context of others' suffering as well. Even though families must live in crowded temporary quarters, propinquity with other victims seems to have some mitigating effects by reducing feelings of isolation. The families who lost members in a terrorist air crash in Scotland have formed an ongoing organization to help each other endure loss and to make sure that the incident is not forgotten.

During disasters, roles are organized around priorities; irrelevant tasks and responsibilities are temporarily discarded. Lowering community and family role expectations increases efficiency in performing essential core roles. At this point, communication networks among individuals, families, community workers, and community service facilities are of great importance. Any disaster disrupts collective behavior, and people involved in the disaster must know with whom to interact, what should be done, and for what purpose.

In the aftermath of natural and environmental disasters, physical needs are dominant, and providing food, clothing, and shelter for victims is probably the most therapeutic initial intervention. Basic survival needs, such as care of the injured, followed by search and rescue missions, have the highest priority. Because professionals may be in short supply, a considerable amount of work must be delegated to uninjured victims and concerned outsiders. Such assignments do much to eradicate feelings of powerlessness. The rationale for advocating crisis intervention in the postdisaster period is that during this time of acute distress, many individuals simultaneously experience the same feelings and reactions. There is irrefutable evidence that disasters provoke great distress in the victims, but the permanence of psychological impairment has not been extensively studied. Lately, there has been some recognition of the need to include mental health counseling in relief programs organized for disaster victims, and judgments have been made that on-site crisis intervention is probably the most efficacious approach. Data accumulated thus far indicate that relatively few disaster victims experience long-term emotional damage, even though substantial numbers report transitory difficulties around problems of everyday living. The value of traditional psychotherapeutic intervention offered in clinical settings is questionable for crisis victims who were functioning adequately before the disaster experience.

Phases of Disaster Reactions

Victims of disasters frequently undergo the following sequence of emotional reactions: a heroic phase, a honeymoon phase, a disillusionment phase, and a reconstruction phase (Burgess & Baldwin, 1980).

The heroic phase appears at the time of the disaster and is characterized by excitement and by people working together to survive the event. During the heroic phase, panic behaviors are infrequent and maladaptive responses are quite low. Fight/flight behavior is rarely evident, and irrationality is notably absent. Dynes and Quarantelli (1976) wrote that "solo or collective panic is so rare as to be an insignificant practical problem" (p. 235). At this time victims adapt by assessing immediate exigencies and cooperating with others to alleviate conditions. In the infrequent cases in which panic was evidenced, there was urgent, severe danger arising within seconds, a limited number of escape routes, and inadequate information, especially with regard to escape routes.

The period following the heroic phase has been labeled the honeymoon phase. This interval is of fairly short duration, generally lasting from two weeks to two months after the first impact of the disaster. During this time optimism runs high, and plans for rebuilding and restoring are formulated. In normal times, a community attends to the production and distribution of goods, social control, social protection, and social needs. During the honeymoon phase, community priorities change: Production of goods is reduced in importance because the objective is to meet basic needs rather than maintain economic productivity. Schools may be closed temporarily, and the media may become a means of communication rather than a source of entertainment. Social activities assume a low profile, but social control and social protection receive high priority. Mutual support among the victims takes the form of regulating and distributing services in an equitable manner unknown in the community before the disaster occurred.

Following these phases of work and optimism comes a period of disillusionment characterized by grief, despair, sleep disturbance, haunting visual memories, and anger at the destruction of life and property. Burgess and Baldwin (1980) suggested that this disillusionment phase might be compared to a second disaster whereby victims must cope with a new social reality replete with losses, destruction, unemployment, and other problems. Occasionally, the victims of disaster present depressive reactions, recurrent fears, nightmares, and guilt for surviving when loved ones died (Lifton, 1969, 1976; Lifton & Olson, 1976). The disillusionment phase may last from several months to a year or more. During this phase rebuilding is begun, but survivors may experience frustration and failure. These negative reactions are compounded by a sense of alienation, loss of confidence, and erosion of basic trust.

The reconstruction phase can be identified by collaborative efforts designed to restore predisaster levels of functioning to the community.

Depending on the magnitude of the disaster, this phase may last a number of years. During this lengthy period, discouragement and apathy may surface if favorable results are slow to appear. At other times cooperation during the reconstruction period causes people to draw closer to each other and perhaps modify their values. An interview with a flood victim seven years after the disaster speaks to this issue: "A house is a very important part of our lives—but it's not the most important part. Let me put it this way . . . a home could never be washed away . . . but a house could" (Ziegler, 1981, p. 9).

War means devastation for humanity; it is the ultimate catastrophe, the disaster that destroys not only human life, but homes, communities, cities, countrysides, business, governments. Many measures used to reduce suffering in the aftermath of a natural disaster are unavailable in wartime because of the complete breakdown of social agencies and institutions. However, many findings related to the mental health of natural disaster survivors are applicable to wartime survivors and, when available, can relieve suffering in the weeks and months following wartime losses.

Families of Holocaust Survivors

In considering the consequences of disaster for families, the special problems of Jewish families who experienced the Nazi Holocaust come immediately to mind. The mass extermination of Jews by the Nazis in World War II destroyed one-third of the European Jewish population. The *Encyclopedia Britannica* (15th edition, 1974) reports that in the concentration and slave labor camps of Germany and its occupied territories, from 18 to 26 million people perished. Only 530,000 people, at most, survived the various camps; of that number, many died shortly after liberation.

Among the various dictionary definitions of the word *holocaust* are the following: devastation, especially by fire, inferno, conflagration, sacramental offering, human sacrifice, and scapegoating. For the civilized world today, the term *holocaust* holds a special meaning derived from the near-extermination of a people by Nazi Germany. One of the significant aspects of this period in history was the worldwide denial of the horrors existing in the camps. Bruno Bettelheim (1952), who survived a concentration camp, has stated that denial was the most common reaction to the Holocaust.

Many questions regarding the consequences of the Holocaust for survivors can be answered incompletely at best. How did the survivors cope during the Holocaust experience and afterwards? What emotional burdens were survivors left with? Individual answers are sometimes hard to elicit, but the concentration camp "survivor syndrome" can be described. The survivor syndrome indicates that the survivor is obsessed with the question of "Why me? Why did I survive?" and ruminates about having survived at the cost of the deaths of others. Survivors wonder whether others would have lived if they had died. Another feature of the survivor syndrome is the inability to mourn for those who were lost. Awareness of a final and irrevocable separation is somehow avoided if the survivor does not mourn; failure to grieve helps survivors avoid pain and somehow keeps the dead person alive.

Several researchers (Solkoff, 1981; Davidson, 1980; Podietz et al., 1984) report various components of the emotional experience of Holocaust survivors, as follows:

- Increased anxiety and fatigue
- Restlessness
- Inability to concentrate
- Mistrust of others
- Guilt for having survived
- Pathological mourning: Inability to mourn or obsessive mourning
- Chronic depression
- Social isolation
- Multiple somatic complaints; psychophysiological disorders
- Dread of the future
- Lack of confidence
- Loss of sense of self
- Anhedonia (inability to experience pleasure)
- Loss of a sense of continuity with the past
- Difficulty in dealing with aggressive impulses: Blocking of feelings of aggression or showing aggressive outbursts against others

During the actual Holocaust experience, denial and repression were prominent psychological mechanisms that the victims needed. Bettelheim (1952) writes:

> Engaging in denial and repression in order to save oneself the difficult task of integrating an experience into one's personality, was a coping mechanism used by the concentration camp survivors. Survivors who deny that their camp experience has demolished their integration, who repress guilt and the sense that they ought to live up to some special obligation, are emotionally depleted because much of their vital energy goes into keeping the denial and repression going. They can no longer trust their inner integration to offer them security, should it again be put to the test, for it failed them once. (p. 33)

Among professional persons who have studied the impact of parental suffering on children of Holocaust survivors, there seems to be little consensus. Early studies emphasize that survivor parents are typically overprotective, controlling, and preoccupied with their past. Though highly valued, children of Holocaust survivors are expected to provide meaning for their parents' lives and to achieve parental goals. As a result, the children are caught in a guilt-ridden web and have difficulty separating from parents. They worry excessively about their parents' health, perhaps reflecting a reaction formation of the anger they feel toward their parents. For parents, the children are supposed to replace those who were lost. The parents tend to act unconsciously in ways that provoke hostility and aggression in the children, and are then unable to deal rationally with these displays of aggression (Barocas, 1973, 1975; Sigal, 1973; Alexandrowicz, 1973).

In contrast to studies that report pathology in the families of Holocaust survivors, other investigators report an absence of psychiatric problems in similar families (Solkoff, 1981). Freyberg (1980) emphasizes that there are a number of factors that may aggravate or ameliorate a child's difficulties at any stage of development. Among these factors are the pre-Holocaust personality of the parents, the quality of the parental relationship, the family's life circumstances, and family dynamics. Solkoff (1981) advises that being the child of a Holocaust survivor is not necessarily a predisposing factor for developing psychiatric problems. Other important factors are the age of parents when incarcerated, duration of incarceration, type of camp where incarcerated, and immediate posttrauma experiences of each parent.

In a comparative investigation, Rose and Gerske (1987) criticize the studies of the 1960s and 1970s on children of Holocaust parents because the studies were done on small samples of children from clinical populations. Because studies of children in outpatient and inpatient settings drew upon a special group, they revealed nothing about the characteristics of healthy children of survivors whose families coped in a constructive fashion. Rose and Gerske report that the major difference between survivors' children and comparison subjects was in the area of independence. Holocaust survivors often do not facilitate the separation of their children because they had no experience with functional differentiation and separation. For them, separation from parents was abrupt and final, with families being killed outright or removed to labor or concentration camps. Their well-controlled research indicates that, as a group, the children of Holocaust survivors have adjusted well despite their parents' experience. They assert further that inferences by clinicians that children of Holocaust survivors are generally maladjusted is a disservice to them.

Therapeutic Guidelines: Disasters

A comprehensive assessment of needs and analysis of resources available to the stricken community are essential to understanding the gravity of the situation. Delivery of services to survivors and rescue of persons still in danger are major areas of concern. Other pressing issues are the identification of community leaders and utilization of persons with special skills and abilities. The importance of mental health counseling through the preimpact, impact, and postimpact stages of disaster can be regarded as a form of psychological intervention that combines primary, secondary, and tertiary prevention. Burgess and Baldwin (1980) wrote that mental health services in the aftermath of disaster are an essential aspect of relief and reconstructive programs. Mental health counseling can be offered in evacuation centers as soon as people are relocated.

The help provided to crisis victims should not be withdrawn prematurely. It must be remembers that high levels of anxiety during and immediately after the disaster impede communication and cognitive understanding. Victims of disaster need to tell their story more than once; repetition of details should receive the careful attention that emotional catharsis deserves. People living in a disaster situation cannot comprehend immediate instructions very well because of the cognitive distortion that anxiety brings. Three months after a flood, one elderly person was discovered living alone in a trailer, incapable of understanding the financial aid forms that had been left by a community worker. He had received instructions at the time of the disaster but at that point was not able to comprehend or to remember what he had been told to do with the papers. One of the most important elements of crisis work is acknowledgment that people in crisis are not ill, but simply people in need for whom the community has a responsibility. Community crisis intervention does not adhere to traditional methods of history taking and scheduled appointments in a clinical setting, but can be undertaken by professionals or paraprofessionals working wherever disaster conditions exist.

In dealing with the consequences of disaster, an important rule is to keep families together if possible. Research in clinical settings and in the laboratory indicates that stress is tolerated more easily if significant persons are present (Garfield, 1979). Separation from families and evacuation from London in World War II seemed to be more harmful for children than remaining and enduring air raids in the company of their families. Studies of combat soldiers have indicated that membership in a supportive group, such as a platoon, does much to reduce battle stress (Bovard, 1959).

Separation anxiety is a universal human experience; loss of loved ones, loss of possessions, and loss of comforting routines are examples of separation that produce feelings of helplessness and hopelessness. In these circumstances, community workers can reduce anxiety wherever possible by providing information about other family members and missing possessions. For many survivors, uncertainty is harder to tolerate than the actual knowledge of what has happened.

Young children are apt to regress and cling to parents or favorite possessions that have been rescued. Such regressive behaviors should be tolerated and understood. Adolescents may display uncharacteristic behavior by becoming withdrawn or belligerent. Either manifestation should be met with consideration coupled with limit setting. Encouraging adolescents to assume responsibilities that are constructive but not unduly demanding may help restore age-appropriate behavior. For adults in the family, loss of home and possessions is a bitter blow. Realization that the rewards of a lifetime of hard work have been swept away may cause depressive reactions with accompanying somatic complaints.

For some survivors, short-term crisis intervention may be insufficient. There are always a number of people who cannot cope with disaster despite relief measures. These individuals do not resolve crisis adaptively but relive their experiences in the guise of nightmares, flashbacks, or intrusive rumination. Some of them react by withdrawing and decreasing their attachment to the living. In some respects, this reaction is a form of post-traumatic stress disorder that can be either acute or chronic in its effects. The disorder has been recognized as an entity in the *Diagnostic and Statistical Manual of Mental Disorders*, third edition, revised (DSM-III-R) (American Psychiatric Association, 1987) and is often applied to combat veterans. Usually the condition is the result of a survivor's inability to integrate the traumatic experience into the pattern of everyday existence. For these individuals, long-term therapeutic intervention may be required, and group treatment is considered to be especially effective when the group is composed of persons with similar residual stress.

A number of variables influence the readiness of victims to accept assistance. People in lower socioeconomic groups are usually more willing to accept physical treatment than psychological counseling. This is a compelling argument for including mental health services in comprehensive disaster programs. Members of ethnic or racial minorities who do not accept the customs of the dominant culture may misinterpret, and therefore reject, help that is being offered. This problem can be dealt with by enlisting the help of racial and ethnic representatives or of religious leaders who are trusted by minority segments of the population. In meeting the total needs of communities beset by disaster, coordinating the relief program is a major undertaking on which successful recovery depends. Human and material resources are too scarce to be wasted on duplicated efforts or uncoordinated missions.

CLINICAL EXAMPLE

Assessment

The Dang family lived in a northeastern city that had a large Southeast Asian refugee population. Mrs. Dang, a 27-year-old Laotian refugee woman, separated from her husband, has appeared numerous times at a busy urban medical clinic with her three sons, ages 2, 4, and 9 years, all of whom had many physical complaints: headaches, stomach aches, earaches, chills, and fevers. Mrs. Dang speaks very little English, so her 9-year-old son acts as spokesman. He understands English fairly well and is always brought along to interpret, even during school hours. The mother, who looks thin and tired, speaks to him at length in a rapid voice in the consultation room, but he translates only a few words to the clinic staff. The nurse clinician and family medicine physician are concerned and eager to be helpful but have become frustrated with the language difficulty and the family's excessive number of emergency visits. At times, the whole family spends many hours at the clinic waiting to be seen, because they arrive without appointments and do not appear acutely distressed. Despite her harassed appearance, Mrs. Dang habitually smiles and appears appreciative. The mother and children are clean and well clothed; Mrs. Dang usually carries a large purse containing numerous important papers: birth certificates, immigration cards, Medicaid cards, and the children's immunization papers. She can always correctly identify each official paper. Recently she appeared with a paper from the school stating that the oldest son had "behavior problems." The report indicated that he had angry outbursts at school; he bit and kicked other children on the playground. The boy had told his mother that the other children called him names. This aggressive behavior is quite uncharacteristic of the boy, who has previously received a great deal of praise in school. It was disclosed in the clinic interview that the husband had deserted the family two months earlier. He remains in the city and lives with another woman. Mrs. Dang, however, did not make any connection between that event and the son's subsequent aggressive behavior. Through the boy, the mother explained that she wanted to change schools for him and asked the nurse clinician to make the arrangements. This solution had evidently been suggested to the mother by a Laotian woman friend.

The Dang family had come as refugees to the United States two years earlier after spending three years in a refugee camp in Thailand and eight months in a refugee camp in the Philippines. Mr. Dang's parents and two siblings were killed in Vietnam during the Vietnam War. Mrs. Dang, whose father was also killed, had a mother and four sisters living in Thailand. She corresponded with them by letter and also had telephoned her mother several times. Both Mr. and Mrs. Dang had obtained the equivalent of a fourth- or fifth-grade education in Laos, and both had worked. Mr. Dang had been employed as a cook and Mrs. Dang as a seamstress. They had come to the United States with few possessions beyond some light clothing and a box of relatives' photographs. In the United States the family followed their old customs. In their home here, Mrs. Dang cooked Thai and Laotian food, which she bought at an Oriental grocery where she purchased fifty pounds of rice at a time. Because they had little furniture, the family sat on a straw rug on the floor and ate from a common soup bowl placed in the center of their dining area. Their small house was kept at temperatures of 85 to 88 degrees, and the children ran around in short-sleeved shirts and bare feet, summer and winter. Their shoes were left outside on the porch by the front door, as dictated by Oriental custom.

The husband's motives for leaving the family were not explained clearly. Apparently, his English was more proficient, and he had obtained a factory job, working long hours. He seemed to spend most of his free time with his Laotian men friends, with whom he sometimes went fishing. Mrs. Dang described him as a caring father. However, the visiting nurse, asked to do an assessment home visit by the medical clinic staff, concluded that she really had not learned much about the marital or parental relationships, even after talking with the family several times.

Planning

The Dang family is sponsored by a local church group in addition to receiving public assistance and food stamps. The family is also involved with numerous social, health, and educational agencies. The first act on the agenda was to call a meeting of the significant professional persons involved to discuss the family's problems as well as their strengths, so that appropriate plans could be made. The meeting was arranged by a family service social worker whose agency had an outreach program for Southeast Asian refugees. In the interdisciplinary meeting, the following plans were developed. The 9-year-old son was referred to a special Laotian counselor who worked in the public school system and was himself a former refugee. The family service social worker agreed to visit the family once a week with an interpreter. ESL (English as a Second Language) classes during weekdays were to be offered the mother through the public school system and transportation arranged for her through a Laotian friend. The church refugee resettlement program arranged to send a male worker to talk with the husband to learn more about his needs and circumstances. The mother gave permission for him to be contacted, since she had a phone number for him.

Implementation

Mrs. Dang was told and reluctantly accepted the decision that a change of schools was not a solution for her son; she was extremely frightened that serious physical harm would come to him if he remained in the school, and it was difficult to reassure her on that score. She did welcome the referral to a Laotian counselor for him and said she would attend meetings with his teacher if an interpreter could be present. This was a hard decision for her, because she seemed fearful of the boy's teacher. Mrs. Dang was proud of her son's academic achievements and expressed the desire to find a job in order to save money for him to go to college. Although she said she wanted to learn English, she was unwilling to be parted from the 2-year-old to attend ESL classes. This youngster was very much attached to his mother. He screamed and refused to stay with a Laotian friend. She was aware that his behavior was becoming more out of control. All she could do was to give him a bottle and hold him close. The 4-year-old son appeared fairly well adjusted and would stay with a friend.

Although Mrs. Dang brightened somewhat at the attention and rallying-around efforts on the part of the community personnel, she continued to be housebound. With all the health care professionals, she remained reserved and did not speak with non-Oriental personnel about her marital troubles. She engaged in extended daily telephone conversations with her Laotian women friends and seemed to turn to them for personal advice and support. Gradually, the 9-year-old son's behavior at school became less aggressive and hostile, and he seemed happier. He liked talking with the Laotian counselor and seemed relieved in the meetings with his teacher, who gave him and his mother special attention through their meetings. The father kept only two appointments with the Laotian counselor but did promise to visit his sons on a regular basis. He did contribute a little to the children's support. His only reason for the separation was that he had found "another woman" whom he liked.

Evaluation

In many Southeast Asian families, the mother of several children is housebound, the older children are used as interpreters, and both husband and wife are reluctant to talk about personal troubles with anyone outside their own cultural circle. They prefer to turn to their own countrymen for advice and comfort. The process of acculturation is a gradual one and is complicated when the refugees themselves have little education in their own language and have a lot of trouble learning English. Neither Mr. nor Mrs. Dang is able to talk about their experiences with loss and devastation in their native country. Professional health care workers cannot realize the extent of the emotional and economic hardships that refugees have suffered before arriving in the United States. It is important to recognize and respect their courage and strength in coming to a strange country where the language and customs are so different. Even the most experienced professional is apt to feel frustrated when dealing with the reticence and evasion that seem to characterize these families. It may be helpful to realize that their experience with hardships has served to reinforce the cultural wariness that characterizes many refugee families. As Mrs. Dang's anxiety and fears lessen, her reaching out may increase. If her motivation is strong enough and her self-confidence is sufficient, she may learn to speak and write better English. This will help her find employment and may even reduce distances between herself and her children. There is always the possibility that she will remain stuck in the old trap and make little progress toward achieving economic independence or accepting mainstream values. Mrs. Dang and all other refugees like her need a great deal of time, patience, and investment on the part of sponsors, health care professionals, and community agencies who can only guess at the refugee experience and who take so many ordinary events in American life for granted.

SUMMARY

This chapter has described how mobility, unemployment, and environmental disasters impact family life. A yearning to be on the move is seen as a uniquely American characteristic. The freedom to move and settle new territories was enhanced when railroads opened up the continent. With more modern transportation available, this also meant more markets for families' farm produce. On a more negative note, the migrant workers were the underprivileged ethnic minorities who suffered poverty and impoverished conditions much like those of eighteenth- and nineteenth-century European peasants.

Federal supervision and control over immigration began in the early 1890s. Between 1892 and 1954, 12 million people came to the United States through Ellis Island. They were persuaded to leave Europe by poverty, anti-Semitism, and overpopulation. Amendments to the immigration laws in the 1970s and 1980s made these laws less restrictive, and the immigration process itself has become less cumbersome, with immigrants now being prescreened and approved by the U.S. embassy in their home country. America is still seen as "the land of opportunity."

The five stages of the migration process were presented in this chapter: (1) the preparatory stage, (2) the act of migration, (3) the period of overcompensation, (4) the period of decompensation and crisis, and (5) the transgenerational impact (Sluzki, 1979). Today the worldwide refugee problem is tragic and disheartening, with an estimated 15 million people uprooted from their homeland, and only 1 percent being resettled each year.

In the second section of this chapter, the impact of unemployment on the family is discussed. Prolonged unemployment of a family wage earner has a disastrous influence on the family's social and economic functioning, as well as serious emotional consequences. Judgmental attitudes toward the poor in England in 1601, when the Elizabethan Poor Laws were established, are not unlike the prejudicial feelings toward the destitute jobless today. The more fortunate members of the public also blame social and economic programs that do not find quick solutions. In this country, advances in technology have caused unemployment to rise as the role of human labor in society has become less important. There is concern about the existence of permanent unemployment in the United States among those persons who, for years, are unable to find jobs.

Prolonged unemployment can have a disastrous effect on the emotional stability of a family; loss of job can mean loss of home, car, and life savings, and dismal future for family members who feel they have no control over their lives. Feelings of worth and self-esteem are linked to employment; for many, personal identify and selfhood are interwoven with their job or profession. An increase in the occurrence of physical illnesses, depression, and even suicide in families, related to chronic joblessness, has been documented. In traditional families, where the husband is the designated provider and head of the family, a wife's seeking employment may attack the husband's feelings of status and competence. The homemaker wife may be poorly equipped to enter the competitive job market. Children are often subject to considerable stress, also, when the parents' emotional and economic security is so threatened.

The next section of this chapter is devoted to a discussion of natural and environmental disasters and their impact on family life. Natural disasters can take many forms, and their impact is influenced by a number of uncontrolled variables. When an environmental catastrophe occurs, individual and social systems become disorganized and dysfunctional; victims struggle to meet their basic needs for food, shelter, and clothing to survive. The unexpectedness of a disaster and the inexperience of the inhabitants in coping with it can drastically alter the outcomes. People who live in an area that is periodically flooded can be better prepared to cope with flood control. Isolated communities can suffer undue hardship because of their inaccessibility to rescue workers.

Disasters impose internal strains on family role enactment because members are not sure what is expected of them or what the future holds. This strain is accompanied by feelings of personal inadequacy. Many times in the aftermath of a disaster, people in a community can become bonded in their efforts to help each other survive. Victims of disasters frequently undergo the following sequence of emotional reactions: the heroic phase, the honeymoon phase, the disillusionment phase, and a reconstruction phase (Burgess & Baldwin, 1980).

War is mentioned as the ultimate disaster for human beings. The last part of this chapter discusses the disaster of the Nazi Holocaust which came out of World War II. It is estimated that 18 to 26 million people died in the Holocaust. Jewish family members who survived the Holocaust have shown some special problems that warrant discussion, the most prominent one being the "survivor syndrome." Those persons who lived through this horrifying experience felt guilty for having survived; had they died instead, they feel, others might have lived. A mistrust of others, a loss of a sense of self, and often an inability to mourn those who were lost, as well as difficulty in dealing with aggressive impulses, are prominent symptoms suffered by these survivors. Bettelheim (1952) noted that denial and regression were necessary mechanisms of defense employed by the survivors, who were too emotionally depleted to integrate the terrors of their experience. There is some controversy among mental health professionals about the impact of parental survivors on their children. Some feel that the fact that only clinical populations were studied gave a negative slant to the picture, while others find in well-controlled research that, as a group, children of Holocaust survivors have adjusted remarkably well despite their parents' experiences.

REFERENCES

Alexandrowicz, D. R. (1973). "Children of Concentration Camp Survivors." *Yearbook, International Association of Child Psychiatry, Allied Professions*, 2: 385–394.

American Psychiatric Association. (1987). *Diagnostic and Statistical Manual of Mental Disorders*, 3rd edition, revised. Washington, DC: Author.

Barocas, H. A., & Barocas, C. B. (1973). "Manifestations of Concentration Camp Effects on the Second Generation." *American Journal of Psychiatry*, 130: 820–821.

Barocas, H. (1975). "Children of Purgatory: Reflections on the Concentration Camp Survival Syndrome." *International Journal of Social Psychiatry*, 21: 87–92.

Berren, M. R. (1980). "A Typology for the Classification of Disasters." *Community Mental Health Journal*, 16 (Summer): 103–110.

Bettelheim, B. (1952). *Surviving and Other Essays*. New York: Vintage Books, Random House.

Bovard, E. W. (1959). "The Effects of Social Stimuli on Response to Stress." *Psychological Review*, 66: 267–277.

Briar, K. H. (1983). "Unemployment: Toward a Social Work Agenda." *Social Work*, 28(3): 211–223.

Burgess, A. W., & Baldwin, B. (1980). *Crisis Intervention Theory and Practice: A Clinical Handbook*. Englewood Cliffs, NJ: Prentice-Hall.

Davidson, S. (1980). "The Clinical Effects of Massive Psychic Trauma in Families of Holocaust Survivors." *Journal of Marital and Family Therapy*, 6(1): 11–21.

Donovan, R., Jaffe, N., & Pirie, V. M. "Unemployment among Low-Income Women: An Exploratory Study." *Social Work*, 32(4): 301–305.

Dynes, R., & Quarantelli, E. L. (1976). "The Family and Community Content of Individual Reactions to Disaster." In H. J. Parad, H. L. P. Resnik, & L. Parad (Eds.), *Emergency and Disaster Management: A Mental Health Source Book*. Bowie, IN: Charles.

Encyclopedia Britannica, 15th edition, 1974.

Fallows, J. (1989). "America Helps Itself by Helping Others." *U.S. News and World Report*, October 23.

Freyberg, J. T. (1980). "Difficulties in Separation–Individuation as Experienced by Offspring of Nazi Holocaust Survivors." *American Journal of Orthopsychiatry*, 50(1): 87–95.

Garfield, C. A. (1979). *Stress and Survival: Emotional Realities of Life-Threatening Illness*. St. Louis: Mosby.

Hall, A. J. (1990). "New Life for Ellis Island and Immigration Today." *National Geographic*, 178(3).

Hartman, A. (1990). "Our Global Village" (editorial). *Social Work*, 35(4).

Information Please Almanac. (1981). New York: Simon and Schuster.

Janosik, E. H. *Crisis Counseling: A Contemporary Approach*. Boston/Monterey: Jones and Bartlett, 1986.

Lifton, R. J. (1969). *Death in Life: Survivors of Hiroshima*. New York: Vantage Books.

Lifton, R. J. (1976). *History and Human Survival*. New York: Vantage Books.

Lifton, R. J., & Olson, E. (1976). "The Human Meaning of Total Disaster: The Buffalo Creek Experience." *Psychiatry*, 39: 1–18.

Macarov, D. (1988). "Reevaluation of Unemployment." *Social Work*, 33(1): 23–28.

McGoldrick, M., & Gerson, R. (1985). *Genograms in Family Assessment*. New York: W. W. Norton.

Podietz, L., Belmont, H., Shapiro, M., Zwerling, I., Ficher, I., Einstein, T., & Levick, M. (1984). "Engagement in Families of Holocaust Survivors." *Journal of Marital and Family Therapy*, 10(1): 43–51.

Rein, M. (1982). "Work in Welfare: Past Failures and Future Strategies." *Social Science Review*, 56: 438–447.

Rose, S. L., & Gerske, J. (1987). "Family Environment, Adjustment, and Coping among Children of Holocaust Survivors: A Comparative Investigation." *American Journal of Orthopsychiatry*, 57(3): 332–344.

Sigal, J. J., et al. (1973). "Some Second-Generation Effects of Survival of the Nazi Persecution." *American Journal of Orthopsychiatry*, 43: 320–327.

Siporin, M. (1976). "Altruism, Disaster, and Crisis Intervention." In H. J. Parad, H. L. P. Resnik, & L. Parad (Eds.), *Emergency and Disaster Management: A Mental Health Source Book*. Bowie, IN: Charles.

Sluzki, C. E. (1979). "Migration and Family Conflict." *Family Process*, 18(4): 379–390.

Solkoff, N. (1981). "Children of Survivors of the Nazi Holocaust: A Critical Review of the Literature." *American Journal of Orthopsychiatry*, 51(1): 29–42.

"The New Refugees." (1989). *U.S. News and World Report*, October 23.

Ziegler, M. (1981). "After the Flood." *Upstate*, November, pp. 9–13.

PART
THREE

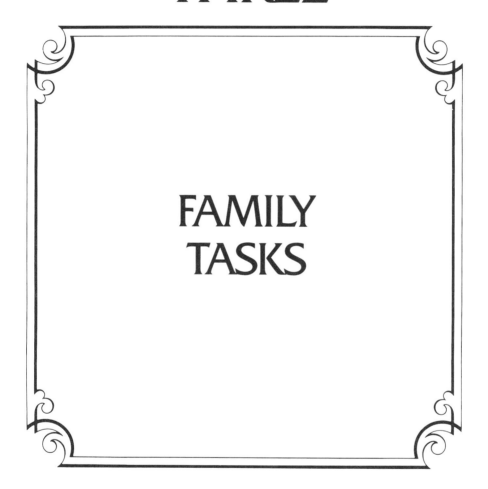

FAMILY
TASKS

CHAPTER SIX

Expanding Families: Life Cycle Tasks and Responsibilities

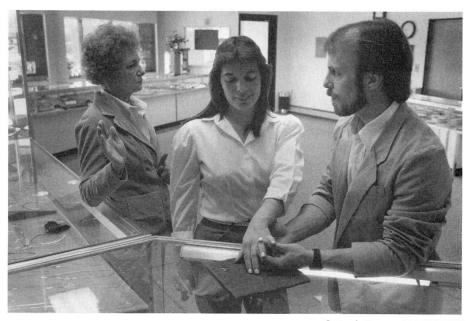

© Frank Siteman MCMLXXXVI

Parenting behavior in humans is certainly not the product of some unvarying, parenting instinct, nor is it reasonable to regard it as merely the product of learning. Parenting behavior has strong biological roots, thus accounting for the very strong emotions associated with it; but the specific form that the behavior takes in each of us turns on our experiences — during childhood especially, during adolescence, before and during marriage, and with each individual child.

John Bowlby

The word *love* has been replaced in professional literature by such terms as *attachment, bonding, object relationships,* and *affiliation.* Even so, *love* has not fallen entirely into disuse. In music, poetry, and drama, it is the emotional state to which we aspire, and the absence of love is considered the least desirable human state. Love's presence does not in itself buy happiness, for the process of loving and being loved is very complex. Although it has positive connotations, love is multifaceted and never automatic or predictable in its consequences. Love is more than passionate desire between two people, for there are important differences between falling in love and staying in love. Ideally, love creates a wish to give to another. It is a mode of relating rather than circumscribed acts limited to sexual attraction or romantic passion.

It is widely assumed that good people are capable of love and bad people are less so. Family members are supposed to love one another. If they cannot return love or have negative feelings about their "loved ones," they are troubled by this. Their negative feelings toward family members may be suppressed, camouflaged, or denied altogether, depending on what is acceptable to the individual and the family.

Love is popularly regarded as the adhesive that keeps families together but, this is a simplistic view that overlooks the many forms, gradations, and effects of love. A family begins when two people marry or commit themselves to a long-term relationship. Marital love between husband and wife differs from premarital and extramarital love in its expression and in its expectations. Parental love differs from marital love in its peculiar mingling of pride, worry, and responsibility. Filial love differs from parental love in its unique blend of gratitude, respect, and condescension, the proportions of which change markedly over time. And fraternal love between siblings is something else entirely, having variable components of camaraderie, egalitarianism, protectiveness, and rivalry. The phrase *pure love* is something of a misnomer, for love is rarely pure but is compounded of many emotions. In actuality, love is made up of many feelings—sexual, social, selfish, and altruistic (Turner, 1970).

Different kinds of love and expressions of love influence and are influenced by the nature of relationships. Thus, love is both a dependent and an independent variable. Feelings of love are involved when two people form a marital dyad, and the nature of love changes as the family enlarges through the addition of new members. This chapter deals with the transitional changes of a couple transformed from a marital dyad into parents. Following this, the chapter describes the changes that accompany the arrival of other children, and the rigors of helping children achieve their age-related tasks. Adoptive and stepparent families are included in the discussion and receive the attention merited by their numbers in contemporary society.

Families expand through birth and adoption, and through remarriage. With longevity increasing, today's families may undergo a period of contraction as children leave home, followed by a period of expansion later on. As aged people become infirm, they may become the in-house responsibility of their children, many of whom are middle-aged or older. This chapter uses a chronological approach in describing family transitions and the role transformations of individual members.

Expansion of a family inevitably brings changes, not merely in the family system but in how the family relates to other systems as well. The entry of any new member alters role enactment and family interaction. Changes caused by loss or contraction are the subject of Chapter Seven, but this chapter is concerned with family expansion. Some hazards are identified, and responsive therapeutic guidelines are suggested for health care professionals working with a family at a particular transitional stage.

CHILDLESS COUPLES

A new family is established when two people make a long-term commitment to each other through marriage or a less formal living arrangement. Although these less formal arrangements sometimes constitute families, in this chapter *family* refers to the stereotypical pattern of a heterosexual couple and their offspring. For our purposes, the heterosexual couple without children is a good starting point for discussing the expanding family.

If a childless married couple live in a community or come from extended families that value procreation, they may undergo social disapproval. Many couples marry without resolving their respective attitudes toward having children. One of the partners may be reluctant to become a parent but may not divulge this before marriage. Or the couple may have agreed not to have children but may hesitate to reveal this to their own parents. Even when both partners agree to be childless, the decision may have adverse results. It usually comes as a blow to their own parents, who had looked forward to grandparenthood. The comments and questions of their parents annoy the couple, especially if one partner is more determined than the other not to have children. Having reached a decision to be child-less, a couple may need help in constructing a life-style that compensates for the lack of children. Many childless couples invest greatly in the marital relationship or devote themselves to jobs or careers. This is especially important if most of their friends in their age group are raising children. Depending on the views of the couple, childlessness may be a source of frustration or of gratification. Couples who are not childless by choice suffer emotional pain that is aggravated by remarks from thoughtless friends and relatives.

Whether they are childless voluntarily or involuntarily, the childless couple must look for other interests and pursuits. They may express their parenting instincts in ways that benefit the community. Although the marital relationship becomes all-important for some partners, others detach themselves from this bond in favor of outside interests. This is more likely to happen if the couple are not childless by choice because the marital relationship itself may be a constant reminder of disappointed hopes, caus-ing one or both partners to withdraw from the relationship. If infertility is the cause of childlessness, practitioners need to know what, if any, steps have been taken to overcome the difficulty. Practitioners should also be familiar with community resources so that suitable referrals can be made.

It is not unusual for one partner in a childless marriage to have increas-ing trouble around the issue as time passes. Tensions between the couple may originate within the relationship or be generated by people and events outside the marital system. Especially for women, the passage of time may bring regrets for a decision made earlier. When being childless brings a couple into treatment, it is essential to identify the origin of the problem and its proportions. A couple may be content in their present state but resentful of interference from extended families. Older couples who face a now-or-never dilemma may need counseling when deciding if they should become parents. The way couples deal with this issue depends on the nature of the marital relationship, the partners' capacity for insight, and their willingness to accept the status quo or to take measures to alter their situation.

PARENTAL TRANSITIONS

Families acquire children in various ways: through birth, through adoption, and through remarriage. The three forms of family expansion differ, but the unifying concepts are family transition and role transformation. Changes in families caused by family expansion are transitional issues because they propel families from one critical life stage to another. As soon as marital partners become prospective parents, a series of boundary shifts and realignments take place. These affect not only the couple but extended family members as well.

Biological Parenthood

Pregnancy is a profound maturational transition, which confirms the vigor and identity of both partners but at the same time places heavy demands on the relationship. The woman is subject to doubts concerning her ability to meet the physical demands of the months ahead and the psychosocial challenges to come. The man, too, is anxious and ambivalent about parenthood even when the pregnancy is planned and welcome. He may be proud of his part in creating new life but also afraid of being displaced in his wife's affection by the newborn child. The current situation reactivates memories of childhood as both partners resolve to do better by their child than their own parents did with them (Stern, 1985).

Most expectant parents have fantasies of what the baby will be like. They imbue the child with unlimited potential, but they also fear the child will be imperfect. Each partner hopes that attractive qualities of their mate will reappear in the child. Weaknesses or defects in oneself or one's mate cause concern lest they be perpetuated in the new generation. As a rule, the expectant mother is given more attention than the expectant father, who is expected to tolerate the whims of his pregnant wife and to gratify her if possible. Unless the marital relationship is rewarding and the wife is sensitive to her husband's needs, his feelings may be ignored (Jordon, 1990).

Pregnancy is a time when prospective parents can forge an alliance that operates as a parental subsystem as soon as the child is born (Sadow, 1984). Even before the birth, thoughtful parents make plans together and begin to function as a team. They talk about possible names for the child, discuss child-rearing practices, and make household arrangements such as preparing a nursery. The gestation period for a baby is nine months; the gestation period for parents is indefinite. Somewhere between conception and the early months of a child's life, parents are formed. Just as children gradually develop a self-concept, so new parents integrate the role of father or mother into their perception of self.

Once a child is born, caretaking duties are thrust upon the new parents. They have little choice in the matter because of the prolonged helplessness of human infants. The relationship of parents, especially mothers, to their children is greatly influenced by the maternal care they once received (Brunnquell et al., 1981). The mothers least likely to abuse or neglect their children are those whose own childhood nurture was adequate or better. One cannot overemphasize the importance of social support for new mothers, especially if given by the baby's father or the mother's own mother. Belsky (1984) calls the parental subsystem "buffered," and explains that three areas—the social network, the mother's nurturing ability, and the child's responses—determine the quality of parenting. Deficiency in any one of these three areas is offset by strength in the others. This means that an irritable, difficult child can be effectively cared for by a mother who herself was well nurtured as a child and who has access to social support. Likewise, an adaptable, happy child can compensate for deficiencies in a mother who was mistreated in early life, has minimal social support, but can manage to nurture an undemanding child.

Parents with high degrees of self-differentiation are less vulnerable to reactivated childhood conflicts and are better able to see their child as unique and separate. Having achieved individuation and differentiation, they look to the child for signs of what the child needs, rather than the memory of their own unmet needs in the past. If their self-concept includes acceptance of the parenting role, they have some confidence in their parenting skills. Partridge (1988) recognizes the value of developing a parental self-concept and describes the psychological domains that make it up.

- *Affective parenting domain:* Parents' feelings about being a mother or father and about caring for a particular child.
- *Cognitive parenting domain:* Parents' perceptions of their role enactment, their rationale for their parenting practices, and the individualized meanings they give to interactions with a particular child.
- *Moral parenting domain:* Parents' recognition of cultural norms and values as these relate to child rearing; evaluation standards they apply to their performance as parents.
- *Integrated parental domain:* Parents' assimilation of past and present experiences in ways that enrich the meaning of interpersonal attachments, of caring for others, and of being cared for by others.

It is obvious from this paradigm that awareness of oneself as a parent considers both the past and the present, and includes emotional, intellectual, cultural, and ethical functioning. Health care professionals are frequently asked to evaluate the quality of parenting that children receive. This is requested of child protective workers, of nurses and social workers planning hospital discharge, in custody disputes, and as part of individual or family therapy. In making these evaluations, the four parental domains previously mentioned broaden the perspective of practitioners and workers.

The First Child

The birth of the first child is described as "a bomb, a salvo in the ever-intensifying marital battle" (Rubenstein, 1989, p. 34). On a cognitive level most new parents expect some restrictions in their lives, but they are unprepared for the enormity of change. Social and psychological consequences of parenthood have been documented by a number of investigators. Rubenstein (1989) describes some consequences of parenthood.

- About half the couples report less overall marital satisfaction after the birth of a child.
- Many couples report frequent bitter arguments about dividing tasks, sharing leisure time, and seeing in-laws and friends.
- Many couples report fewer expressions of affection such as kissing, hugging, praising, or complimenting each other.
- Many couples report less sexual interaction and less pleasure in making love.

Belsky (1984) finds that couples who value romance and sex in marriage rather than partnership are more likely to report marital dissatisfaction after becoming parents, especially if they have not been married long. It is older couples who seem better able to cope with transition to parenthood, even though couples who defer parenthood often complain that the birth of a child disrupts their well-ordered lives. Younger couples and those with less education seem to have more relationship problems after becoming parents. Evidently, no timing pattern for having a first child is totally advantageous.

After a couple become parents, gender role enactment increases. This may be attributable to the parental self-concept each partner has developed. When a woman becomes a mother, her perception of herself as a wife and a worker is overshadowed, while a man's perception of himself as a husband and a worker is strengthened by parenthood. Thus, for women the role of parent seems to be dominant, whereas for men the role of parent is secondary (Belsky, 1984). Husbands seem to help more with child care than their fathers did, but this is an area of contention. Turner (1970) observes that fathers who involve themselves in child care are "draftees," not volunteers. Interestingly, Rubenstein (1989) reports that fathers in dual-career families help more with feeding the baby and changing diapers, but the more services they perform, the more discontent they express with their marriage. It is older mothers who are more apt to receive help from husbands; younger mothers are more apt to receive help from their own mothers. Compared with husbands who are the sole wage earners, men in two-salaried households are more likely to quarrel with their wives about child care and to be the target of criticism from the wives.

Many women who say they want more help from their husbands behave in ways that curtail assistance. One problem is that new mothers need help, but at the same time they want to be in charge. Thus, they scrutinize and criticize the way the husband handles the baby and performs household jobs. Asking a husband to dress the baby or put the baby to bed for a nap invites him to get involved. But if the wife then objects to the outfit the husband chooses or the blanket he uses to cover the baby, many husbands will withdraw and let the wife manage without help.

Therapeutic Guidelines

Childbirth education classes welcome the attendance of prospective fathers, and most of them participate willingly. It is ironic that so much preparation centers on labor and delivery, which last only a day or so in a couple's life, while so little deals with the weeks and months following the birth. Tulman et al. (1990) studied a group of women for a six-month period after they had delivered healthy babies. They found that a woman's ability to take care of her baby and resume her usual activities improved steadily from three weeks to three months after delivery, but did not change significantly between three and six months postpartum. Six months after delivery, 6 percent had not entirely assumed child care activities; nearly 20 percent had not fully assumed household activities; 30 percent had not fully resumed their usual social and community activities; and more than 80 percent had not resumed their usual self-care activities. Of the 97 subjects in the study, 57 returned to work or school within six months after delivery; 60 percent of them had not resumed their usual level of activities at work or school.

Along with guidance through labor and delivery, couples need information about the effects of parenthood on their relationship. A husband who knows that new mothers are not interested in resuming sexual intercourse soon after childbirth will be more understanding of his wife's reactions and less apt to feel rejected. New parents also need help with issues of task allocation, the role of in-laws, and the integration of marital and parental role enactment. Efforts should be made to reinforce the significance of father in the parental subsystem. Even witnessing the baby's first bath, which is usually demonstrated to mothers in the hospital, should be open to fathers and to the baby's siblings if there are any. Parenting is a family affair, and families function better if there are no left-out members.

With dependable contraception, many (though not all) births are planned. Because many couples defer childbearing until their educations are complete and their careers established, they may be in their late thirties or early forties when their first child is born. These older parents require different kinds of services. They tend to be well informed and to know what services they need. Because they are more vocal than younger parents, they seem, to be more demanding. They are assertive enough to shop around for the services they want and may ask that customary policies be adjusted on their behalf. Usually they have waited so long to have a child that the experience is very precious to them. Once they are convinced that health care professionals are competent and well intentioned, they appreciate assistance, although they may be reluctant to give up autonomy.

In working with new parents before and after the birth, practitioners should keep in mind the four psychological domains that constitute the parental self-concept. Parents cope better with the birth of an infant if they make plans for meeting their new obligations. This means helping them to anticipate the duties and rewards that are in store for them. The following questions describe practical matters that should be considered in advance.

- Is the father or another selected family member available to help the mother for a few weeks after the birth?
- Is there enough money for extra expenses?
- What adjustments have been made for living on less income if the mother does not return to work?
- What arrangements have been made for child care if and when mother returns to work?
- What preparations have been made in the home to make room for the child and the equipment that will be needed?
- What thought has been given to the allocation of household chores and child care duties?
- What changes or restrictions will be experienced by the couple after the child is born? Discussion should include limits on personal freedom and leisure, discretionary income, sexual activity, and the marital relationship in general.

The period of infancy brings joy to parents as well as stress. Within a few weeks after the birth, the mother starts to understand what is needed by signals the child gives her. After the initial adjustment period, the husband may expect his wife to expand her interests beyond the infant and pay more attention to him. Her first reaction may be that he is unreasonable, that she has too much to do and cannot leave the baby. If the marital relationship is healthy, the mother will realize that it is safe to delegate some tasks to others and that the child will survive some separation from her. A child's progress is heightened when parents are able to balance the child's needs and their own. Each day brings new accomplishments to the growing infant, and mutual pride draws the parents together. As the baby learns to laugh, walk, and talk, it finds a place in the family system. Gradually the couple learn to relax and enact their new roles as if they had always been parents.

Adoptive Parents

Access to dependable contraception and legal abortion has reduced the number of infants in the United States available for adoption. Changing attitudes have made it more acceptable for single mothers to keep a child. As a result of the scarcity of infants, the adopted child today is likely to be past infancy and may be of a different race or nationality from the adoptive parents. These older children may have had several foster parents or been subject to distressing experiences of one kind or another. Such factors compound the adjustment problems faced by adoptive parents and the children they take into their homes.

For many years, persons concerned with adoption procedures tried to "match" the child with the adoptive parents, but this seems less practical today, when many couples are willing to cross racial and national boundaries to find an adoptable child. There is an erroneous belief that black children are seldom adopted by black families. In fact, for many generations, black families have taken children into their homes with and without legal adoption. At present, many children of all races are being raised by grandmothers and other relatives who must take the place of drug-addicted parents. Many adoptions now result in biracial families as Caucasian families adopt nonwhite children of American or foreign lineage. Many children adopted by American families are of Japanese, Chinese, Vietnamese, or Korean ancestry; a sizable number of these children may themselves be biracial.

The practice of adopting children of another race, nationality, or ethnic group often works well. But it also has the potential for adjustment problems unless parents fully accept differences in the adopted child's appearance and temperament and are prepared to deal with issues as they arise. Some years ago black social workers issued a position paper warning of the damaging effects on black children of being adopted by white parents (Berman, 1974). This seems an extreme viewpoint, but transracial adoptions do require concerted efforts on the part of the parents. For one thing, the family must deal with careless remarks from outsiders about the child or the parents. Even when parents manage to insulate the child from such experiences, there will be moments when the child feels different and perhaps inferior. Gibbs (1987) states that biracial children, adopted or biological, usually have good relationships with other children in elementary school but that friendships deteriorate in secondary school. In a period when peer conformity is valued, children in biracial families are rejected by their adoptive parents' groups and also by their own because of the incongruity between their appearance and that of their family.

In trying to shield children who come from other racial or ethnic groups, adoptive parents may become overprotective. The children often respond either by becoming very dependent on the parents or by disdaining protection and rebelling against parental control. The problem may be especially severe for black children adopted by white families because of societal messages blacks receive that they are inferior. In a study of mixed-race families in London, Benson (1981) found that virtually all the children, aged 3 to 16 years, rejected their black identity either behaviorally or verbally. Gibbs (1987) reports research findings that biracial children have fewer identity problems if they live in a racially mixed community rather than a predominantly black or white neighborhood.

Over the last decade more than five thousand unaccompanied Indochinese children have resettled in the United States. The official U.S. policy is that unaccompanied minor children entering the country should maintain ethnic ties during the assimilation process. However, 90 percent of

Indochinese children entering without family have been placed with white families for adoption or foster care, and only 10 percent have been placed with families of their own ethnic group. In contrast, other countries elect to keep unaccompanied minors with their ethnic peer group, either in hostels or small group homes. Australia, for example, places such children in hostels until they are released to the care of families in their ethnic community. Porte and Torney-Porte (1987) report that Indochinese youngsters living in group homes or with white families were significantly more depressed than their counterparts in foster care with families of their own ethnic group. Those in ethnic foster care felt freer to enter the mainstream culture and emulate the behavior of mainstream teenagers. Although the important adults in their lives were not Americans, youngsters in ethnic homes had less trouble adapting to life in the United States, evinced less depression, had better academic records, and believed they had more control over their lives. The research data indicate that the day-to-day presence of adults with a similar ethnic background is a bridge that helps children move comfortably between their old culture and the new one they have entered.

A risk that is present in any adoptive family but is more frequent in biracial adoptive families is the tendency of parents to blame any questionable action of the child on heredity. This absolves the parents of responsibility for deficient parenting, but it labels the child alien. When a child's behavior is attributed to heredity that the parents do not share, the child is victimized. Many children living with their biological parents become scapegoats for various reasons, but an adopted child may be especially vulnerable because of unshared genetic inheritance.

Family theorists whose perspective is psychoanalytic explain how some parents unconsciously generate and perpetuate a child's negative behavior so as to express their own unconscious urges. The child who is an incorrigible truant, for example, may be reprimanded by father and wept over by mother, but may continue the behavior because one of the parents derives vicarious pleasure from the child's action. Giffin et al. (1968) explain the dynamics in the following words:

> The entranced facial expression apparent to the child describing a stealing episode, a sexual misdemeanor, or a hostile attitude toward a teacher conveys to the child that the parent is achieving some pleasurable gratification. No amount of subsequent punishment will act as a deterrent against the recurrence of the acting out. A child wishes to do the thing which he senses gives the parent pleasure, even though he may be punished. (p. 675)

It is important in working with families that have a child who is "different" to identify scapegoating and victimization. Family communication may signify to the selected child: (1) Don't do things you are forbidden to do and (2) If you persist in doing forbidden things, I will forgive and protect you.

Therapeutic Guidelines

Adopting parents are placed in a supplicant position in that they must meet certain standards before being permitted to adopt a child. This need to pass a test of sorts threatens the confidence of a couple who may already be dealing with their inability to have a natural child. Once a couple adopts a child, they must decide when and what to tell the child about its background. Another concern is that a friend or relative may disclose information to the child before the parents do so. There is no set rule regarding this; much depends on the child and the adoptive parents. Moore and Stern (1980) believe adoptive children should be told when they are about 6 years old. When the child is older at the time of adoption or is of a different race or ethnic background, disclosures may have to be made shortly after adoption.

When very young children learn they have been adopted, they may feel anxious. If they have lost one set of parents, they wonder if they might not lose another. Disclosures should be carefully timed and planned. The question adoptive parents must answer is whether the child is of a suitable age and temperament to grasp the information and deal with it. Some adoptive parents fear that the child will love them less because they are not the biological parents. If the parents are unsure of how to proceed, the issue is important enough to discuss with an expert so that the parent–child relationship is not jeopardized.

The genetic inheritance of an adopted child is often in doubt because records lack complete information. Agencies and workers may not conceal problems deliberately but may simply be unaware of genetic problems. There is no doubt that deficient information in this regard causes disquiet in adoptive parents that biological parents do not experience.

When adopted children come from the same racial and ethnic group as the parents, it is easier for the community to accept the child as an integral family member. Even here, however, adoptive parents may have unanswered questions about the child's background and heredity. Their questions proliferate if the adopted child does not meet parental expectations through the years. At one time details about an adopted child were shrouded in secrecy, but this is less true today. Adoption agencies are more forthcoming about a child's preadoption history and his or her natural parents. Some states give adopted children access to their early records when they reach age 14 or more. It is now believed that adolescents who have been adopted are better able to resolve their identity crisis if they know about both sets of parents. One reason that experts advise telling children during their latency years is to avoid adding a complicated identity crisis to the turbulence of adolescence.

The growing numbers of biracial and transnational adoptions mean that health care professionals must be sensitive to potential problems. Usually the children in such adoptions are older, and their socialization has already begun. When they become part of a new family, they must quickly adjust to family patterns that may seem very strange to them. Participation in a support group where common problems are shared can be very helpful for couples contemplating the adoption of a child who is different from themselves. Research shows that contact with fellow ethnics is desirable for children adopted by nonethnic families. Children who are part of mixed-race families benefit from living in integrated neighborhoods, where they encounter families representing more than one race. Assimilation into mainstream society is a goal, but preserving ethnic and racial ties avoids disengagement from any single group, promotes self-esteem in the adopted child, and maintains a healthy balance between the familiar and the unfamiliar.

Families who adopt a child of any age and of any race or ethnic background embark on a serious mission. In effect, a stranger enters their family, and this requires adaptation from everyone concerned. Child and family need a variety of support services, as well as understanding from relatives and neighbors. The gamut of services includes counseling, education, help with practical matters, and group meetings where common experiences can be shared.

Clinical Vignette: Adoption Problems in a Racially Mixed Family

Fourteen-year-old Doreen was born to a white mother and a black father. Her natural parents were unable to care for her and she was made available for adoption when she was 3 years old. Prior to that time she had been placed in a series of foster homes; two of the foster families were black and one was Caucasian. At age 3 Doreen was adopted by a white professional couple. Throughout grade school her adjustment was good, but her behavior changed after entering ninth grade. She no longer wanted to wear the conservative clothes her mother considered appropriate, and she dressed and acted in ways that identified her with the black counterculture. Her parents realized that Doreen was caught up in an adolescent identity struggle that was racial as well as personal, and for a time they were permissive. When her angry rebellion disrupted the household, when she refused to go to school and began stealing from her parents, they brought her to a clinic for disturbed children and adolescents, despite her protestations.

Doreen's parents suspected that she was abusing drugs and alcohol. She had taunted them many times with the fact that she was sexually active and promiscuous. Besides Doreen and her parents, the family included a younger sister, who was Eurasian and had also been adopted. In family meetings Doreen said that she had always felt inferior to her sister, who, she insisted, was favored by the parents. It was clear from Doreen's statements that she felt herself to be an outcast. She resented her multiracial family and felt that her family system was "weird and freaky." Doreen's parents had never kept information about their origins secret from the girls. Her sister was the child of a Vietnamese mother and a white solder. Doreen was the child of a woman who had disappeared from sight and a father currently serving a prison sentence for drug abuse and armed robbery.

It was evident that Doreen had chosen or been chosen to enact the role of the family's bad girl. Unhappy at home and at school, she had joined the company of rebels and nonconformists who formed their own deviant group. Doreen identified with her biological father, who had broken society's rules, and was estranged from her adoptive parents, whom she regarded as totally conventional. In conflict about so much of her life, Doreen was trying to resolve her racial and personal conflict by sympathizing with her natural father. This also punished her parents and sister for their unspoken ambivalence about her racial mixture.

Family therapy continued for about a year, and Doreen remained in individual treatment for a year longer, with the option of returning whenever she felt the need. Family sessions dealt with the fact that the parents in this family were ambivalent in many respects and that this confused both girls. The parents were upwardly oriented and materialistic, but they also were nonconformists. Proof of this is the fact that they deliberately formed a multiracial family. Their decision, in effect, contributed to the alienation of both girls, who had not formed a strong sibling subsystem because they seemed to have little in common. Through therapy, Doreen learned that her adoptive parents were not so conventional after all, and that her rebellion owed something to them as well as to her outcast father.

Doreen verbalized her anger at adoptive parents who had not prepared her for life as a black person but had taught her to pretend to be white. Surprisingly, in this anger she was joined by her sister, who accused the parents of being hypocritical in matters of race. "They pretend that everyone is the same color, but they're not, and we're not. Mom and Dad need to help Doreen learn how to be black as well as white, and I need to learn to be yellow as well as white." This statement, which was both an accusation and a plea for help, became the thrust of the family sessions.

For all adopted children, the questions they ask as they get older are "Who am I?" and "Where do I fit in?" In order to cope with identify conflicts, they tend to adopt one of two behavioral extremes, alternating between dependency and counterdependency. They may handle anxiety by becoming fiercely independent, resenting parental controls to the point of verbally abusing their parents. This was the behavior pattern chosen by Doreen. On the other hand, they may exhibit inhibited behavior and avoid peer interaction or limit it to specific activities such as sports. According to Gibbs (1987), it is the purpose and flexibility of the behavior rather than its form that makes it adaptive or maladaptive.

Sibling Relationships

As Toman (1976) reminds us, there are advantages and disadvantages to whatever place one occupies in the family constellation. There is one demand that only children do not face, and that is the need to accept a younger brother or sister. Most children react with mixed emotions to the entry of a brother or sister into the family system. This is true even when parents go to great lengths to make the transition easy for the older child.

Because it is hard for anyone to adjust to many changes within a short period of time, the rate of change in the family should be leisurely and unhurried so that the older child has time to become accustomed to new arrangements. For this reason, many child experts advise telling children about an expected birth early in mother's pregnancy, before changes in her contour are apparent. Young children are proud and excited at the prospect of being big brothers or sisters, but they also worry about being replaced and look for reassurance. Some preschoolers are afraid of being "traded in" for the new baby, much as daddy trades in a used car for a new one (Kutner, 1989).

Even though parents carefully describe what new babies look like and how they act, children expect the new baby to be an instant playmate, preferably one of their own sex. Although many young children regress when a baby joins the family, some older children make a giant developmental leap, becoming more proficient at tasks like tying their shoes or putting toys away. There are a variety of things parents can do to increase a child's comfort in sharing home and parents with a new baby. During the pregnancy and after the birth, parents should continue customary rituals and routines. This is not a good time to stop telling bedtime stories or playing favorite games with children. Often it is meaningful to show older children family pictures and talk to them about what they were like as infants. This provides an opportunity to talk about what the new baby will be like. All children are somewhat interested in asking about when and where the baby will be born, but not all of them want to know the details. Here parents should take their cues from the child, answering questions but not offering more information than the child requests.

Involving the child in preparing a place for the new baby and choosing items for the nursery or layette is helpful, but wise parents will remember to get the older child some inexpensive items for his or her own room. Bringing a gift home from the hospital for the older child is another excellent idea. Because preschoolers have no sense of time and are afraid that mother may never return, they enjoy having a calendar on which to cross off the days until she returns home. All too often, the flurry of gifts and preparations makes the older child feel forgotten. Older children need to feel included and to be reminded that the same hubbub and joy accompanied their own imminent birth as well.

Sibling Rivalry

It is hard for parents to endure quarreling among their children, and it helps to know that there are positive aspects to sibling quarrels. Conflict among siblings is unrelated to their actual affection for one another. It may be reassuring for parents to hear that some quarreling between siblings arises from the fact that they can bicker without being rejected by one another. Moreover, the reasons children fight are complicated. In some instances children fight in order to prove their independence and individuality. This is considered the reason that siblings of the same sex and near the same age fight so often. Another reason brothers and sisters quarrel is to discharge anger toward an adult that cannot be expressed directly (Kutner, 1989, 1990). Constant bickering among their children makes life difficult, but there are some measures that make the situation more bearable for parents.

- Try to anticipate and avoid situations that trigger sibling quarrels. Some children, for example, cannot work with a sibling without arguing. Many times the same child can work well alone or with an adult. The solution is to designate tasks and activities so that siblings need not work in tandem unless they choose to do so.
- Avoid trying to determine which child is to blame for a quarrel. Unless a parent was present, it is impossible to decide how a dispute began or who is at fault. If blame is assigned to one child, the dispute is aggravated, not settled. The wisest course is to separate quarreling children without disciplining one more than the other. Scolding or punishing only one of the combatants escalates their disagreement.
- Help quarreling children find alternative ways to settle their dispute. This might include sharing, taking turns, or bending the rules of a game. Alternative behaviors they discover on their own then become part of their problem-solving repertoire. Here parental involvement should be limited to guidance, not to punishing or arbitrating.

ELDERLY DEPENDENTS

Many couples in later life find themselves facing the problem of what to do about an elderly relative, usually a parent, who can no longer live independently. For most American families, nursing home placement of the relative is a last resort. As the physical and mental health of the elderly relative deteriorates, there follows a period in which the relative lives a semi-independent existence. Often they can manage on their own if family members perform supplementary services or if they have recourse to community agencies. When the time comes that an elderly relative can no longer live alone, the decision of a majority of families is to bring the relative into the family home. This commitment is indefinite in duration; many families of progressively impaired relatives accept responsibility for long periods of time, up to a decade or more. Figure 6.1 shows the rising percentages of people in the United States aged 75 years or older.

Family home care is "the provision of personal, non-professional services and support by one or more members of a family to someone who is

FIGURE 6.1. Population
Percentages of Men and Women
in the United States Aged 75
Years or More

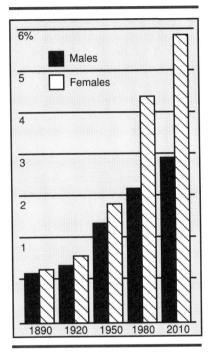

6%

■ Males

☐ Females

5

4

3

2

1

1890 1920 1950 1980 2010

Source: U.S. Census Bureau.

dependent as a result of physical, mental, or emotional impairment or disability" (Perleman, 1983, p. 2). This definition excludes parent–child interactions when neither is impaired, and implies a shared household. Most families go to great lengths to avoid institutionalization of elderly relatives. Despite rising numbers of elderly persons, there has been no proportional increase in the nursing home population. In the 1960s, before Medicaid was instituted, about 4 percent of the elderly lived in nursing homes; by 1980 the proportion had increased to 5 percent (Shanas, 1981). Usually it is the worsening of mental rather than physical functioning that compels families to seek institutional care. In comparing nursing home residents with their counterparts living independently or with their families, Hagestad, Smyer, and Stierman (1984) found little difference in the physical health of the two populations, although the nursing home residents had more mental impairment. The most notable difference between the two groups was the unwillingness or inability of families to give the extensive help that community or family-based living arrangements required.

Family home care is extraordinarily difficult, especially for the primary caregiver. Usually this is a woman, most often a daughter or daughter-in-law. If the caregiver is in early middle age, she may still be raising her own children and may have an outside job as well. Therefore, these women must struggle to enact filial, marital, and parental responsibilities simultaneously. Fatigue and discouragement are all too common among these caregivers, who see no end in sight and must deal with conflicting feelings of anger and guilt for being angry. If the caregiver is beyond middle age, she may have health problems of her own and lack time to take proper care of herself. A critical issue for caregivers is the indefiniteness of the situation and the knowledge that it can only get worse. A mother of small children knows that they will enter school before long; parents of adolescents, remembering their own youth, know that sooner or later teenagers become sensible adults. But the individuals taking care of an elderly relative cannot foresee their release. They have not experienced old age first hand, and they find the terrain frightening because it is unknown but waits around the corner for everyone.

There are, of course, enormous differences in the health of senior citizens. Among the 65-to-74 age group, 98 percent live independently or with family members. In the 75-to-84 age group, 94 percent live independently or with family members. In the over-85 age group, 77 percent live independently or with family members. This means that only about one in five persons even in the oldest group has been placed in a nursing home. This is a testimony to the obligations being assumed by family members (Eckholm, 1990).

Black, Hispanic, and other minority families do not place elderly relatives in nursing homes in proportion to their numbers in the general population. Asians are another ethnic group with a tradition of offering family home care to their elderly or disabled relatives. Old age stereotypes hinder the development of programs needed by families who are providing home care. Fiscal stringency is another factor restricting program development. Yet families need help immediately in the form of respite care, nursing services, homemaking assistance, and guidance through the maze of policies and legislation that has been implemented. Even the most devoted family reaches a point of exhaustion in trying to care for frail elderly members. The family may be divided over what should be done; relationships deteriorate, and everyone feels fragmented and trapped. It is at this stage that family caretakers tend to seek assistance from health care professionals.

When the family has provided care for weeks, months, or years, they feel miserable about considering a nursing home placement. They believe their efforts have failed, and the placement decision underlines their failure. Kermis (1986) writes that in nursing home placements a health care professional has two clients, the elderly person who is being institutionalized and the family that is making the decision. Kermis also claims that a psychological as well as a financial means test has been imposed on many caretaking families. Just as the elderly person must use up all financial resources to be eligible for Medicaid, so families must deplete themselves physically and psychologically, until nursing home placement is the only answer. Ideally, support services should have been available all along so that families do not reach this desperate point. At present, the home services available to caretaking families are a Procrustean bed. The services are not made to fit the families; instead, families must adapt to fit the services.

Home care services should be individualized and flexible, changing as family needs change. Coordination is essential to ensure that the elderly person and the caretaking family receive what is needed at the precise time it is required. Kermis (1986) divides home care services into three categories: *core services*, those most frequently needed; *specialized services*, those sometimes needed; and *general services*, those widely used that require modification in order to fill the needs of caretaking families and the elderly person. Table 6.1 shows the three categories of home care services; Table 6.2 shows funding sources.

Therapeutic Guidelines

Bringing an elderly person into one's home represents a major transition for all concerned. Life transitions occur whenever present circumstances are disrupted in ways that demand massive reorganization of one's life (Selder, 1989). In addition to help with practical matters, caretaking families require empathic understanding from every health care provider who becomes involved. Uncertainty is part of the human condition, and the care of an elderly relative is fraught with uncertainty. Caretakers need to know as much as possible about the condition of the elderly person, including what to expect now and in the future. Uncertainty is increased if one cannot share

TABLE 6.1. Categories of Home Care Services

Core Services	Specialized Services	General Services
Medical	Dental	Pastoral
Nursing	Audiological	Legal and protective
Social	Ophthalmic	Conservatorship
Homemaker	Speech therapy	Financial
Health aide	Psychotherapy	Shopping
Nutritional	Podiatric	Transportation
Pharmaceutical	Inhalation therapy	Personal contact
Medical equipment/supplies	Occupational therapy	Respite care
Physiotherapy	Rehabilitative therapy	

Source: Adapted from Kermis (1986).

TABLE 6.2. Sources of Home Care Reimbursement

Medicare
Medicaid
Social Security Act (Title XX)
Older Americans Act
State Community Services for the Elderly (varies from state to state)
Developmentally Disabled Assistance Bill of Rights (P.L. 94-103)
Health Revenue Sharing and Nurse Training Act (P.L. 94-63)
Blue Cross and other private insurers
State departments of mental health (varies from state to state)
Veterans Administration

Source: Adapted from Kermis (1986).

the caretaking experience with others who will understand. A number of support groups are available to families caring for relatives with Alzheimer's disease, cancer, or strokes, among other disabling illnesses. These groups provide a forum for sharing information and emotions. Not being able to talk about the caretaking experience makes families feel isolated and unappreciated.

When a family accepts responsibility for the home care of an elderly person, they change the existing order of their lives in drastic ways. In order to adapt, families must first acknowledge that the relationship with the elderly person that formerly existed must be relinquished. Reminding caretakers of this may be a way of reducing bitterness and resentment at having to care for a parent toward whom one has ambivalent feelings at best. An effective therapeutic strategy is to help caretakers acknowledge the new reality in which they live, to recall the past if they choose, but to focus on meeting demands of the present. In addition, family members need encouragement to take time for themselves, especially in maintaining important roles beyond caretaking; primary caretakers may lose touch with friends unless they are encouraged to preserve relationships. All too often the primary caretakers seem to embrace martyrdom by refusing to delegate tasks or ask other family members for help. Taking care of oneself and pursuing outside interests can be presented as a service performed on behalf of the elderly relative. By attending to some of their own needs, families are able to give a better quality of care and for longer periods of time. Thus, coping with this stressful transition is improved by continuing to live as normal a life as possible and engaging in accustomed activities. One middle-aged daughter of an elderly mother said that she felt isolated in a world inhabited only by herself and her mother. At the same time, her husband and children were complaining that the woman was oblivious to any needs except those of her mother. When this happens, the primary caretaker has built her own prison and has shut herself off from sources of support. The primary caretaker is inclined to live mostly in the past or the present. But reliving the past may be unproductive if it invites comparison with present difficulties. The present circumstances are not easy, and caretakers often say they just take one day at a time. Although this may help the caretaker to avoid dwelling on the most onerous aspects of care, it also robs the caretaker of a future. This inability or unwillingness to contemplate the future creates a climate of hopelessness and grim endurance. Respite intervals should be planned so that the primary caretaker has something to look forward to besides endless responsibility.

In summary, health care professionals need to provide practical suggestions and cognitive information to caretaking families. Additionally, they must offer empathy, opportunities for verbalization of the family's feelings about their situation, encouragement to continue customary role enactment, and permission to find enjoyment. Far too many families caring for elderly people at home sacrifice their own comfort and morale. With the number of very old people growing year by year, more and more families face the reality of taking care of an elderly relative. Figure 6.2 projects the extent of the issue over the next few decades.

Family caregiving is usually delegated to a female household member. Brody (1985) suggests that women may have an internalized model of care giving based on mother–child interaction. With this in mind, it is easier to understand the role strain experienced by women who find themselves caring for a relative who once performed mothering functions for the caregiver. Many of the caretaking women report changes in their feelings toward the elderly relative (Pett et al., 1988). When the personality of the relative deteriorates because of physical or mental decline, the relationship patterns that once existed may change beyond recognition. Constant interaction with an elderly, deteriorated relative makes caregivers afraid of their own

FIGURE 6.2. Projected Care Need of Persons over 65 Years

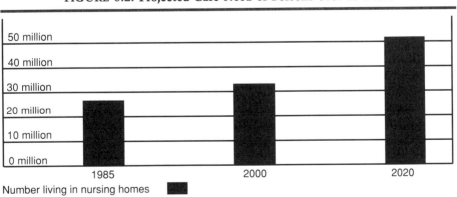

Source: Adapted from Eckholm (1990).

aging and of the possibility of inheriting the disability suffered by the relative. A few caregivers respond to these fears by guarding their own health and trying to enjoy life; more of them respond by devoting most of their energy to being caregivers. For some, there seems to be a need to compensate for their feelings of aggression by enacting the role of filial devotion to the hilt (Pett et al., 1988).

The consequences of caring for an elderly relative denote a great need for psychological support. Short-term counseling, crisis intervention, and psychotherapy are indicated for overstressed caretakers and their families. Cognitive therapy that includes realistic expectations and family or group therapy based on a transgenerational approach can be very useful. Family intervention should also include teaching less involved family members to be more supportive of the primary caregiver. Several researchers indicate that support groups alone are insufficient for resolving disparate family conflicts and expectations (Glosser & Wexler, 1985).

STEPPARENTS

According to the latest available census reports, there were almost five million children in the United States living in stepfamilies. This estimate is probably too low because it does not take into account those children living in households where a biological parent is living with but is not married to a new partner. Nor does it include children who have stepsiblings or half-siblings living in other households. Their numbers will increase in the next decade, and society will have to modify its proceedings to suit the special requirements of these families.

Every stepfamily is made up of members who have suffered loss of one kind or another, through death or divorce. Each member may be at a different stage of becoming reconciled to the loss. This means that when a parent marries again, reactions can be intense. Stepfamilies not only begin in an atmosphere different from that surrounding first marriages; they also evolve differently. Every partner brings to marriage an unwritten contract of their expectations; in remarriage the contract may be extensive, containing ideas of child rearing, money management, and task sharing (Visher & Visher, 1989). Only recently have stepfamilies been given attention by researchers and other professionals. Preparatory classes are available for pregnant couples, for adopting parents, and for single parents, but programs for stepfamilies are rare, even though the difficulties faced by these families can be severe.

Joint custody is more common than it once was, but mother more often than father is the custodial parent. Because she has been a single parent before remarrying, the mother usually is in charge of the children at first. She tends to continue the practices she has always used. In the new family she acts as the interpreter and mediator; she explains the stepfather to the children and the children to the stepfather. This gives the mother considerable power but also impedes family integration. Because he is not the biological parent, the stepfather initially asks mother how she wants him to act toward the children. In response, mother may suggest that they make no immediate changes and gradually get used to one another. If the stepfather is willing to move carefully and makes friends with the children, family integration is facilitated. In some cases, however, the stepfather, who, after all, is a new husband, may forcefully assert himself in a manner that makes rivals rather than friends of the children.

Occasionally, the stepfather behaves harshly toward the children, especially if they do not make him feel welcome. Unless this behavior is interrupted, the mother will be torn between the children and her new husband. In this sequence of events the family becomes disorganized. Everybody makes rules but no one adheres to them. Family members reach high levels of conflict, communicating by shouting or by not talking at all. The stepfather and mother are locked in symmetrical relationships in which both vie for control.

Mothers who are accustomed to father being the household disciplinarian may appear to yield control, but this is not a genuine gesture if the mother enforces only those rules that she agrees with and sabotages the rest. For example, the couple may agree on the amounts of the children's allowances or on the chores they will do, whereupon mother will add to the allowances or excuse the children from certain chores without the knowledge of the stepfather. Other mothers who find it hard to handle their children may allow the stepfather to be totally in charge. This may also have adverse effects on stepfather–stepchildren relationships and may make children idealize their formerly intact nuclear family (Moore & Stern, 1980).

Because stepfamilies establish intimate family relationships that are not biological and have not evolved over the years, sexual boundaries may become blurred. This weakening of sexual boundaries may be exacerbated by the climate in the home during the remarried couple's early romantic interactions. Weakened sexual boundaries may lead to sexual fantasies or to the expression of anxiety through quarreling or distancing maneuvers, all of which may be used as defense against sexual arousal. Pubescent teenagers may be attracted to stepsisters or brothers, or a stepparent may be drawn to a child. Accurate data on sexual abuse in families is not readily available, but there is general belief that stepfamilies are less likely to permit or collude in the perpetuation of incest behavior than nuclear families. Sexually abused children seem less guilty or ambivalent when the abuser is not the natural parent but a stepparent. In stepfamilies the child is inclined to blame the mother for bringing the abuser into the family and to want to escape from both mother and stepfather (Sager et al., 1983).

The disintegration of the intact nuclear family distresses the children who are involved, and who rarely have a voice in parental decisions to separate, divorce, or remarry. The adults in the picture may suffer to varying degrees, but they have control of their future in ways that children do not. Parents can do a number of things to help children accept the prospect of parental remarriage. Visher and Visher (1979, 1988) advise parents to be solicitous but to pay more attention to building a strong marriage than to considering children's feelings. They note that many re-married couples hesitate to establish a strong alliance with the new spouse out of concern for the children. Yet a strong alliance gives children two parents on whom they can rely. Experts advise the biological parent to enact the primary parenting role with support from the stepparent (Kutner, 1988). More behavior problems seem to occur when the stepparent immediately takes over major parenting functions and the biological parent abdicates.

The younger the children, the more readily they accept the stepparent. Even among younger children there are differences; elementary school boys seem to have more difficulty adjusting to divorce, whereas girls have more problems with remarriage. Younger children are inclined to express their anger, but their older siblings may withhold emotional involvement with the new family. Under the anger there is sadness about the remarriage. Children of divorced parents cherish the hope that their parents will re-unite, and remarriage destroys that hope (Fassler, 1988). After a parent has remarried, children consider it important to see their biological parents together occasionally. It is reassuring for children of divorce to see their biological parents in the same place without fighting (Krementz, 1988). This persuades children that they can depend on both biological parents in times of emergency.

The child of biological parents who have divorced and married new partners lives in a state of flux. Even after remarriage the biological parents must communicate from time to time about their children. Custody may be awarded to one or both of the natural parents. Even when one parent has sole custody, visitation rights mean that children must adapt to two differ-ent households, which may have very different standards and customs. Differences become more troublesome when one parent derides the other parent and the other household. Children seem able to fit in if the biolog-ical parents refrain from criticizing each other and allow the child and the other parent to define the terms of their relationship, at least in the early months of remarriage.

The remarriage of a parent is undoubtedly hard on the children. The father's relationship with his new wife reveals aspects of his personality with which children may be unfamiliar. This means that the remarried parent may seem different. The same is true of the mother whose remar-riage causes her to emerge as a sexual being. At the time of divorce, a son's identification with his mother may be reactivated. This is strengthened when mother looks to a son for support. As a result of her remarriage, it is harder for a boy to suppress knowledge of the mother's sexuality. Clinical evidence shows that it is the relationship between stepmother and stepdaughter that is more difficult. Bohannon (1984) explains that, during the oedipal romance, daughters give up father so as to identify with mother. Divorce tells the girl that her father is discarding or being discarded by the mother with whom she identified. When father remarries, the girl is left with a sense of being mistaken about her parents and of confusion about the whole identification experience. Thus, it is not surprising that many stepdaughters greet a father's remarriage with doubt verging on suspicion.

Couples contemplating remarriage are already aware that marriage and parenting are exceedingly complex. If one or both have been divorced, they have been introduced to failure and dread its recurrence (Goldberg, 1985). As a result many of these couples arrange for premarital counseling. The overall goal of counseling is to prepare the couple for remarriage and stepparenting, if there are children. Usually premarital counseling involves only the couple, but child-centered issues arise; the counseling sessions can prepare the couple for those issues most likely to come up. At this time it may be necessary to review custody and visitation arrangements and to discuss obligations to former mates and to custodial and noncustodial children. In stepparent families there may be several children at different developmental stages. Stepparents need information on what to expect from the children in terms of their age-related tasks. If stepparents realize that adolescents in all probability are struggling with separation and independence, they will be less disappointed when adolescents are reluctant to become close to parents or stepparents.

No new family springs effortlessly into existence, and this is especially true of remarried families, where every member has already experienced much turmoil. Among the common problems faced in remarried families are the following.

- The new husband or wife who marries a single parent may be less than eager to welcome stepchildren as part of the package.
- Former mates may accept the remarriage of a former spouse but dislike being replaced as their children's parent.
- Children are reluctant to give up fantasies that their natural parents will reconcile, and therefore see stepparents as obstacles.

Children of divorce feel that adults have let them down. Having lost one parent through divorce (or death), the children now fear that the remaining parent will abandon them after remarriage. The most adaptive behavior in stepparent families begins with the natural parent in charge of the children, provided the natural parent has functioned as the primary custodial caregiver. The stepparent initially accepts existing arrangements in the home and respects the prior authority of the natural parent. Without making immediate changes, the stepparent endeavors to make friends with the children. Ideally, changes are made through consensus, with all members participating. With minor adjustments, the same adaptive patterns can be used in remarried families where some children belong to the mother and some to the father.

Competition is prominent in many stepparent families. Stepsiblings are bound to have some problems in living together, and must allow time for relationships to develop. The stepparent family is more open than other systems, for it must allow access to biological parents who do not live in the stepparent household. The biological parent outside the home may distrust a stepparent's interest in or affection for the children and may need reassurance on this score. The biological parent is apt to be ambivalent about this issue, hoping that the stepparent is fond of the children but not wanting to lose a primary place in their affection. It is necessary for both biological parents and stepparents in the remarried family to remind everyone concerned that the new family will be the joint creation of parents and children, and that the process will take time. Individual and family issues in the stepparent family need to be negotiated, either in private or with the help of a professional counselor. Even if the parent and the prospective stepparent discuss child-rearing practices before remarriage, adjustment problems are likely to surface. Discrepant opinions of role enactment and acceptable behaviors must be worked out if the stepparent family is to remain functional. Difficulties are less likely to arise from resistance to being part of a new family if there are no unrealistic expectations that peaceful accommodation will occur without hard work.

Clinical Example: The Scapegoated Stepchild in a Remarried Family

Bruce and Amanda have been married for five years, and both have been married before. Living with the couple are Amanda's 8-year-old son, Billy; Bruce's 10-year-old daughter, June; and 5-year-old Annie, who was born of the current marriage. Bruce owns a hardware store with a dozen employees. He is a generous, paternalistic employer who says proudly that he is like a father to his staff. Amanda is a few years younger than Bruce. She is a quiet, rather self-effacing woman who is a full-time housekeeper and an active worker in her church. She is conscientious about everything she does and describes herself as a worrier and a perfectionist.

Bruce married Amanda when Billy was 3 years old and she had been divorced for six months. Her first husband had walked out when Billy was a baby, saying he was too young to settle down yet. At the time of her marriage to Bruce, Amanda was having trouble dealing with Billy. When Bruce saw the temper tantrums and the struggles between Billy and his mother, Bruce asked Amanda if she wanted him to help her control Billy. Amanda welcomed the offer; she realized that she had indulged Billy after his own father left, and she wanted peace restored. However, Amanda was unprepared for Bruce's idea of discipline. At first he spanked Billy, but when this had little impact he began beating Billy with a strap. Amanda protested, but Bruce told her she was too soft with the boy. His methods made sense to him because he had been beaten in the same way by his parents and his grandfather.

The punishments had an effect on Billy, who became quieter and less rebellious, obeying his stepfather's rules except when he "forgot." Both Amanda and Bruce say that he forgets the rules pretty often but is improving.

Billy has not seen his natural father in four years. He knows that his father is a musician who plays in a band and travels from town to town. Billy says that he could live with his father if he did not travel so much. He likes music, and his mother has told him he can join the school band as soon as he is old enough. When Billy was 6, his stepsister June joined the family when her mother (Bruce's first wife) remarried. June has not seen her mother since then because the distance is great and her mother cannot afford to visit. Bruce has not allowed June to visit her mother because he feels she belongs where she is. June is never beaten because Bruce does not believe in hitting girls, and anyhow, "June always knows when to quit."

Amanda enforces most of Bruce's rules but is more permissive. She allows June considerable latitude and is very indulgent of Annie "because she is still a baby." She wonders if Bruce isn't too strict with Billy, but she doesn't protest much because she feels that Bruce knows more about raising a boy. Testing at school had shown Billy to be exceptionally bright, but his school performance is poor. He has few friends and never brings playmates home from school. The two girls seem happy and well adjusted. Billy is apathetic except about music; he no longer has temper outbursts, but he seems listless and depressed. School personnel have suggested counseling for Billy or therapy for the family if Billy's academic and emotional status does not improve. Because the school personnel impressed Amanda with the gravity of the situation, she prevailed upon Bruce to attend counseling sessions with her and Billy. It bothered her that her son was being labeled a problem child, but she accepted Bruce's decision that the girls should not participate.

Assessment

In the family meetings the practitioner observed that Billy was an alert, handsome little boy who was reserved but eager to please. Although Bruce speaks directly and firmly to Billy, the boy avoids eye contact and answers in a muffled voice. If he is slow in answering Bruce or the practitioner, Amanda answers for him. Although the two girls were not present, the practitioner was able to see that one child-rearing method was being used for them and a much harsher one for Billy. Amanda stated that she was uncomfortable when corporal punishment was inflicted on Billy, but added that he had been a "handful" and that she didn't want him to grow up irresponsible like his father. She praised Bruce for being a good provider and for his steadiness.

The mother in this remarried family had given her husband total authority over her son. In the sessions she admitted that before marrying Bruce, she had found Billy uncontrollable. In fact, one of the reasons she married shortly after her divorce was to give Billy a father. Bruce had behaved in ways that allowed Amanda to become very close to the girls. The alliances within the household excluded Billy, who was the scapegoated child. Although Bruce was not introspective, he could acknowledge that Billy was the only child in the home who was not related to him by blood. Amanda wields little power in her own right, but she functions as an intermediary between Bruce and all the children. She protects Billy as much as possible, to the point of deceiving her husband. Once when Bruce insisted that she beat Billy, she faked a beating from behind a closed bedroom door. After Bruce has punished Billy, she provides candy and other treats to comfort him.

Planning

The signals from school personnel alarmed both parents. They persuaded Amanda to intervene more directly on behalf of her son. She knew that Billy was precocious in many ways, and she blamed herself for letting the home situation harm him. Bruce was not accustomed to being confronted by Amanda, and he found himself consenting when she said firmly that there would be no more beatings of anyone in the family. Although some progress was made at initial family meetings, the practitioner urged the parents to bring the two girls as well. Amanda promptly agreed, and Bruce went along with her. She seemed to know that her son had not been given equal treatment, and she was determined to change this.

Intervention

The family practitioner agreed to meet without the girls only to begin treatment. As soon as she realized that omitting the girls would again label Billy as the bad child, she insisted that everyone attend. In this she was joined by Amanda, who established a therapeutic alliance with the practitioner. Efforts were directed toward strengthening Amanda's parenting role. Currently Bruce was the primary parent for Billy, and Amanda was the primary parent for the girls. With encouragement from the practitioner, Amanda compared her tender parenting of Bruce's daughter with the stern measures used on Billy. She accepted much of the responsibility for putting Bruce in charge of Billy in the early years of the remarriage. What was needed were shared parental functions, not allocation of parenting along gender lines. June and Annie needed more involvement with their father.

Billy needed more involvement with his mother and a different kind of involvement with father.

Evaluation

The changes in the family made Billy feel less isolated. He drew closer to his sisters, remained wary of father, but felt more protected by mother. Amanda and Bruce were encouraged to substitute more rewards and fewer punishments to elicit positive behavior. Physical punishment of any sort was outlawed because, as Amanda said, there has been too much of that already. Amanda became more active in school events and welcomed any friends that Billy brought home. Bruce made arrangements for June to visit her mother over summer vacation. Amanda hesitated to let Billy visit his father because he was so transient. However, she wrote to her former husband and told him that Billy seemed to have inherited his father's musical talent. She invited Billy's father to visit when he was in the area and enclosed a letter from the boy. This started a friendship by mail in which Billy wrote about daily events and his dad sent souvenirs and postcards from interesting cities. The turn of events was not wholly welcome to Bruce, but he didn't resist too much. In family meetings he paid tribute to the kind of wife and mother Amanda was to all the children. Without saying it directly, Amanda had become a force to be reckoned with in the household; this benefited all the children and ultimately strengthened the remarried relationship.

SUMMARY

Families expand in several ways, and each expansion is a major transition for family members. Families expand through the birth of a child, the adoption of a child, and the formation of a remarried family. In later stages of family life, expansion occurs when an elderly relative, unable to live independently, joins the household. Occasionally an adult child who has left home returns to the family of origin for extended periods of time.

The birth of a first child and of any subsequent children changes marital partners into parents whose role enactment acquires new dimensions. Parenthood is stressful for both men and women, but the expectant or new father may be overlooked unless attention is paid to including him in plans and preparations. Today adoption often involves an older child who may be from a different ethnic or racial background than that of adoptive parents. Some experts find that children placed with families of different race or ethnicity benefit if they are given continued access to other families and individuals like themselves. Far from impeding integration, such access is thought to promote adjustment to new customs and expectations.

Sibling relationships are often the cause for parental concern. It is important to prepare children for the birth of a sibling and to involve them in preparing for the new baby so they do not feel excluded. Sibling rivalry at some point is almost inevitable, and is aggravated if parents get too involved in settling differences. Encouraging children to settle arguments on their own is better than having parents make judgments and issue ultimata. Because siblings can quarrel without risking permanent separation from one another, their disagreements and reconciliations can prepare them for handling problems with other children outside the home.

Elderly parents and grandparents who can no longer live on their own encroach on the lives of adult family members in many ways, ranging from health supervision to providing a home for the elderly relative. This is a burden that the vast majority of families accept. Their responsibilities in this area can be very heavy because supplementary home care services are inadequate. Nursing home placement is a difficult decision for families and a painful adjustment for the elderly person. If home care services were more extensive and more available, placement in nursing homes might be delayed for years.

Stepparent families are complex systems with considerable potential for problems. Counseling before the marriage takes place is advisable for couples with children who contemplate forming a stepparent family. Even if premarital counseling does not take place, the prospective couple should discuss household arrangements and interactions with the children's biological parent(s). Child-rearing views regarding discipline and stepsibling relationships benefit from discussion and negotiation. Every member of a stepparent family brings shared and unshared experiences that cannot be ignored. Anticipatory guidance in the form of extensive discussion and preparatory counseling is highly recommended to couples planning a remarriage that includes stepparenting.

REFERENCES

Belsky, J. (1984). "The Determinants of Parenting: A Process Model." *Child Development*, 51(1): 83–96.

Benson, S. (1981). *Ambiguous Ethnicity*. London: Cambridge University Press.

Berman, C. (1974). *We Take This Child: A Candid Look at Modern Adoption*. Garden City, NY: Doubleday.

Bohannon, P. (1984). "Stepparenthood: A New and Old Experience." In R. S. Cohen, B. J. Cohler, & S. H. Weissman (Eds.), *Parenthood: A Psychodynamic Perspective*. New York: Guilford Press.

Brody, E. (1985). "Parent Care as a Normative Family Stress." *The Gerontologist*, 25(1): 19–29.

Brunnquell, D., Crichton, L., & Egeland, E. (1981). "Maternal Personality and Attitude Disturbances of Child Rearing." *American Journal of Orthopsychiatry*, 51(4): 680–691.

Eckholm, E. (1990). "Haunting Issue for the U.S. — Caring for the Elderly Ill." *New York Times*, March 27, p. A-1.

Fassler, D. (1988). *Changing Families: A Guide for Kids and Grownups*. Burlington, VT: Waterfront Books.

Gibbs, J. V. (1987). "Identity and Marginality: Issues in the Treatment of Biracial Adolescents." *American Journal of Orthopsychiatry*, 57(2): 265–278.

Giffin, M. E., Johnson, A. M., & Litin, E. M. (1968). "The Transmission of Superego Defects in the Family." In N. W. Bell & E. F. Vogen (Eds.), *The Family*. New York: Free Press.

Glosser, G., & Wexler, D. (1985). "Participants' Evaluation of Educational Support Groups for Families of Patients with Alzheimer's Disease and Other Dementias." *The Gerontologist*, 25(2): 232–236.

Goldberg, M. (1985). "Repetition vs. New Beginnings." In D. C. Goldberg (Ed.), *Contemporary Marriage: Special Issues in Couples Therapy*. Homewood, IL: Dorsey.

Hagestad, G. O., Smyer, M. A., & Stierman, K. (1984). "The Impact of Divorce in Middle Age." In R. S. Cohen, B. J. Cohler, & S. H. Weissman (Eds.), *Parenthood: A Psychodynamic Perspective*. New York: Guilford Press.

Jordon, P. L. (1990). "Laboring for Relevance: Expectant New Fatherhood." *Nursing Research*, 39(1): 11–16.

Kermis, M. D. (1986). *Mental Health in Late Life: The Adaptive Process*. Boston/Monterey, CA: Jones and Bartlett.

Krementz, J. (1988). *How It Feels When Parents Divorce*. New York: Knopf.

Kutner, L. (1988). "For Children and Parents War Isn't Inevitable." *New York Times*, June 30, p. C-6.

Kutner, L. (1989). "Small Rituals May Ease Anxieties." *New York Times*, September 14, p. C-3.

Kutner, L. (1990). "Sibling Fights Can Help Children Later On." *New York Times*, February 1, p. C-8.

Moore, J. A., & Stern, P. N. (1980). "Entry of Children into the Family System." In J. R. Miller & E. H. Janosik (Eds.), *Family-Focused Care*. New York: McGraw-Hill.

Partridge, S. (1988). "The Parental Self-Concept: A Theoretical Exploration and Practical Application." *American Journal of Orthopsychiatry*, 58(2): 281–287.

Perleman, R. (1983). *Family Home Care: Critical Issues for Services and Policy*. New York: Haworth.

Pett, M. A., Casserta, M. S., Hutton, A. P., & Lund, D. A. (1988). "Intergenerational Conflict: Middle Aged Women Caring for Demented Older Relatives." *American Journal of Orthopsychiatry*, 58(3): 405–417.

Porte, Z., & Torney-Porte, J. (1987). "Depression and Academic Achievement among Indochinese Unaccompanied Minors in Ethnic and Nonethnic Placements." *American Journal of Orthopsychiatry*, 57(4): 536–547.

Rubenstein, C. (1989). "The Baby Bomb." *New York Times Good Health Magazine*, October 8, pp. 34–41.

Sadow, L. (1984). "The Psychological Origins of Parenthood." In R. S. Cohen, B. J. Cohler, & S. H. Weissman (Eds.), *Parenthood: A Psychodynamic Perspective*, New York: Guilford Press.

Sager, C. J., Brown, H. S., Crohn, H., Engel, T., Rodstein, E., & Walker, L. (1983). *Treating the Remarried Family*. New York: Brunner/Mazel.

Selder, F. (1989). "Life Transition Theory: The Resolution of Uncertainty." *Nursing and Health Care*, 10(8): 437–451.

Shanas, E. (1981). "The Elderly: Family, Bureaucracy, and Family Help Patterns." In A. J. Gilmore, A. Svanborg, M. Marois, W. Beattie, & J. Protrowski (Eds.), *Aging: A Challenge to Science and Society*. Oxford: Oxford University Press.

Stern, D. (1985). *The Interpersonal World of the Infant*. New York: Basic Books.

Toman, W. (1976). *Family Constellation: Its Effects on Personality and Social Behavior*. New York: Norton.

Tulman, L., Fawcett, J., Groblewski, L., & Silverman, L. (1990). "Changes in Functional Status after Childbirth." *Nursing Research*, 39(2): 70–81.

Turner, R. H. (1970). *Family Interaction*. New York: Wiley.

Visher, E., & Visher, L. J. (1988). *How to Win as a Stepfamily*. Baltimore, MD: Dember.

Visher, E., & Visher, L. J. (1989). *Stepfamilies: A Guide to Working with Stepparents and Stepchildren*. New York: Brunner/Mazel.

CHAPTER SEVEN

Contracting Families: Life Cycle Tasks and Responsibilities

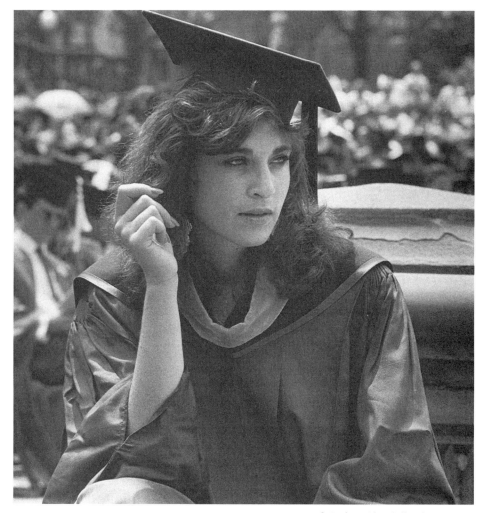

Loss may strengthen survivors, bringing out creativity, spurring them on to accomplishment, or it may leave behind a destructive legacy, all the more powerful if it is not dealt with.

Monica McGoldrick

This chapter deals first with the family whose membership decreases through the normal life cycle changes. It begins with a discussion of the launching of children through the various developmental stages: infancy, preadolescence, adolescence, and young adulthood. This section ends with a description of the symbolism of the wedding of the young adult and its relationship to separation and individuation. Emphasis is on the *mutuality* of the launching task; that is, both parents and children have certain tasks they must accomplish in the "letting go" process. Parents must give overt *and* covert permission to be separate, and children must take some risks in developing relationships outside the family. It is recognized that both parties will experience anxiety and ambivalence in these endeavors. The chapter stresses that an individual's achievement of a genuine personhood in his or her own right takes a lot of hard work and is not necessarily brought about when the young person goes off to first grade, leaves for college, takes a job, marries, or even moves five hundred miles away. The achievement of personal autonomy is a long-term process, which starts early in life. It may become stuck along the way despite a family's strengths. Parents may falter in their attempts to help their children move on in life because of their own unresolved separation issues with their families of origin. Parents and adult children may move apart and come back together again many times before the psychological emancipation is complete. The family bonds may remain strong and can continue to facilitate the separation process provided the *bonds* do not become *bondage*.

The second section of Chapter Seven deals with the failure of the marital subsystem. It begins with a description of some important myths about marriage and gives some reasons that marriages fail. Divorce and its painful aspects are discussed in some detail: the psychological trauma and the impact on children, friends, and extended family. Divorce mediation as a viable method of resolution is presented. The chapter explores single parenthood from both parents' points of view and also looks at the life of divorced mothers who do not have the custody of their children following divorce. The section ends with an outline of the family's issues/tasks following divorce: the need to stabilize a living situation for *all* parties, loyalty issues for the children, and the importance for the divorced parents of agreeing and being clear about their mutual responsibilities. The emotional tasks of mourning and healing are presented, and the section ends with a discussion of why some families do not heal after divorce, but remain "stuck" in their development.

The last part of this chapter is concerned with losses in the family through death: the death of a child, of a spouse, of parents in the formative years, and of aging parents. Once again, the family needs to experience the stages of mourning before it can readjust, regroup, and get on with the business of living. The meaning of the funeral ritual is discussed, as it also has symbolism that aids in the family's task of expressing grief and saying good-bye to the deceased person.

LAUNCHING: THE SEPARATION OF CHILDREN

The separation from family of origin is a process that involves a number of developmental stages over the years. Both child and parent must go through these stages in order for the child to achieve genuine personhood. If the parents had trouble separating from their own families of origin, they may bring their unresolved problems into the relationship with their children. Some families of origin help their children accomplish various developmental tasks, until the time comes for the child to make the major break and leave home for good, whether for college, a job, or marriage. At this time a family that previously functioned well may become dysfunctional as parents and the young adult reinforce in each other the fear of separation. The separation may occur, but it may be complicated by ambivalence and contradiction.

Infants Grow to Be Toddlers

Aside from birth itself, the most important step in the differentiation of infant from mother occurs when the infant becomes aware of being separate from the mother; this realization comes at approximately 4 to 6 months of age. At this point of differentiation, the concept of *boundary* becomes significant. Prior to that time, the mother and infant experience a mutual and necessary symbiosis. The infant eats, sleeps, eliminates, and is totally dependent on the mother. Many fathers today also play a major role in this early period with their nurturance and availability. One young father once said proudly, "I can do everything except nurse the baby!"

The establishment of the boundary mentioned earlier is extremely important. At some point the infant needs to learn to tolerate some frustration of his or her wishes. When? How much frustration? How long to let the baby cry before picking up the infant? Many volumes have been written on the subject. Young parents struggle with these questions from generation to generation. How the new parents will behave is multidetermined by a long list of variables: how they were treated as young children, their own level of self-confidence, their attitudes about being parents, and what they know about a child's developmental stages, to name a few. If consistent nurturance and caring are present for the infant, plus a mutually helpful marital bond, chances are that infant and parents will survive relatively unscarred. When children begin to walk (or, more accurately, when they start to crawl), the infant–parent world changes markedly. What parent has not experienced fear when the toddler takes his first steps *alone*, *down* a few stairs? Curiosity and a wish to explore and examine his or her world become an important part of the toddler's experience to which the parent must respond by giving permission and by aiding the explorations.

Preadolescence: School and a Widening Social World

Because so many mothers in families are employed today, many children are hustled off to day care by eight weeks of age, and even younger infants are cared for by persons other than the mother. According to U.S. Census Bureau figures for 1987, 56 percent of all women were employed in that year. Of women who were married, most worked. This is in strong contrast to 1940, when only 27.4 percent of women were employed, and even more so to 1890, when only 18.9 percent did. Children attend nursery school at varying ages prior to age 5, when they enter kindergarten. Thus, entrance into first grade may not be the first major step away from home and family.

The child brings part of the new world of school home to parents and, in so doing, shares experiences with the parents in order to obtain their recognition and approval. For their part, parents need to learn to share their authority with caretakers and teachers, who are important and essential to the child's development. Strong friendships can develop among schoolmates in the early grades. Sleepovers, the sharing of interests as well as of secrets, and strong alliances against *perceived* unfair authorities are part of the latency-aged child's world. Other children's parents and church and synagogue teachers also become important adults in the child's world. For the child not fortunate enough to have a biological family, there are others who have influence and who *can* enrich the child's experiences: welfare workers, foster care parents, adoption workers, and other personnel in health and social institutions, as well as adoptive parents and stepfamilies.

Adolescence: Biological and Emotional Upheaval

The appearance of puberty signals the end of childhood, but there is no clear dividing line between these developmental stages. The state of sexual maturation brings with it the development of primary and secondary sexual characteristics. It is well known that girls attain full growth earlier than boys. Although menses may begin, this does not mean that the young girl's uterus is ready to support a pregnancy. The bodily changes that take place in both girls and boys bring with them an awkward self-consciousness. Acne, with its ugly infections and scarring, as well as painful menses for some girls, are very likely to hamper the teenager's wish to grow up. Individuation at this point is often accompanied by feelings of ambivalence, fear, confusion, and loneliness (Blos, 1962). Extremes of emotion are experienced and expressed. Unresolved childhood problems often reappear and need to be dealt with and resolved if possible. Parents of adolescents are often either near or in their midlife period, where they must address their own pertinent life cycle issues and changes. It is also a time when extended family members (grandparents) are growing old, may be ill, and may die. So the business of separation or letting go may have considerable significance for the parents of the adolescent. Their task is to let go of the adolescent, encourage independence, and untie the parent–child bonds. But they have ambivalent feelings, too. And how can they respond to a teenager who one minute wants total freedom, and the next minute regresses to the dependent behavior of a 6-year-old? There is confusion on all sides. Adolescence is truly a drama of extremes in emotion and behavior, which tries the family's emotional maturity and flexibility. Nathan Ackerman (in Carter & McGoldrick, 1980) adds an optimistic note when he states that many adolescents have a resilience and a sense of humor that is readily available and can be extremely helpful with all the upheavals and unsteadiness they exhibit. To complicate matters further, today's world offers complex choices. Modern birth control methods offer the opportunity of sexual activity at an early age without fear of pregnancy. But there is still teenage pregnancy, and most adolescents have not achieved the emotional maturity to deal with sexuality in a responsible fashion. Also, the ever-present threat of AIDS adds to the anxiety about promiscuous sexual behavior. Also ever-present is the threat of alcohol and drugs, with peer pressure a strong influence on the impressionable teenager.

Young Adulthood: Job, College, Career

For young adults, a job can mean some independence and freedom from parental dependence and authority. Poor families may need the young adult's earnings to support family members. Freedom may not yet be in sight; parents, or a single parent, may decide how much money to extract and how it is to be spent. At first, the young adult may not earn enough to live separately, and an agreement needs to be reached about payment of room and board. In some cultures, parents who have immigrated to the United States prefer that working adult daughters live at home until they marry. Some families may own and operate a family business in which a number of adult children work. This may not mean a continued regressed dependence on family and parents. Whether or not the young adults are independently functioning persons with some autonomy in their own right depends on the nature of the relationship between the older family authority figures in the business and the offspring.

The young person's graduation from high school and entrance into college become important milestones in a family's life. An individual's educational achievement has particular social and emotional significance for the family. When a child's education exceeds that of the parents, parental pride may be insufficient to overcome the disparity of interests between parents and child. The child who is unwilling or unable to attain the parents' academic standards may also experience alienation from parents. Young adults' career choice may be heavily influenced by the overt *and* covert wishes of their parents. The selection of an occupation or profession may be fertile ground for rebellion against the parents; such a resistance may also be seen as a testing ground for parental recognition and approval. It takes maturity and a genuine letting go for parents to acknowledge *and* accept an adult child's choice of a very different field of interest in which to earn a livelihood. This is especially true when a career choice also means that the adult child may have a different style of living and a social group of persons with different cultural and educational backgrounds from that of the parents. Wise parents who genuinely care about their children and want to maintain contact with the adult child *can* achieve this, provided the basic family values are not *too* much threatened or thrown aside.

Marriage and the Wedding

The marriage of any of their offspring is a significant event in a family's life cycle. For both the couple and the families of origin, it is a transition that brings them into a new era of their history. For the couple, it is a transition from old loyalties to new bonds and allegiances. Their relationship now has legal sanction, which brings both rights and responsibilities. For the families of origin it can be a time of *both* loss and gain, although the loss is more keenly felt. The marriage of a young adult gives family relationships a different dimension. The siblings and extended family of both bride and groom now have in-laws. More open family systems welcome and incorporate in-laws into the bosom of the family, allowing family relationships to be broadened and enriched. More closed family systems view in-laws as outsiders, to be regarded with suspicion. Most families are somewhere between these two extremes. If they live at a great distance, many families of the bride and groom do not meet until the wedding, when family tensions are high.

The wedding ceremony, no matter how simple or how grand, has symbolized the joy and romance of the occasion, and problems often are denied or set aside (Carter & McGoldrick, 1980). The period of wedding preparation often reflects the family process. Planning involves numerous minute details: who makes arrangements, who gets invited, to stay where, who pays, what people wear, gift giving, photographs, flowers, where the ceremony will be, who performs it, what vows are to be spoken (some couples write their own), where the reception will be, who stands in the receiving line, in what order, what food is served, what the music for entertainment will be — this is just a modest list of the particulars. Heightened parental tensions are usually related to a sense of loss and anxiety about the change in the family. The family organization will be different, and parent–child roles will change. The power of human emotional passions heightened at this time should not be underestimated. Parental feelings about the marriage ceremony should be considered, whenever possible (McGoldrick, 1980). Marriage *is* a family affair, whether family members are present or not. Those persons who marry without family or friends present have their reasons. Most often the issues in such situations are family disapproval, premarital pregnancy, previous divorce, an impulsive decision to marry, or an inability or unwillingness of the parents to meet the cost of a wedding.

Today, in many religious wedding ceremonies, both parents escort the bride and both participate in "giving" her to the groom, a custom that some consider archaic, feeling that it is no longer useful to think that a woman is being "given" to a man. This is a change from earlier tradition, when it was the father who "gave the bride away" to the groom — a gesture in itself highly significant. The father relinquishes his daughter, now a sexually mature woman, to her chosen mate. What is most important is that parents of both must give their overt *and* covert emotional permission for the bride and groom to be married, to be intimate, and to begin to establish their own family. Despite the mixed feelings they experience before and during the wedding ceremony itself, families do have a resilience and do experience joy and comfort afterward. Such families enjoy a different closeness with the newly wedded couple and look forward to grandchildren, their connection with the future.

Therapeutic Guidelines

It is important to know the developmental stages of children's growth. What is normal or expected behavior for a 6-month-old, a 2-year-old, an 8-year-old? For example, why are the "terrible two's" so named, and why is it important for a preschooler to have some choice about the clothing he or she wears? Separation from parents and individuation are a gradual, step-by-step process that extends over many years. It is also important to understand the parents' resistance to letting children go. This is a very complex task for both children and parents and is not easy to accomplish. Parents may be conflicted and ambivalent, but they rarely entertain conscious desires to impede the growth of a child. One should remember that adolescents yearn for independence and autonomy at the same time they want to be cared for and dependent. Their confusion exacerbates the confusion of the parents. Adolescence is an emotionally painful growth period, and parenting can be painful, too. Change is also frightening for the participants. One should not expect the separation of adolescents from parents to be quick, painless, or clean-cut. Most adolescents need to rebel against the rules, regardless of what they are. Yet, teenagers would flounder even more if no rules or standards were available. It is important for health professionals not to overidentify with either the adolescent or the parent. One needs to establish rapport with both generations and help the parents to be in charge without being unfair or abusive. Parents sometimes need to be stricter and always need to be clear and explicit about rules. Parents need to be mutually supportive if they are to present a united front and prevent triangulation. If parents cannot agree, they may need some time and extra help to problem-solve their differences.

Family tensions usually surface at the time the young adult child marries. This is because the marriage represents a loss for the family and a change in the family's structure and function. Change is usually met with resistance and ambivalence. Strong families can weather such changes and get on with life's tasks, whereas dysfunctional families may need professional help before they can get back on the track.

THE FAILURE OF THE MARITAL SUBSYSTEM

Myths about Marriage

The myths are plentiful about what marriage *is* and what it is *not*. These myths serve to obscure the reality of the marriage relationship and prevent the marital partners from viewing each other in proper perspective as human beings with needs and strengths, as well as vulnerabilities. The perpetuation of myths about marriage blocks growth and change, and often breeds distance and resentment between the partners. Some myths are conscious and readily available for exploration, while others are unconscious and less available for definition and evaluation. All of us carry from our families of origin myths and values about marriage, as well as about male and female roles in marriage. Conflicts often stem from differing views and expectations about roles. These views are emotionally laden and often difficult to talk about in a logical and reasonable fashion.

What are some of the prevailing myths about marriage? Several warrant mention here. Some people believe that problems will be resolved automatically when love is present (Lederer & Jackson, 1968). This belief implies that no conscious effort or action is required to establish and maintain a stable, working marital relationship or to resolve differences. Some marital partners assert there is a way of behaving that guarantees satisfaction and bliss. Others have confidence that if only the right spouse is located, the mysteries of life and love will be solved (Jourard, 1975). Another false notion often expressed is that one partner will always know intuitively, without discussion, how the other feels and what reassurance or advice is needed in every situation. In other marriages, "negative" beliefs are held, such as the expectation that one partner will *not* be able to understand or meet the other's emotional needs. In this stance, it is believed that no one can be trusted to give without extracting a heavy price in return. Therefore, one should be as self-sufficient and independent as possible, asking little or nothing of the partner. Along with this conviction, which is usually learned in the family of origin, there is often a smoldering resentment in the spouse who expects nothing, asks nothing, and hopes for nothing. The partner who does not trust, who is unable to give emotionally, may despise and reject the spouse who makes demands. As might be expected, spouses who perpetuate this negative system have considerable difficulty creating a healthy give-and-take relationship.

Why Marriages Fail

Marriages fail for many reasons. According to Lederer and Jackson (1968), alienation between the married pair is usually precipitated not by deliberate malevolent behavior but by what the partners omit to say and do. In this paradigm, failure in marriage is attributed to two destructive omissions: (1) the failure of spouses to identify, determine, and mutually assign areas of competence and responsibility, and (2) the failure of spouses to evaluate their differences realistically.

Sooner or later, most couples become involved in power struggles over decision making, indicating that they have not established the allocation of tasks involved in living together. Incompatibility between partners is often a matter of unresolved differences. A marital relationship will generally become unsatisfactory when one partner cannot allow the other to think, act, or respond independently. The ability to be in touch with one's feelings, to express them, and to enjoy a degree of autonomy is necessary for the maintenance of individuality. Individual feelings and thoughts form the essence of what makes a person separate and distinct from others. An individual who is denied this right by a partner is predisposed to marital dissatisfaction. The behaviors of both partners require continuous accommodation, but feelings and thoughts are not synonymous with behavior.

There are other reasons that marriages fail. Couples may not know each other well when they are married. Those who marry very young and have not completely separated from their families of origin often enter the marriage relationship with romantic, unrealistic illusions about married life. These persons usually hope to achieve a sense of personal identity through marriage. Among the immature attitudes surrounding marriage is the need of spouses to project onto each other images from past relationships. These images may represent the kind of person one partner wishes the other to be, or the way in which one partner wants the other one to change. Some partners gradually relinquish these illusions and accept each other as persons in their own right. But when partners cannot give up their illusions, disappointment and anger will follow. The anger can grow to enormous proportions over the years. Fortresses are erected that isolate the partners; ammunition is stored for repeated battles. The marital relationship becomes a war game characterized by vindictiveness and suffering. Such a system may become entrenched and endure for years. Physical violence may erupt as a partner becomes a wife or husband abuser, and the marriage assumes the characteristics of a sado-masochistic relationship, in which vicarious and erotic pleasure is derived from inflicting and/or receiving pain. Some of these marriages last until a partner dies. Others end, usually when one partner no longer experiences pleasure of any kind and terminates the relationship. Marital partners mature and grow at different rates; one may change rapidly, while the other remains transfixed in an early developmental stage. In times of stress or crisis, one spouse may regress emotionally and, for complicated reasons, be unable or unwilling to grow or advance. The chasm between the partners then widens; they drift apart, realizing they no longer have much in common, and end the relationship.

Adultery is frequently the reason for the dissolution of a marriage. When one spouse finds out that the other is having an affair, the discovery may precipitate a crisis that can be used in marital counseling to look at what is wrong in the marital relationship. Occasionally, both partners can learn and grow from the experience. In some marriages, the extramarital affair takes place with the tacit approval the other partner, who may wish to withdraw from the sexual relationship. At other times, the discovery of an adulterous liaison is taken as the final act of treason that severs the relationship beyond repair.

Lederer and Jackson (1968) emphasize that the crumbling of a marriage relationship takes place so gradually over the years that most couples do not perceive what is happening until their problems have reached enormous proportions. It is important to analyze what takes place in the alienation of spouses from each other. Misunderstanding, misinterpretation of actions and motives, a gradual decrease in verbal communication between spouses, or an increase in the frequency of verbal battles all become causes for and effects of alienation. Feelings of hurt and resentment accumulate. Avoidance of any constructive verbal communication causes isolation and emotional distance in the marital dyad. Physical distance often follows also, with the husband staying away from home or the wife seeking relationships or attachments elsewhere.

Separation

The final separation of the couple may come only after prolonged periods of distress, many painful encounters, and mutual recrimination and vindictiveness. Often, episodes of separation are followed by attempts at reconciliation, which may be spasmodic and temporary. Not all separations are planned; some spouses desert impulsively and never return. Regardless of the forms that alienation assumes, each partner involved in a failed marriage suffers loneliness, humiliation, loss of self-confidence, guilt, and depression.

In some marriages alienation persists for years before the separation takes place. Why does it take some couples so long to separate permanently even after years of a stormy and painful relationship? And why do couples renew acrimonious communication even after the divorce? Weiss (1975) writes that these behaviors are due to the nature and persistence of attachment feelings. Once the marital attachment is formed, no matter how stormy or destructive the relationship becomes, some residue of the attachment survives, and it is extremely difficult to discount.

There are primitive aspects of attachment. One is reminded of the original attachment to the mother and the symbiotic tie of the infant and mother in the early months of life, which is necessary for the infant's survival. Some troubled couples stay stubbornly attached, regardless of the intense emotional pain they may suffer. One depressed woman said she remained for thirty years in a loveless marriage fraught with many battles because it was "better than being alone." For some, whose ego or feeling of self is so fragile and poorly formed, being alone means being adrift and unconnected—a state more frightening than being attached in an unhappy marriage. For others, the storm of battle gives them a reason to exist. These partners experience tremendous excitement and anticipation as their emotional energy is spent gathering ammunition for the next combat.

Divorce

In the early 1900s, divorce was unusual, infrequent, and shameful, a family disgrace to be hidden and not discussed. In 1984 it was estimated that almost half of marriages in the United States would end in divorce (Weingarten, 1986). Divorce is an open acknowledgment that a marriage has failed. It represents a change in the family system that is extremely difficult for every member. Parents and children alike may feel trapped, defeated, and frightened. Divorce introduces a profound disruption in the family life cycle. Families must undergo several additional stages of the family life cycle to reestablish balance and order in their lives (Walters et al., 1988).

Legal Aspects

Even under the best conditions, divorce generally involves an expensive legal process and a court procedure. Although the grounds for divorce vary from state to state, an agreement must be reached and a settlement made about property, alimony, child support, and custody. The community and the courts generally assume one partner to be the guilty party and the other the innocent one.

The process of divorce and the concept of custody are undergoing major changes in this country. No-fault divorce and custody of children shared jointly by both partners are common in numerous states. These are fair and admirable changes; nevertheless, making divorce and custody agreements remains a complex process, which requires careful attention. Fersch and Vering (1976) state that legal requirements regarding divorce, custody, and support are often in opposition to emotional realities. Most contested divorces are handled by lawyers in the traditional adversarial legal system. The issues of "justice" in divorce cases are so complex as to be almost indecipherable. The law requires that partners fit their difficulties into a limited structure. The law does not say, for example, that the partners should examine their relationship and give an honest statement to the court about its failure (Fersch & Vering, 1976). If the couple goes to court to secure the divorce, the process can become a prolonged battle royal. The mutual accusations and highly charged exchanges are of the most hostile and vindictive kind. The hurt and blame, as well as the emotional damage that follows such scenes, can last for many years. The resultant scars are slow to heal and, as one would expect, have a marked impact on the children and extended family as well.

Divorce Mediation

As one way of trying to eliminate such destructive forces in the divorce procedure and to avoid long court delays, a process known as divorce mediation has developed in the last decade. By definition, it is a process in which the divorce partners agree to meet with a third person, or persons, to resolve differences through mutual compromise and face-to-face discussions. It is not a clinical or diagnostic procedure, nor is it considered psychotherapy. In this process, it is not felt that a suppression of all affect is good. The expression of feelings on the part of both partners, though *not* a prolonged catharsis, is encouraged. It *is* the hope and goal of the divorce mediation that neither partner will be the loser, be blamed, or be exploited. There is no coercion on the part of the mediators, who try to show the partners that everyone in the family can profit from coming to a resolution of issues outside of court. Mediators are nonjudgmental and generally encourage arbitration in a constructive emotional atmosphere. Divorce mediation requires training and skill on the part of the mediators. In some states, such services are often now suggested by lawyers and courts.

Not all couples seeking divorce can agree to participate in such a process, and clearly, it is not to be viewed as capable of solving all the problems of divorcing couples. Although it has proved successful with a wide variety of persons, certain cautions are suggested. The problems to be settled vary considerably and depend on the following factors: the couple's resources, how long they have been married, what stage of the family life cycle they are in, and whether children are involved and at what ages. Also, such a process may not work; prolonged and intense emotional upheaval is seen as a serious threat to the rational process of negotiation (Weingarten, 1986).

Psychological Aspects

Needless to say, divorce has a major emotional impact on the couple and their children, as well as on extended family and friends. Families of origin and friends take sides, line up with first one and then the other, and are generally confused. Someone must be to blame! In their search for an explanation, people feel there has to be a victim and a culprit. People seldom know all the facts. Anyway, facts are obscured by the strong emotions expressed by the partners involved. Robert Weiss, who led support groups for the separated and divorced, speaks vividly of the persistence of attachment. Such a well-entrenched bond is not easily broken and is strongly resistant to dissolution. Even long after divorce, when couples who have been at a distance for years with little or no contact meet again or have communication, the old feelings of attachment are reawakened and remind the couple of their strength (Weiss, 1975). A woman in the process of a nasty divorce once said, "Even though this is god-awful to go through, if Richard would ever ask me to marry him again, I am sure I would say 'yes.' "

Health care professionals are increasingly aware that the major losses brought about by divorce must be addressed. People must *feel* the pain of these losses before they can be set aside, and mourning the losses is indeed a painful process. There are stages of denial, protestations of anger, and periods of depression and despair. The goal of the grieving process for all losses is to achieve a sense of acceptance or detachment. Only when this stage has been reached are people able to get on with life's tasks.

Impact on the Children

The breakup of a marriage and the loss of family as it was known takes a heavy toll on the children, particularly young children, regardless of how well separation is handled by the parents. Atkin and Rubin (1976) state that young children understand and interpret what happens with their parents in relation to themselves. Children can be full of self-blame when parents quarrel, and they often feel they are the cause of problematic situations. Parents, for their part, may be certain that they have hidden marital discord from the children, but family interviews almost inevitably reveal the opposite. Small children are not easily deceived. They quickly notice and are affected by tensions in the atmosphere at home. Nonverbal responses such as reddened eyes, hostile glances, angry silences, or false politeness between the parents are indications of friction that children do not fail to observe. Longfellow (1979) states that how a child deals with the experience of

separation and divorce is largely influenced by the child's level of development. Factors that play a major role are the child's personality traits, ability
to cope with stress, and areas of strength. Longfellow states that younger
children are more hurt by the negative aspects of the divorce because they
have less reasoning ability to help them understand and cope with the
experience.

Adolescents, by contrast, were found to have a better understanding of
their parents' incompatibility and to be worried about *their* future marriages
(Wallerstein & Kelly, 1974). Longfellow hypothesizes that the ability to
reason in adolescents made easier their adjustment following divorce,
whereas the inability to do so made more difficult the adjustment of preadolescent children. Although divorce is fairly common nowadays, for some
adolescents a parental divorce is a great source of embarrassment; some
even keep it a secret for years. There is no doubt that marital discord has a
negative effect on children and that separation and divorce may lessen this
stress. If the discord continues after the divorce, and particularly if the child
is used as a pawn by the fighting parents, the child is more likely to
experience adjustment problems.

Some adult children become devastated over the breakup of their parents' marriage, which may have lasted twenty or thirty years or longer. This
is particularly likely to be true if the children have idealized their parents'
relationship and if the parents have been successful in concealing the seriousness of their deep-seated troubles. The parents may have made a secret
pact to stay together "until the children are grown." A long-term affair of
one of the parents may blossom into a remarriage, leaving the adult children
angry, confused, and quite unable to integrate all of the "sudden" changes.

Sole Custody and Single Parenthood

For many years, traditionally, the custody of children, particularly young
children, has been awarded by the courts to the mother, unless it has been
demonstrated that she is unfit or incompetent. Today, with the father much
more actively involved in parenting from birth on, that is not so often the
case. "Equal rights for fathers" organizations have sprung up in many places,
and many more fathers today try to get sole custody of their children. If he
can prove in court that the mother is morally or mentally unfit, the father
will be awarded custody.

For either custodial parent, the burdens of single parenthood are great;
one parent cannot be two parents. Loneliness, hurt, and the struggle to put
one's life back together still must be faced, as well as the ever-present
financial problems. Many single-parent mothers are so overburdened that
their emotional availability to their children is highly limited for many
months past divorce. Visitation poses problems as well, particularly if the
separated or divorced parents have different sets of values and rules. In their
own upset emotional state, children do not know what to think or believe

and are at high risk of developing serious emotional and behavioral problems.

A divorced mother may need to supplement support payments (if she gets any), but may be inadequately prepared to enter the job market. She must either accept a reduced living standard or find a way to obtain a marketable skill. Should she take courses or find a job, she will incur the additional expense of child care. A divorced father who pays child support or alimony has less money for his own needs. He, too, may be forced to accept a less comfortable standard of living. Divorced homeowners may have to give up the family residence and move to less expensive quarters, which may be in different neighborhoods or communities. Renting in a lower-class neighborhood is very different from owning a home in middle-class suburbia. The deserted mother without access to support payments may have to apply for public assistance. Economic privation adds to the adjustment problems confronted by separated or divorced couples. Unless the father is around, or the parents have joint custody, the employed single mother is very overburdened. She has little or no time for herself and must be the sole decision maker, the sole disciplinarian—the sole "everything."

The single father is likewise overburdened. If he is employed, he is more likely to hire a housekeeper or ask a female relative to move in. The divorced father without custody must adjust to a totally different life. He is no longer head of the household and experiences feelings of anger and sadness about not being able to protect, comfort, or care for his children. He becomes an income source rather than a provider (Weiss, 1975). A reduced income due to alimony payments and child support often means a lower standard of living for him, also. He, too, must face the loneliness, despair, and all the leftover emotional fallout from the tumultuous period prior to the divorce. If he takes a live-in woman friend as a way of coping with the sadness of being alone before he has worked through the transition to being single again, he may only compound his personal and parenting problems.

What about mothers *without* custody? Much has been written about *fathers* without custody (Weiss, 1975; Atkins & Rubin, 1976; Rosenthal & Keshet, 1981). The U.S. Census Bureau tells us that the number of mothers without custody has almost tripled in the period from 1970 to 1983. Greif (1987) states this group is the least studied and understood, perhaps because they are hard to find or because of a judgmental attitude toward them. Because there is little research about mothers without custody, this article is reported here in some detail. The author did a comprehensive national review of 517 mothers without custody. The article contrasts the mothers who were satisfied with those who felt guilty and uncomfortable. The study looked at the noncustodial mothers who had not remarried and who, for the most part, were Caucasian and Protestant, with some college education and with an average age of 39. They had lived without their children for approximately four years. The children were living with their father rather than other persons or in institutions. The income of these mothers, including alimony, was above the national average for women who lived alone, as well as for mothers alone with children. Most, but not all, had given up custody without a court battle. Traditionally, mothers are supposed to raise their children; if they do not, people conclude they are unqualified or incompetent in some way. These women usually have limited financial means and are ostracized by disapproving family and friends. The findings in this research provide a deeper understanding of mothers without custody and also have implications for therapeutic work with them. What came from the study was a clear division of three groups of mothers: those who felt comfortable with their noncustodial role, those who were uncomfortable, and those who experienced mixed reactions.

In summary, those mothers who seemed content with their role were those women who shared some responsibility for the marital breakup, had a satisfactory relationship with their children, and had achieved some personal success in a job or career. These mothers also had good social supports. The noncustodial mothers who were more discontented suffered from poor self-esteem and strong feelings of failure. They had poor job and social skills. They blamed the father for the marital breakup and saw themselves as the victims. This was particularly true if these mothers had lost custody in a court battle. They had no other identity or role than that of "mother," whereas the more satisfied mothers had broadened their personhood to include other interests and skills. The implications for the therapeutic work with these unhappy mothers emphasizes helping them in several ways: to mourn and work through their loss, to learn job and social skills, and if possible to develop constructive communication and better relationships with their children (Greif, 1987).

Joint Custody, Coparenting

Joint custody, a new concept in divorce law in the last decade, will be examined here, as well as its connection with divorce mediation (discussed earlier in this chapter). Joint custody is a statute in divorce law in some thirty states (Elkin, 1987). Essentially, it means a shared willingness on the part of divorced parents to work together for the benefit of the child or children. Elkin describes the growth of this concept in a society that has failed to recognize the needs and rights of children in the cases of divorce. Fathers have been delegated to an inferior role, with little authority and responsibility except for support payments. Recent research emphasizes the importance of the father's role in the child's development, and fathers are showing us that they can be as nurturant as mothers. There has been increasing concern among persons in the legal profession and the behavioral science field that custody and visitation matters need to be studied and laws revised. With other two million parents divorcing each year and over one million children living in other relationship groups, it has been estimated that nuclear families make up only 10 percent of all families living in the United States (Elkin, 1987).

Elkin describes joint custody as involving an equalization of power, authority, and the responsibilities of parenting. There are several benefits for both children and parents: Children feel less abandoned and are reassured that both parents care for them and will continue to plan for their welfare. Parents have time for themselves and some relief from twenty-four-hour sole care and responsibility. Elkin makes clear several criteria each *for* joint custody and *against* joint custody. In order to be effective in the joint custody arrangement, parents must be able to separate husband/wife roles from parental roles, be committed to making the plan work, have good communication and be flexible in giving the children's needs some priority over their own, and be able to negotiate differences. He does not recommend joint custody arrangement for: parents who have a history of addiction; families where violence, neglect, or mental pathology has been present; or severely disorganized families. Obviously, it will not work for parents who cannot meet the foregoing criteria. And, Elkin concludes, it is not for all divorced families.

The Family's Tasks Following Divorce

Following the divorce, the family's structure changes markedly and so the roles of family members are altered also. In summary, the major tasks are as follows:

- Marital partners need to give up their commitment to each other. Growth and maturity can take place if each assumes some responsibility or "owns" his or her part in the failed marriage. The divorced person may choose a second partner who resembles the first spouse and repeat the mistakes of the first marriage. Or the divorced spouse can grow and change, learn about himself or herself in the process, and find a more satisfying and lasting second intimate relationship, or continue life without a partner.
- Divorced parents need to clarify their parenting roles with the children, as well as come to an agreement about their mutual responsibilities.
- A stable living situation for *all* family members needs to be established, to include a home base and economic security. This may mean a move to a different residence and community, as well as a change in schools for the children. Reliable income may come from alimony, child support, earnings from the employment of both parents, or public assistance.
- Last but not least, there is the timely task of emotional healing. Mourning takes place when the pain of the loss is experienced and shared among the family members. As in divorce mediation, constructive communication among family members can spell progress, while persistent feelings of anger, hurt, and blame can mean the process of reorganization and "regrouping" has become stuck. Psychological help from professional persons can often facilitate the healing process but does not necessarily speed it up. New support systems for *all* family members need to be

developed through extended family, friends, schools, and religious organizations. The services of appropriate social and health agencies can be sought when needed.

Loyalty Issues and Children's Tasks

Children are angry, hurt, confused, and ambivalent about parental divorce. Some children experience relief when the quarreling parents finally do separate. Despite all the intense emotional distress, children can retain loyal feelings for both the parents and the original nuclear family for many years. As has been mentioned, divorce brings a heavy emotional burden to the children and a challenge to the health care professional who works with divorced families. What are the emotional tasks of children whose parents divorce, and how long does it usually take to complete these tasks? Judith Wallerstein (1983) and colleagues in northern California conducted a ten-year follow-up study of 60 divorced families with children to learn about the long-term impact of divorce on the child. There were 131 children in the study, aged 3 years to 18 years, at the time of the final parental separation. Most, but not all, families were white and middle-class. By the ten-year mark, the researchers had had contact with 51 of the families and 98 children. The study presents a discussion of the six psychological tasks facing the child; this is in addition to the ordinary tasks of growing up. These tasks are the following (Wallerstein, 1983, pp. 233–242):

1. Acknowledging the reality of the marital rupture
2. Disengaging from parental conflict and distress and resuming customary pursuits
3. Resolution of the loss
4. Resolution of anger and self-blame
5. Accepting the permanence of the divorce
6. Achieving realistic hope regarding relationships

These are formidable tasks indeed. Each one may not be completely worked through, especially the third through the sixth, which the individual may be working on for years to come. Some brief details about the six tasks follow:

Task 1. Acknowledging the reality of the marital rupture: The child's age, developmental stage, needs, problems, and personality influence his or her comprehension of the parental divorce. The young child may experience frightening fantasies about being left and can be overwhelmed by intense emotions of sadness and rage. All of the children in the study had completed the first task by the end of the first year of the parents' separation.

Task 2. Disengaging from parental conflict and distress and resuming customary pursuits: The child's anxiety and sadness about the parental separation need to be put aside, but this is very difficult to accomplish because the home atmosphere may be highly chaotic, and the child may feel too unhappy and worried to invest much emotional energy outside the home. Schoolwork usually suffers, and commitments to extracurricular activities seem to wane. In families where the siblings could be supportive to each other, some pain was eased. By a year to eighteen months after the parental separation, most children in the study had reinvested in school and outside friendships.

Task 3. Resolution of the loss: The resolution of the loss is perhaps the most difficult of the tasks. The nucleus of this charge is that the child must recover from his or her deep feelings of rejection and fears about whether he or she is lovable. All children feel rejected when a parent leaves. Frequent communication with the departed parent and responsible, consistent contact between the child and the departed parent help to dispel the child's fears.

Task 4. Resolution of anger and self-blame: Resolving children's anger and self-blame following parental divorce takes years. The experience of intense anger generated by parental divorce often goes hand in hand with school truancy and failure and with delinquent acting-out behavior in adolescents. Relinquishing the anger can pave the way for forgiveness, and only then is the young person able to get rid of the feeling of helplessness and experience some sense of relief.

Task 5. Acceptance of the permanence of the divorce: The fantasy that divorced parents will remarry each other is prevalent among most children. This is especially true for children who were quite young when the parental divorce took place. Older children more easily give up this wish for reconciliation.

Task 6. Achieving realistic hope regarding relationships: This is the task that integrates all the coping abilities of the person who struggles with pain and fears about a parental divorce. Many young adults of divorced parents are afraid of intimate relationships and marriage for fear of failure. The core question of their ability to love and *be* loved and to trust another person must be resolved. These young adults must find ways to establish and maintain their feelings of self-worth; they must have successfully separated themselves from the parental conflicts and found their own independent direction. Wallerstein (1983) concludes: "It is likely that even when these tasks are successfully resolved, there will remain for the child of divorce some residue of sadness, of anger, and of anxiety about the potential unreliability of relationships which may reappear at critical times during the adult years" (p. 242).

Families Who Don't Heal and Remain "Stuck": The Persistence of Pain around Unresolved Issues

Weiss (1975) describes the stages a family goes through in the recovery process: the initial stage of shock and denial; second, a transition period in which the partners and children experience great emotional distress; and, finally, the recovering phase in which the family gradually begins to put the pain of the past in perspective and get on with the tasks of living. Economic and emotional stability is restored. Involvement in routines at school and work bring diversion, and new friends and attachments enter the picture.

Some families, however, do not heal, but remain "stuck" in the first or second phase indefinitely. Some partners spend years waiting for the departed spouse to return, unable or unwilling to accept the finality of the divorce. These separated and divorced marital partners cope poorly and do not resolve the loss by working through the normal mourning stages. They remain in a regressed emotional state, are embittered and vindictive, and let the whole world know how they have been wronged. They inflict their sorrows and grievances on anyone who will listen, and their lives are built around a career of being the poor wretched victim.

Many divorced spouses suffer in silence, but their behavior speaks of their unrelenting despair and anguish. Some become martyrs and find other people who reinforce this posture. Their lives thoroughly disrupted, plagued with financial worries, lonely and overburdened with the care of children, many single-parent mothers stay on welfare forever, never seeking the education or training needed to prepare them for the job marketplace. If alcohol or drugs were abused previously, the abusing partner may now become dependent.

Children who are subjected to such an environment naturally do not do well, either. They may blame themselves or be blamed by either parent for the family breakup. Children's behavior problems can escalate into trouble with the law, so that the family comes to the attention of school authorities and of other social, health, and legal agencies who try to help. The poor adjustment of these families is not surprising, because most of them were dysfunctional in many areas prior to the marital split.

Therapeutic Guidelines

It is important for the health care professional to allow for feelings of loss, grief, hostility, and disillusionment on the part of all family members when there is divorce and a breakup of the family. The emotional tasks are painful, overwhelming, and take a long time to be accomplished. Whenever possible, divorce mediation should be considered; see the discussion in this chapter to review the contraindications. Support, custody, and visitation issues should be worked out in the finest detail. If a court procedure takes place, it can have a lasting negative impact on all family participants, particularly on the children, should they be required to testify. Single parents (both mother and father) need a lot of support. The health care professional should not be a judge, encourage the blame game, or expect a single parent to be a miracle worker. It should be remembered that children may have very different reactions with regard to experiencing feelings of blame, loyalty, and anger. The health care professional should not expect everyone to feel alike, or to experience the process in the same way.

Prolonged behavior problems in children and the appearance of serious depressive symptoms in any family member may warrant a referral for psychiatric evaluation and treatment.

Clinical Example: Family Reaction to Desertion by a Parent

Bella Sills, her husband, and their four boys moved from the mountains of West Virginia to an industrial town. The move was prompted by the prospect of a job for her husband. Bella and the children had problems adjusting to the change. They missed their friends and relatives in the rural mountain surroundings they had left. The new neighborhood had a mixed population of black, white, and Hispanic families. Bella felt out of place, and her three school-aged sons had frequent fist fights with other children. Bella's husband found a job shortly after their arrival; then Bella discovered that her year-old baby had intestinal parasites. The cost of health center visits for him and the other boys taxed the family's meager resources.

A community nurse visited to help Mrs. Sills care for the baby and coordinate treatment for the other boys. The nurse observed that Mrs. Sills was increasingly short-tempered and distracted. With encouragement, the mother revealed that her husband had recently lost his new job, had been drinking heavily, and had deserted the family with no plans to return. The family was nearly out of food, the rent was overdue, and there was no money in the house. "And to make things worse, I got the kids under foot all the time. They have no shoes to wear to school. I say go play and they play for ten minutes. And Billy has started to wet the bed again."

Assessment

Mrs. Sills was angry and very frightened. She felt abandoned by her husband in a hostile environment, and she had some realization that her children felt the same way. The oldest child, 10-year-old Billy, had been his father's favorite, and he keenly felt the loss. His mother had told him, "You're the man of the family now," and this added to his worries. The onset of enuresis—the behavior of a much younger child—was his way of telling mother that he wasn't ready to be grown up. Before leaving, Mr. Sills had violent quarrels with his wife. In one argument he told her that she and the children "were dragging me down." The children, of course, overheard this.

Billy thought he had done something wrong to make his father leave. He accepted his father's statement as truth, interpreting it as a sign of his own worthlessness. Billy's 8-year-old brother heard the message that Billy was now the man of the house. He reacted by becoming Billy's shadow. He looked to Billy for direction and reassurance. This made Billy doubly anxious. He wanted to be just a brother, not a substitute for absent dad. The 5-year-old boy asked endless questions about his father's whereabouts and clung closely to mother. The youngest child continued his usual routine of looking for "Da" and calling his name in the evenings when his father was usually home from work.

Planning

The community nurse took the initiative to make appropriate referrals for the family. She knew that Mrs. Sills needed to express her feelings in ways that would not upset the children, and she arranged an appointment with a mental health practitioner. The children needed shoes and other clothing; Mrs. Sills needed guidance in filing an application for welfare benefits and food stamps. Mrs. Sills was uncertain whether to stay where she was or return to rural West Virginia where she had access to an extended family system.

Intervention

Mrs. Sills was reluctant to apply for welfare, but she had no alternative. In her old environs there was a tradition of mutual assistance that made official entitlements unnecessary. The mental health professional assigned to Mrs. Sills was a female social worker with whom she felt comfortable. Although she was psychologically unsophisticated, Mrs. Sills was able to make a connection between Billy's bed-wetting and her husband's desertion of the family. This made her even angrier at her husband, but she began to reassure her children. Realizing that they were afraid that she also would abandon them, she promised not to leave them. "I'm not leaving you — we're a team. And Daddy didn't leave because of you. He's mad because he lost his job and mad at himself for leaving West Virginia. He loves you even if he's not here. And he knew that we'd be able to take care of each other just fine."

Evaluation

The family struggled to readjust after Mr. Sills left. Her social worker urged Mrs. Sills to accept the role of the single parent she had become, and not to consider Billy a parent substitute in any way. This approach decreased the anxiety and insecurity felt by the three older boys. As Billy felt safer, his enuresis became very infrequent. His 8-year-old brother again treated Billy like a playmate and looked to his mother for leadership. The 5-year-old boy asked fewer questions about his father, but when he did ask, his mother answered honestly and at length.

The predicament of Mrs. Sills and the children was aggravated by uncertainty. The father had not died, and the parents were not divorced; yet the family had suffered a real loss. It was hard for them not to grieve, but also hard for them to grieve fully when Mr. Sills might return to them. Therapeutic intervention encouraged them to talk about their missing father but to strengthen the family as it now existed. The older boys and their mother participated in making a decision to stay in the new neighborhood rather than return home. Mrs. Sills was persuaded that there were advantages to staying where they were. She had negotiated the welfare system successfully, and the boys had become accustomed to their new school. At Mrs. Sill's invitation, her younger sister agreed to live with them for a time, and this pleased the boys as well as their mother.

LOSSES IN THE FAMILY THROUGH DEATH

In all cultures, death is a significant happening, like other important events in a family's history such as birth, puberty, and marriage (Fulton, 1965). "Death is an intensely poignant event, one which touches the deepest sources of human anguish, and one which each of us yearns to be spared" (Engel, 1964). A profound love that is lost is profoundly mourned; the pain of the loss is acute and can be debilitating. Acute and profound grief can play havoc with the mourner's reason and sense of reality.

A number of persons have written about the experience of death and dying and its implications for the dying person and the family. In 1917, Sigmund Freud presented the first original work about the psychology of the grieving process in his paper, "Mourning and Melancholia." Erich Lindemann (1944), a psychiatrist in Boston, discussed the management of acute grief. Currently, much attention is being paid to the subject of death and dying and to helping the dying person and the family. Dr. Elizabeth Kübler-Ross's book, *On Death and Dying*, published in 1969, an outstanding contribution to this field, originated out of an interdisciplinary seminar on death at the University of Chicago. She says the dying patient can teach us much about living and the meaning of life, and those who can learn from the dying person perhaps will have fewer anxieties about their own demise. There is increased interest in how people die and concern about whether to prolong life for the terminally ill when death is imminent. We have advanced medical technology for saving life, but we are less advanced in our knowledge about how to deal humanely with the dying process. Family therapist Murray Bowen (1976) says that thoughts of death, or of staying alive and avoiding death, are man's main preoccupation. Yet people shy away from talking about death. Many people die isolated and alone and cannot approach others about their dying. Bowen describes three processes in operation around the terminally ill patient: (1) the intrapsychic process within the person, in which there is always some denial of death; (2) the closed family relationship system; and (3) closed physician and medical staff communication system. Incurable disease is discussed with patients and families in greater depth now than in times past, but much remains to be accomplished in teaching professional staff to deal with the difficult process of death and dying.

Death of a Child

One reads frequently in newspapers about the death of a child through an automobile accident, a drowning, the mistaken ingestion of poison, or cruel abuse from parents. Or one learns of a child stricken with a hopeless disease, an infant who was stillborn, or a child who suffered an unexplained "crib death." Such events arouse horror and disbelief. How untimely, how tragic such a loss appears, and how unfair to those involved. One recognizes that old people die, but a child's death stirs the strongest indignation. For a family, a child represents the future. The death of a child from accident or illness cannot fail to cause a major emotional upheaval in the family. The extent of its impact depends on several factors: the child's age, the length of time the child has been part of the family's history, the child's role in the family and his or her relationship with the other family members, and the circumstances surrounding the death.

The loss of a child through death leaves an unfilled place in the structure of the family system, particularly when the child was an only child, or the oldest or youngest child. The death of an only child robs the marital couple of their parenting role, and they must revert to being a childless couple. The death of the oldest child has special significance for the parents since this was the firstborn, the child with whom parenthood was first experienced. A youngest child's death is significant also, since this child was the baby of the family, and often an especially favored child. Sibling positions shift with the death of a child. A usual consequence of the death is that the remaining offspring become more precious, but devalued compared to the virtues of the dead child. The effect of these shifts depends on the nature of the parental relationship, parent–child relationships, sibling relationships, and intrafamilial relationships within the entire system.

Following the death of a child, there is an adjustment of functions of the surviving family members. A major question for the family is the way in which the dead child's role and functions will be distributed. For example, in a poor family, should the next sibling in line be delegated to replace the oldest sibling in working to contribute toward the economic support of the family? If the youngest and favored child has died, who now will be the favored one? If the scapegoated child has died, who must fill the role of being exploited, filling the gap between distant or hostile parents, or acting as a repository for the family's hostile feelings?

Professional persons are often in a quandary about how to deal with fatally ill children and their families. Significant advances have been made in the diagnosis and medical care of the terminally ill child, but our affective support has not kept up with our technical skills. It is difficult to know what to tell a dying child and family and how to time certain disclosures. The inclusion of siblings in discussions poses problems for all health care practitioners. Friedman (1974) states that the young child does not search for a diagnosis but, rather, for assurance that he or she will not be abandoned. Older children can cope better with their disease if they know the diagnosis. Many older children seem aware of their diagnosis, even when they are not told. The inability of any dying person to discuss illness and pending death with parents, relatives, and friends may increase feelings of anxiety, confusion, and isolation. Children and adults who sense that they have an incurable disease may feel deceived by family members who deny or give false hope. Siblings cannot help noticing a discrepancy between an inadequate explanation given to them and the treatment the dying brother or sister receives in the form of extensive medical attention and special privileges. It follows, then, that the special status of the ill child may be resented by the confused siblings. This in turn will make the mourning process more complicated, since siblings will feel guilty about having resented the treatment accorded the dying child.

Research has indicated that parents of a dying child, instead of growing closer to each other in their suffering, experience an increase in their own difficulties (Yalom, 1989). The marital relationship of the parents is put to a serious test when a child faces terminal illness. Under such severe stress, the strongest of marital relationships will be shaken. Parents can become closer under this strain and help each other, but the effects of the tragedy will clearly depend on the strength of the marriage. If the marriage is already unstable, the death of the child probably will not pull the parents together in a lasting way. Even a strong marriage will be tested, but it is more likely to weather the turmoil and pain. It is fortunate if there are other children in the family to assure the couple of their continuing parental role. Couples who are capable of having more children may also be able to deal more easily with their despair. The loss of a child through death has a major social impact on a family system. Upon the death of an only child, the parents become a childless couple among friends with children. Envy is added to feelings of sadness and loss. Extended family members may also experience painful loss when a child dies. For example, a grandmother may have a deep sense of deprivation at the death of a grandchild who represented a link to the future.

Death of a Spouse

The death of a spouse brings a very different type of alteration to the family system. Whether death occurs after sudden or prolonged illness, or by accident, the loss of a spouse has tremendous impact on the surviving partner and all the other family members. Death involves leaving and being left. Who is to say which causes greater suffering? In the case of a terminal illness, the task of the dying person is clear, whereas the tasks of the survivors are less so.

After the death of a spouse, there are many psychological tasks to be performed by the rest of the family. The surviving parent may become overly preoccupied with his or her own distress and be unable to give much to the children, whose grief around the loss may be equally intense. Frequently, the persistent needs and demands of the children help the surviving parent to become less self-engrossed and to deal with pressing realities. People who suffer a loss eventually learn that the passage of time considerably diminishes the acute feelings of sorrow and loss.

The work of mourning the loss is the first order of psychological business for the family. It is a complex but necessary process. Immediately following the death of a spouse, there may be a period of disorganization in family life. This is to be expected, and most families eventually settle back into familiar routines of daily life in the weeks following the funeral. "Normal" stages of the mourning process, as discussed by Engel (1962), include: (1) the stage of shock and disbelief, in which the reality cannot be accepted; (2) the stage of developing an awareness of the loss, in which the bereaved person begins to face the emptiness, the painful void; and (3) the stage of restitution, in which the "work of mourning" takes place: mourning with family and friends, the funeral ceremony, and the preoccupation with the loss.

The circumstances surrounding the death have much to do with the nature of the grieving process. The process is also affected by the relationships within the family before the death, which have the power to mitigate or exacerbate feelings of loss. A conflictual and highly ambivalent relationship with the deceased family member can complicate and prolong the mourning process for an individual or for the whole family. Family members who never had the chance to resolve a hostile and guilt-ridden relationship when the relative was alive are likely to experience a painfully prolonged mourning process, which may last for years, unless the person seeks therapeutic intervention.

Both public and private mourning are necessary in the working-through process. Sharing the painful feelings of the grief and allowing friends to offer comfort relieves feelings of isolation. A person also needs to grieve privately; the pain of the loss needs to be experienced and felt. When feelings are denied or pushed aside, emotional complications may follow.

Death of Parents

Parents of a Family in the Formative Years

At times, mothers and fathers die at an untimely age, from either accident or illness. Loss of a parent also follows when a parent commits suicide, is institutionalized for a long period, or deserts the family. The prolonged absence of one parent changes the structure and function of the family system. The family's task then is to cope with the loss in a way that allows for growth, individuation, and the acceptance of eventual separation. One-parent families do survive whether or not the remaining parent chooses to bring another person into the family unit as the spouse and stepparent. The death of both parents of a young family is a major catastrophe for the children and the family system.

The grieving process varies for each individual in the family because the relationship of each with the deceased person was different. Children need to mourn and to see their parents mourn. When a parent does not let children witness weeping as a reaction to death, children may feel they are not permitted to show feelings and that crying is forbidden. In family system terms, the nature of the family's grieving indicates how well the family will heal when there has been a real working-through process. If pain and grief have been avoided, the grief will remain an unresolved problem.

In the family system, the original parental subsystem no longer exists when one parent dies. The remaining parent is left to raise the children alone. Roles need to be reorganized. Decisions have to be made about who will assume what responsibility for whom and when. In the case of the death of both parents, surrogate parents—either extended family members or foster parents via an outside agency—need to fulfill the parental role. Group homes and children's institutions, sponsored by church, or federal, state, and county funds, are available. Sometimes children who have lost both parents are legally adopted by relatives or foster parents.

A young, surviving parent may confront a changed social status even when economic conditions are unchanged. The new status is not always clear to the surviving spouse, who may continue to feel very much married. The widowed parent may try to find a niche in the former social group of couples and families. Single parents, whether widowed, separated, or divorced, have access to groups like Parents without Partners, which are formed to meet the social needs of single parents seeking relationships with persons like themselves.

Older Parents

People in their middle years (between 40 and 60 years of age) can expect their parents' retirement, advancing infirmity, and finally death, although these events do not always take place within a short period of time. Old age is sometimes viewed as a completion of the life cycle, which brings a sense of closure. Life review and reminiscences are often a part of the effort of the elderly to look back on their lives and accomplishments.

Parents grow old, and one of them eventually dies before the other. In some instances a widow or widower past 60 years of age remarries and lives out the remaining years happily with a second spouse. More often, however, the surviving aging parent continues to live alone or with an adult child's family. In our culture, emphasis is placed on independence from parents. Old people are not delegated to a position of honor as in more traditional societies. Most couples' houses are not big enough to accommodate the older person's need for privacy. Three generations living together can be complex, and adjustments are required from everyone when an older parent joins the household of a married son or daughter. The decision to provide a home and care for aging parents is a difficult and stressful one. Many factors — personal, social and economic — must be carefully weighed in making the decision.

Some widows may continue to live alone for years, taking care of their own physical and social needs and trying desperately to remain independent and not become "a burden" to their children. Widows who were extremely dependent on their husbands may become even more dependent and helpless when they have to face life alone. Some widowed men continue to live in an apartment or house; others, not possessing housekeeping skills, move in with children or other relatives, or into a residence for the elderly. In actuarial terms, far more women than men outlive their spouses. Women are often somewhat younger than their mates, and their life expectancy exceeds that of men.

The surviving older parent struggles with the loss of the spouse in addition to facing old age alone. If the relationship was of long duration, the loss is severe. Old persons have been known to say that part of them died with the spouse to whom they were devoted for 40 or 50 years. The social world of the old person gradually narrows as relatives and friends die or move away. Older persons tend to reduce their social activities and become less involved with people.

Subsidized housing for the elderly is a boon for those with limited incomes. The enormous cost of medical care and nursing homes for the elderly can cause catastrophic loss of life savings; for some, the only recourse is to apply for public assistance.

The death of a parent is a milestone in life for a person of any age. With it comes a real break with the past, and the original family system enters another phase of its life. As long as their parents survive, middle-aged adults are not conscious of representing the older generation. But with the death of elderly parents, middle-aged adults feel their own mortality drawing closer. Occasionally, they begin to see themselves as more vulnerable and their own children as ascendant.

The Funeral Ritual

There have been funeral rites in some form as long as there has been civilization. In primitive societies, the funeral ritual may have taken place in several stages. First, there was the disposal of the body by cremation or burial. Then, for varying lengths of time afterwards, there were other ceremonies and celebrations that took place to offer the mourners an opportunity to express their intense feelings and grief. In some societies, there was a fear of coming in contact with the body; in others, there was lavish preservation of bodies in tombs filled with treasures and quantities of food. Ambivalence, denial of death, and contradictions appear in many of these primitive death rituals (Mandelbaum, 1965).

Family therapist Murray Bowen says that today funeral customs serve to repudiate death and to preserve conflictual emotional relationships between the deceased and the living. He states that avoidance of death and the dying represents people's fears about their own demise, as well as the wish to avoid both their own intense emotion and that of others. Bowen says that the funeral rite was most effective in facilitating the grieving process when the person died at home with family and friends present, and when these family members and friends built the coffin, cleansed and dressed the body, and buried the dead themselves. In his opinion, children are not hurt by the revelation of death but are upset by the family's anxiety about it. The following example is a case in point. A 4-year-old boy overheard his family's discussion of plans for his grandmother's funeral. The conversation had been conducted in hushed tones in the next room, as it was felt he was "too young" to be included. He came running in and asked, "How can she be all right in the ground in a box?" This same boy, several years later, asked to be taken to see his grandmother's grave and at that time asked many questions about her illness—"What did she have on in the coffin?"—and about the funeral service. If the expression of his curiosity had been invited at the time of his grandmother's death, he would not have felt the need to hold in his feelings and, perhaps, nurse his fears. A 15-year-old boy asked to see his mother in the surgical intensive care unit where she was in a coma following brain surgery for a malignant tumor. She was not expected to live. The boy's request sobered his family when he stated, "I have to prepare myself."

The funeral service or ritual in any culture or religion serves the function of gathering family and those close to the deceased, so that they can say goodbye to the dead, pay homage, and comfort each other. The absence of any ceremony or recognition of such a need, in our view, represents a denial of death and a lost opportunity for the mourners to be comforted.

Clinical Vignette: Traumatic Death of a Child

The Davis family, consisting of husband, wife, and three children, lived in a trailer on the outskirts of town. One winter night an overworked heater caught fire. Awakened by fumes, Mr. Davis managed to lead his wife and two daughters to safety. When he returned for his son, both of them became trapped inside and died in the fire. At the time of the accident, Mrs. Davis seemed to be in shock. Even after a few days, she reacted stoically to her loss. The little girls cried and were comforted by their grandparents. But even during the funeral rites, Mrs. Davis remained dry-eyed and composed.

After the tragedy Mrs. Davis moved in with her parents but was uncommunicative even with them. She refused, however, to let her daughters out of her sight. They slept in the same bed with her and were no longer allowed to attend the nursery school they had enjoyed so much. Two months after her losses, Mrs. Davis showed no signs of working through her grief. She was gentle enough with the children but showed no joy or spontaneity. The children began to avoid her and spent as much time as possible with their grandparents. Mrs. Davis did not really interact with the children but seemed comfortable only when they were within sight.

Mrs. Davis's parents were sympathetic, but as time passed they became very concerned. With the encouragement of the family pastor, Mrs. Davis was finally prevailed upon to accept help. An appointment was made with a psychotherapist in the area. The thrust of therapeutic sessions was acknowledgment by Mrs. Davis of her enormous loss and expression of her grief. Like other survivors, Mrs. Davis felt guilty and deserving of punishment. Her lack of spontaneity and joy in her surviving children were part of her need to atone. Her therapist pointed out to her that neither she nor her daughters deserved to suffer further. However, her intense ties to the girls and the reduced social interaction she imposed on them and herself was counterproductive for everyone. Responding to suggestions that she consider the social and emotional needs of her girls, she made attempts to widen their social contacts. She agreed to let them return to nursery school and resume a more normal existence. It was evident that her losses continued to overwhelm Mrs. Davis and that it would take a long time for her to accept what had happened, but she was responsive to making efforts on behalf of her daughters. Her therapist believed that in responding to the normal developmental needs of her daughters, Mrs. Davis's own grief would lessen. The process for this overcontrolled, overwhelmed woman would probably be very long.

Therapeutic Guidelines

In assessing the impact of death for a family, it is important for the health care professional to become acquainted with a number of factors: the age of the deceased person, the nature and cause of death, the family's position in the life cycle, and the position in the family held by the deceased person. Equally important in this evaluation is knowledge of the deceased person's relationships in the family. The more complicated and difficult the relationships with the deceased person, the more problematic the mourning process can be. The pain and sadness of the loss can be avoided by the survivors in several ways. Anger can be projected onto others, particularly onto doctors and hospital personnel who did not "do enough" to save the life of the deceased person, or who should have tried this procedure or that medication. The family may not have adequately worked through deaths that occurred in the past; perhaps feelings of grief and mourning for others are already deeply repressed. The family members do not have the emotional stamina required to deal with another loss. Overwhelming bitterness, emotional apathy, or an inability to *feel* the pain of a loss may signify a pathological process, and a referral for psychiatric evaluation is needed.

The health professional should encourage the family to talk about the deceased person and their feelings of grief, but should remember that all family members may not be able to do so. Many family members express feelings of guilt—"I should have done this or told him that"—and these feelings are not unusual. Feelings about old, unresolved problems with the deceased person will surface at this time, also, and will need to be discussed. Understanding the processes of grief can help the health care professional to communicate with the family members and console them. It should be remembered that some people are ready to die and do not fear death; they fear only life, particularly when all life holds for them is the agony of pain, discomfort, and further isolation. Most families who become ready to let go of a terminally ill relative want that person to die in peace and with dignity. Other families who are not so ready to say goodbye need a lot of compassion and support.

SUMMARY

This chapter, "Contracting Families: Life Cycle Tasks and Responsibilities," has dealt with the loss of family members in three parts: (1) the launching, or the normal separation of children in the family life cycle; (2) losses through marital separation and divorce; and (3) losses in the family through death. The main theme throughout emphasizes the impact of losses in the family system on its structure and function, and on family tasks in coping with these losses. It also stresses that coping with loss is an individual matter, that family members experience loss differently and mourn differently, but are interdependent in that *how* they mourn loss and adjust in life afterwards is heavily influenced by *how* others in the family grieve and cope after the loss.

The section on launching considers separation and individuation as a step-by-step process, from infancy to adulthood. It discusses family tasks with infants, preadolescents, adolescents, and young adults. It comments on the symbolism of the wedding ceremony and its relationship to separation and individuation, with the explicit direction that the *parents* need to give *emotional permission* for the young adult to leave the family nest, marry, and have other love objects.

The section on separation and divorce speaks of the myths of marriage and why marriages fail. It discusses the aspects of divorce in some detail: the legal aspects and divorce mediation, the psychological aspects, the impact on children, and single parenthood. It deals with joint custody and the family's tasks following divorce.

The section on losses in the family through death mentions significant contributions of some writers on the subject of death, from Sigmund Freud to the current-day psychiatrist and family therapist Murray Bowen. The chapter addresses specifically the deaths of a child, a spouse, and parents (both younger and older parents), and the impact of these losses on the family as a whole. At the end of this section is an exploration of the meaning of the funeral rite for the family, as well as a commentary on its importance in the mourning and letting-go process.

REFERENCES

Ackerman, N. W. (1958). *The Psychodynamics of Family Life.* New York: Basic Books.

Atkin, E., & Rubin, E. (1976). *Part-Time Father.* New York: Vanguard Press.

Blos, P. (1962). *On Adolescence: A Psychoanalytic Interpretation.* New York: Free Press of Glencoe.

Bowen, M. (1976). "Family Reaction to Death." In P. J. Guerin, Jr. (Ed.), *Family Therapy.* New York: Gardner Press.

Carter, E. A., & McGoldrick, M. (1980). *The Family Life Cycle: A Framework for Family Therapy.* New York: Gardner Press.

Elkin, M. (1987). "Joint Custody: Affirming That Parents and Families Are Forever." *Social Work,* 32(1): 18–24.

Engel, G. L. (1962). "Psychological Responses to Major Environmental Stress. Grief and Mourning: Danger, Disaster, Deprivation." In G. L. Engel (Ed.), *Psychological Development in Health and Disease.* Philadelphia: W. B. Saunders.

Engel, G. L. (1964). "Grief and Grieving." *American Journal of Nursing,* 64(9): 93–98.

Fersch, E. A., Jr., & Vering, J. A., III. (1976). "Divorce: Legal Requirements vs. Psychological Realities." In H. Grunebaum & J. Christ (Eds.), *Contemporary Marriage: Structure, Dynamics and Therapy.* Boston: Little, Brown.

Freud, S. (1953/1917). "Mourning and Melancholia." In *Complete Works* (Vol. 14). London: Hogarth Press and Institute of Psychoanalysis.

Friedman, S. B. (1974). "The Fatally Ill Child." In S. B. Troup & W. A. Greene (Eds.), *The Patient, Death and the Family.* New York: Scribner.

Fulton, R. (Ed.), (1965). *Death and Identity.* New York: Wiley.

Greif, G. L. (1987). "Mothers without Custody." *Social Work,* 32(1): 11–16.

Jourard, S. M. (1975). "Marriage Is for Life." *Journal of Marriage and Family Counseling,* 1 (July): 199–208.

Kübler-Ross, E. (1969). *On Death and Dying.* New York: Macmillan.

Lederer, W. J., & Jackson, D. (1968). *The Mirages of Marriage.* New York: Norton.

Lindemann, E. (1944). "Symptomatology and Management of Acute Grief." *American Journal of Psychiatry,* 101: 141–148.

Longfellow, C. (1979). "Divorce in Context: Its Impact on Children." In G. Levinger & O. C. Moles (Eds.), *Divorce and Separation: Context, Causes, and Consequences* (Chapter 17, pp. 287–306). New York: Basic Books.

Mandelbaum, D. G. (1965). "Social Uses of Funeral Rites." In R. Fulton (Ed.), *Death and Identity* (pp. 338–360). New York: Wiley.

McGoldrick, M. (1980). "The Joining of Families through Marriage: The New Couple." In B. Carter & M. McGoldrick (Eds.), *The Changing Family Life Cycle: A Framework for Family Therapy,* 2nd ed. New York: Gardner Press.

Rosenthal, K. M., & Keshet, H. F. (1981). *Fathers without Partners.* Totowa, NJ: Rouman and Littlefield.

Wallerstein, J. S. (1983). "Children of Divorce: The Psychological Tasks of the Child." *American Journal of Orthopsychiatry,* 53(2): 230–243.

Wallerstein, J., & Kelly, J. (1974). "The Effects of Parental Divorce: The Adolescent Experience." In E. Anthony & C. Koupernik (Eds.), *The Child in His Family.* New York: Wiley.

Walters, M., Carter, B., Papp, P., & Silverstein, O. (1988). *The Invisible Web: Gender Patterns in Family Relationships*. New York: Guilford Press.

Weingarten, H. R. (1986). "Strategic Planning for Divorce Mediation." *Social Work*, 31(3): 194–200.

Weiss, R. S. (1975). *Marital Separation*. New York: Basic Books.

Yalom, I. D. (1989). *Love's Executioner and Other Tales of Psychotherapy*. New York: Basic Books.

PART
FOUR

FAMILY
PATTERNS

CHAPTER EIGHT

Heterosexual Families: Patterns and Variations

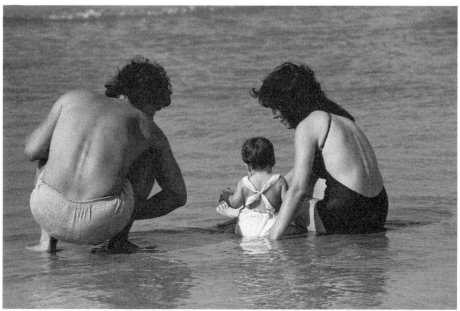

© Frank Siteman MCMLXXXV

Don't shut yourself up in a bandbox because you are a woman, but understand what is going on and educate yourself to take part in the world's work, for it all affects you and yours.

Louisa May Alcott

Every human relationship is basically heterogeneous because each person brings to the relationship a unique set of expectations, perceptions, behaviors and defenses. In heterosexual relationships, differences are compounded by social and biological forces that affect the growth and development of men and women. In virtually all families the socializing experiences of children are influenced by the gender of the child. Even in families dedicated to equal treatment of sons and daughters, subtle distinctions are made and are reinforced by society at large. This means that when a man and woman marry or establish any meaningful relationship, there are discrepancies in their expectations of each other based on their respective histories. To some extent this has always been so, but it is especially true today, when traditional role performance based on gender is no longer a guiding principle of family life (Dionne, 1989).

Until recently, marital roles and responsibilities were recognizable and well defined. Gender stereotyping assigned the male to the role of provider, with the woman functioning as nurturer and caregiver. Indeed, persons considering marriage often asked themselves, "Will he be a good provider?" or "Will she be a good homemaker and mother?" Beginning in the 1960s, sex role stereotypes weakened, partly as a result of the entry of many women into the work force, and partly because of the efforts of the women's movement. With the weakening of old rules, couples had to adapt as best they could to changes proposed by people who wanted marriages that were emotionally rewarding rather than task-efficient. In traditional marriages, role enactment was specific and the partners more or less conformed. In present-day marriages, however, ambiguity and confusion characterize the role enactment of heterogeneous couples.

The reshaping of marital roles causes problems for couples who are no longer guided by old signposts but must construct their own. With more emphasis on emotional gratification, ideas about what constitutes a successful marriage have changed. At one time the accumulation of property and the successful rearing of children were enough to sustain marriages that were emotionally sterile, but this is less so today. Undoubtedly a price was paid by countless husbands and wives in order to preserve traditional marriages. Many wives who seemed outwardly happy were inwardly frustrated by their daily routine of cooking and cleaning, but they believed they had no alternative. Husbands trapped in the role of primary provider felt compelled to stay in jobs that held no prospect of recognition or self-fulfillment. For the husband who left every day for work, home was a haven made possible through his own efforts. For the wife, home was not a haven but a workplace where her contributions were often taken for granted. Still, as long as they stayed together, both partners enjoyed social approval for a marriage that was an effective working relationship (Friedan, 1986).

Divorce is a significant and often traumatic event for the persons involved, but it is no longer accompanied by great social stigma. Nevertheless, successful heterosexual marriages continue to be crucial to the well-being of society. It is appropriate, then, for health care professionals to recognize hazards and safeguards that contribute to the success or failure of marriages. The intent of this chapter is to look at phases and patterns of heterosexual marriage, to connect these to various events in the marital life cycle, and to offer therapeutic guidelines for health care professionals working with heterosexual couples.

DEMOGRAPHIC DATA

For purposes of clarity, *marriage* is defined in this chapter as a legalized sexual union of a man and woman, accompanied by a public commitment of their willingness to assume certain rights and responsibilities over time. *Divorce* is defined as the legal termination of a marriage; *remarriage* is defined as the marriage of an individual who was previously married to someone else.

In years past marital status was viewed in absolute terms: One was either married or one was not. A person who was not married was likely to be single or widowed but rarely divorced. Today the designation of marital status is more complex. Couples may establish a cohabiting arrangement in which they live together without legal ties. Unwed, separated, or divorced persons, usually women, may be raising their children in single-parent households. Additionally, there are frequent changes in marital status as cohabiting couples marry or married persons divorce and remarry someone else.

High divorce rates in the United States are cited as indicators of the decline of marriage and family life, but this is misleading. It is true that divorce rates have risen, but at the same time death rates have declined. Marriages are ended through death as well as through divorce and separation. Thus, the overall rate of marital dissolution attributal to death and divorce has been stable for the last one hundred years. Perhaps the most profound change is popular acceptance of divorce as the solution to an unhappy marriage rather than a personal moral failure. Spanier and Furstenberg (1982) wrote that divorcing partners do not oppose the idea of marriage or family life per se but reject only their own unsuccessful marriage. They do not condemn the institutions of marriage and family, but only their own mate selection and disenchantment with a particular partner. There is a strong presumption that in spite of high divorce rates, more people in the United States are married than in any other industrial country. Americans on the whole are optimistic about marriage. When one marriage proves disappointing, they opt out in order to try again.

The idealized family pattern is the nuclear family in which father is the sole breadwinner and mother stays home to take care of the family. In actuality only 13 percent of families in the United States follow this pattern. Families in which both husband and wife work outside the home constitute 16 percent of all families, and this proportion is increasing. About 21 percent of all family households consist of widowed, separated, or never-married persons. No children are present in about 23 percent of the nation's families, either because the partners are childless or because the children have been launched. Single-parent households, usually headed by a mother, account for 16 percent. It is axiomatic that learning the composition of a particular family is an essential task for caregivers, since problematic issues frequently relate to who lives or does not live in the household (Bjornsten & Stewart, 1985).

Most persons in the United States marry before reaching age 30, but recent demographic trends show a delay in marrying, so that most marriages now take place between 25 and 44 years of age. Educational and career choices for women have probably contributed to later marriages, as has later childbearing. Over the last forty years about 25 percent of all women were married before reaching 20 years of age. Teenage marriages are less frequent among men because men tend to choose wives younger than themselves. Women today are inclined to bear far fewer children than in the past. In 1900 the average woman in the United States bore six; today she is likely to have one or two. In general, white families are smaller than those of other races. Families where parents have more education have fewer children than less educated couples; women employed outside the home have fewer children than full-time homemakers do. Table 8.1 shows lifetime births expected by wives between 18 and 34 years of age. Percentage distribution is given by race, age, education, and labor force status.

The childbearing and child rearing responsibilities of nineteenth-century women spanned two or more decades. Today, women often defer childbearing until they feel ready or until they have established themselves professionally. When they do choose to have one or two children, these activities are compressed within a few years rather than a few decades. This development, combined with the greater longevity of women today, means that most couples will spend some twenty years together without children in the home. Characteristics that made the partners effective in the earlier stages of married life may prove inadequate at this later time. If the marriage is to remain functional, the couple must move from child-oriented activ-

TABLE 8.1. Lifetime Births Expected by Wives, 18 to 34 Years Old (Percentage Distribution)

| Number of Births | Race | | | Age | | | Education | | | Labor Force Status | |
	White	Black	Spanish Origin[a]	18–24	25–29	30–34	Not High School Graduate	High School Graduate	College: One Year or More	In Labor Force	Not in Labor Force
None	5.8	4.2	3.5	5.2	5.3	6.4	3.6	5.2	7.3	8.2	2.5
One	12.3	14.0	8.5	11.8	12.9	12.6	11.3	12.3	13.3	15.3	8.9
Two	51.5	40.7	40.5	54.9	51.9	46.2	40.0	51.3	54.9	52.2	48.9
Three	21.4	23.3	28.1	20.9	21.3	22.4	26.1	22.8	17.8	17.7	26.5
Four or more	8.9	17.9	19.5	7.1	8.6	12.4	19.1	8.5	6.7	6.7	13.3

Source: U.S. Bureau of the Census, Current Population Reports, Series P-20, No. 358, 1980.
[a]Persons of Spanish origin may be of any race.

FIGURE 8.1. **Percentage of Married Men and Women by Age Groups**

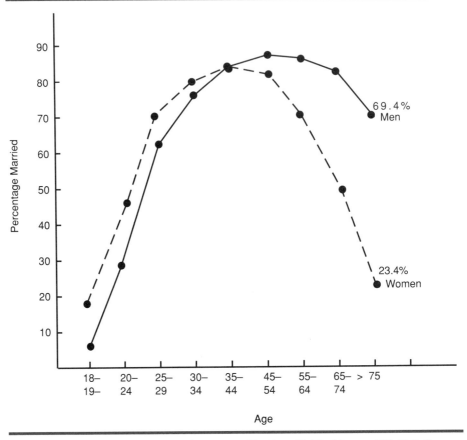

Source: Reprinted from U.S. Statistical Report, Table 49, p. 38 (Washington, DC: U.S. Government Printing Office, 1980).

ities to couple-oriented activities. New ways of interacting must be adopted that enable husband and wife to renew mutual interests and attend to each other's emotional needs.

Differences in the longevity of men and of women have led to far greater numbers of widows than widowers. After age 44 correspondingly fewer women than men are married because so many of the husbands have died. As of 1982, 80 percent of men past 65 years were married, but only 40 percent of the women. Even sadder, 83.7 percent of older men lived in families, but only 56.8 percent of older women did. One reason for this is that widowers are more likely to remarry than widows, perhaps because they have more choices (Segraves, 1985). Percentages of married men and women by age groups appear in Figure 8.1. Percentages of widowed men and women by age groups appear in Figure 8.2.

FIGURE 8.2. Percentage of Widowed Men and Women by Age Groups

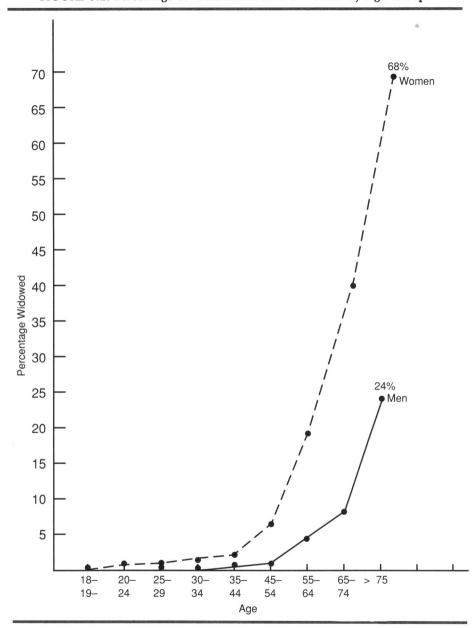

Source: Reprinted from U.S. Statistical Report, Table 49, p. 38 (Washington, DC: U.S. Government Printing Office, 1980).

DIFFERENT VISIONS, DIFFERENT VOICES

Every marriage is actually two marriages, the marriage as seen through the eyes of the husband and the marriage as seen through the eyes of the wife. Not only are perceptions of the marriage different for each partner, but, as Gilligan (1982a) remarked, they respond differently, speaking in a "different voice." Men and women may inhabit the same world, but their vision of the world is influenced by gender. The social conditioning of boys differs from that of their sisters. This is true even in these transitional times, when equal treatment of the sexes is demanded by feminists and enforced by law.

The work of two major theorists, Lawrence Kohlberg (1968) and Carol Gilligan (1982a), sheds light on the psychological development of boys and girls. Kohlberg is a social scientist who formulated a theory of moral development based on a longitudinal study of males aged 10 to 28 years. He found that as boys mature, they learn to make moral choices based on abstract ideas of right and wrong. In making their choices, boys are guided by rules concerning justice and lawfulness. The sequence of moral development is fixed, progressive, and hierarchical, moving from lowest to highest levels. Not everyone reaches the highest level of moral development, but those who do base decisions on an impersonal system of ethics. Kohlberg's method consisted of presenting a hypothetical moral dilemma to subjects and asking them to choose a course of action and justify their choice.

The moral development schema of Kohlberg was widely accepted, but it raised some troublesome questions. When female subjects were presented with a moral dilemma, they did not use principles of justice and law to determine if a course of action was right or wrong. Instead, the girls moved the moral dilemma to a personal realm. They speculated as to who might be helped or hurt by a certain action and made choices on a level that, for Kohlberg, represented a lower stage of moral development (Gilligan, et al. 1989).

Gilligan, a former student of Kohlberg, does not reject his theory but reinterprets it. First, she asks whether the last stage of moral development he presents is necessarily highest or best. In other words, choices based only on law and justice may or may not represent the highest form of morality. Gilligan's work makes it possible to contend that the interpersonal concern girls show in relationships is not inferior but merely different. One might go further and add that the concern girls have for caring may complement and even challenge the masculine preoccupation with rights and justice. The word *caring* has special connotations for Gilligan. She adds to the stereotype of the caring, nurturing female the ability to be responsible for oneself as well as others (Prose, 1990).

One moral dilemma devised by Kohlberg and presented to subjects is a situation in which a man with a sick wife cannot afford to buy a life-saving drug. The question Kohlberg asked is whether the man should steal the drug after the druggist refuses to lower the price. Gilligan presented this situation to two 11-year-old children, Amy and Jake. She found that the boy answered the question that was asked: "Should the man steal the drug?" Amy answered a different question, which was not asked. She was less interested in *whether* the man should steal the drug than in *how* he should *behave* in this predicament. As Gilligan noted,

> these children see two very different moral problems—Jake a conflict between life and property that can be resolved by logical deduction, Amy a fracture of a human relationship that must be mended with its own thread. Asking different questions that arise from different conceptions of the moral domain, they arrive at answers that fundamentally diverge, and the arrangement of these answers as successive stages on a scale of increasing moral authority calibrated by the logic of the boy's response misses the different truth revealed in the judgment of the girl. To the question "What does he see that she does not," Kohlberg's theory provides a ready response; to the question, "What does she see that he does not?" Kohlberg's theory has nothing to say. (Gilligan, 1982b, p. 206)

Until Gilligan's work appeared, it was assumed that self-direction and autonomy were the ultimate in personality development, and that maturation emphasized separation and individuation. Gilligan (1982a, 1982b) states that for girls maturation depends less on separation from mother and more on the continuity of attachment. In psychoanalytic language, boys must renounce connections to mother in order to identify with father. This is less necessary for girls, because identifying with mother permits ongoing attachment between mother and daughter. Gilligan identifies two distinct moral languages that are gender-related. There is the language of logic that preserves individuation and the language of caring that preserves interpersonal attachment. As women advance educationally and professionally, they tend to follow male modes of moral development. Although women seldom lose all interest in interpersonal relationships, their care and concern for others is diluted by growing regard for impersonal, abstract justice (Prose, 1990).

Applying theories of moral development to heterosexual couples helps explain discontents arising between partners. A common complaint of wives is that husbands are uncomfortable with emotional intimacy and are reluctant to talk about aspects of the marital relationship. Wives accuse their husbands of simply not talking to them. This comes as a surprise to husbands, who believe they do talk with their wives. What few couples realize is that talking means one thing to the wife and another to the husband. The wife is comfortable talking about feelings, but this is a topic the husband approaches reluctantly. The wife wants to hear that she is loved and appreciated. The husband believes his love is expressed by what he does, not by what he says. For him, sharing activities with his wife or helping around the house are meaningful expressions of affection. Although she may appreciate such actions, the wife seeks verbal assurances of his devotion. Many wives feel neglected because the tender communication of the courtship gives way to mundane conversations about trivial matters. Foreplay for women includes nonsexual attention, and many women object to men who maintain emotional distance but then expect their partner to respond to sexual overtures. Each blames the other for deficiencies, but neither is at fault. Both partners have an authentic vision of the marriage as they experience it, and each speaks to the other in an authentic voice. When problems develop because the partners have different perceptions of what is happening, one recourse is to help each partner understand the other's perceptions and listen to the other's voice (Goleman, 1986).

When couples reach an impasse regarding their different interactional styles, a common reaction is for the husband to deny the existence of the problem and for the wife to be preoccupied with it. A therapeutic response by a health care professional is to state that a problem for one partner inevitably becomes a problem for both. Admitting a problem exists is a first step toward dealing with it. For example, a husband may insist that his wife overreacts in certain situations, although she denies this. Without making a judgment, the health care professional can explain that if the wife's behavior troubles the husband, then it should be discussed. Similarly, a wife may complain that her husband withdraws rather than talk about disputed issues. The validity of the complaint need not be questioned, but the cause and effect of the husband's withdrawal need to be explored. The fact that the wife voiced the complaint requires that the problem be acknowledged. Reminding the partners that men and women often disagree about how to think and act is reassuring for the partners and an effective step in negotiating compromise.

Verbalization of feelings in a marriage is important to women, perhaps because socialization of girls encourages talking rather than doing. If the husband believes that cleaning the kitchen or putting the children to bed indicates devotion, it may be necessary to comment on the indirect nature of his messages while recognizing his intent. When studying male and female differences, Gilligan et al. (1989) noted that for boys the greatest threat is loss of autonomy, whereas for girls it is the loss of a relationship. It follows from this that independence is highly regarded by men, whereas closeness is highly regarded by women. It is possible to encourage the wife to interpret the husband's positive actions as signs of his love and simultaneously encourage the husband to be more direct. Asking the husband to describe things he does around the house that are expressions of love enables the wife to make connections between what the husband is doing and what he is feeling. A truly gratifying marriage is one in which the husband learns to fear closeness less and the wife learns to fear separateness less. Describing their behavioral differences and the reactions of each partner to these differences is helpful. An emotionally expressive wife and a laconic husband deserve equal consideration from each other. The goal of counseling is for the couple to accept some differences in their interactional styles, to tolerate some differences, and to compromise on those that are extreme.

The "battle of the sexes" is a phrase coined long ago. Even couples in happy marriages face discrepancies in their expectations of each other. During courtship men are more apt to verbalize feelings, but after marriage they are more reticent. Courtship for some men is a chase or conquest with the woman as the prize. Once the prize is won, men turn to other pursuits, investing themselves in work, hobbies, or friendships with buddies. The change in behavior leaves wives dissatisfied and husbands bewildered. It is possible that husbands and wives disagree simply because they label certain behaviors as intrinsically good or bad, without trying to understand the gender-related perspective of their partner.

LIVING TOGETHER

Throughout the 1940s and 1950s conservative attitudes toward sex and marriage prevailed. In the 1960s conservatism gave way to radicalism that extended into relationships between men and women. Premarital and extra-marital sexual encounters became commonplace. For women, dependable contraception made sexual intercourse less risky. Liberal attitudes toward sex outside marriage encourage couples to live together in quasi-marital relationships accepted by the community. It is difficult to determine exactly how many people are living together in a premarital or extramarital relationship because reporting is unreliable and the status of the participants changes.

In previous times, when sexual abstinence outside marriage was advocated, people married for reasons that were mostly sexual. This was probably more true of men than women, because socialization of women included suppression of sexual feelings. Moreover, the consequences of sexual activity were heavier for women than for men. An important consequence of today's sexual freedom is that most people who marry now have previous sexual experience and high standards for sexual satisfaction. Cohabitation or living together without marriage is not a new idea, nor is it restricted to any country. In some primitive societies marriage occurs only after the female has presented the sexual partner with a child. In other societies a formal betrothal takes place after which sexual encounters are permitted. Usually, but not always, the betrothal is followed by legal marriage. Even so, the extent of cohabitation today is a new phenomenon in Western society.

Supporters of cohabitation once expected the practice to lead to more stable marriages because the couple knew each other well, but this has not proved to be the case. In the United States couples who lived together before marriage, divorce or separate in greater numbers than couples who marry without having lived together (Barringer, 1989). Sexual liberation seems to have had two major effects. Previous sexual experience would presumably reduce the chances of marrying the wrong person for the wrong reasons. On the other hand, previous sexual experience may create excessive expectations, leading to impatience when these expectations are not met (Segraves, 1985). It is possible that persons who live together without marriage are reluctant to make a formal commitment, and this reluctance predisposes them to separate or divorce. Persons who live together without marriage are strong enough to resist family or religious pressure. The same strength may lead them to terminate marriages that are disappointing. Perhaps couples who live together without marriage are less influenced by desire for stability and permanence and more influenced by desire for immediate gratification. Sometimes the couple living together may realize that the relationship is deteriorating and turn to marriage as a magic cure, much as a troubled husband and wife may decide that having a baby will end their marital problems. In some instances living together helps couples understand each other and fosters satisfactory ways of interacting, but marriages of couples who have lived together seem to be more fragile, at least from a statistical standpoint.

Living together without marriage is now part of the life cycle pattern in the United States, taking place both before marriage and after divorce. No one suggests that cohabitation leads to unhappy marriages, but neither is it a prerequisite for a happy marriage. Research indicates that it is usually a short-term arrangement leading either to marriage or to termination of the relationship. Barringer (1989) reports the following research data on the living-together phenomenon:

- The number of heterosexual couples living together without marriage is on the increase, especially for people who marry more than once. In the 1980s, 60 percent of persons who married for a second time cohabited, usually with the person who became the second spouse.
- Cohabitation usually lasts one year, ending when the couple separate or marry. One-fourth of cohabiting couples marry within the first year, one-half within three years. Only 10 percent of cohabiting couples stay together ten years without marrying or separating.
- One-half of all high school dropouts live with a partner before their 25th birthday; one-quarter of all college graduates live with a partner before their 25th birthday.

Additionally, research shows that living together is rarely a permanent arrangement and may or may not denote a lasting commitment. Although living together may lead to a strong marriage, the transitory nature of cohabitation seems to persist even after the couple marry.

HETEROSEXUAL MARITAL DEVELOPMENT

Introductory Phase: Romantic

Early in the marriage, the partners tend to idealize each other. Behaviors that would seem objectionable in others are attractive in the idealized partner. Other people become less important; each partner feels lonely and incomplete without the other. The physical attributes of the partner are exciting and attractive. They enjoy an active sex life that is meaningful to both of them. During the romantic phase of the marriage, one partner may be jealous and possessive. The other partner may not object to possessiveness if it is kept within bounds. However, extreme possessiveness by one partner may be resented by the other, who then yearns for more freedom. The possessive partner may insist on exclusive rights to the other to the extent that claims of work, relatives, and friends become an issue. In the romantic phase the relationship has a Romeo and Juliet quality; other interests and other people recede into the background. The phase varies in length and intensity depending on the personalities and emotional needs of the couple. If one partner chooses to adopt a more distant interactional style before the other is ready, adjustment problems ensue. The partner who wishes to continue the closeness of the romantic period feels threatened and enacts the role of pursuer. He or she may try to control the time and activities of the other. This causes the distancing partner to feel threatened and to increase attempts to maintain personal space. These attempts take the form of looking for an escape hatch, which may consist of working late or arranging schedules to permit breathing space.

Some partners want more than emotional closeness; they try to dominate the partner. Teasing, directing, and manipulating are used to avoid giving the partner equal rights and equal decision-making powers. The role chosen by the dominant partner is that of a parent who is wiser and more capable. Because domination strategies are disguised as affectionate and well-meaning, the partner treated as a child finds it hard to oppose the parent/spouse. In parent/spouse interactions, a delicate balance may operate for a while, but the situation is hazardous. A classic example of child/wife and parent/husband is depicted in Ibsen's play *A Doll's House*. In the play, Nora, the wife, grows up and finds her marriage intolerable. In Dickens's novel *David Copperfield*, the child/wife Dora conveniently dies so that the maturing hero can marry Agnes, who is more his equal.

Sometimes it is the wife who assumes the role of parent and treats her husband as a willful, errant child. This is a script often enacted with an alcoholic husband; the parent/wife forgives, punishes, and rescues the husband, acting more as a parent than a spouse. The reaction of a wife whose husband suffers a serious illness such as a cardiovascular accident often takes the form of behaving as his mother and allowing him to become regressed and dependent entirely on her.

Working Phase: Productive

The working or productive phase of marriage is a middle period lasting twenty years or more. In this period the couple is occupied with two major tasks: rearing children and making a living. In some marriages more emphasis is given to one of these tasks than to the other. In many marriages the two tasks are interrelated and carried out simultaneously.

Dual Careers

Family life has been dramatically changed by several forces. One is an economy that encourages, even necessitates, two incomes to support a household. Another is the feminist movement, which erased the guilt women felt for pursuing their own interests and careers. Demands of women for equal rights have opened new employment opportunities, so that more women are doing work they enjoy. Relationships between health, marriage, and working wives have been investigated. Bjornsten and Stewart (1985) report that working married women have fewer health complaints than single working women or full-time homemakers. Perhaps it is the healthiest and most capable women who combine marriage, motherhood, and a job. This means that the lesser symptomatology of working wives may reflect higher coping skills already present when they accepted jobs, whereas the greater symptomatology of homemakers not in the labor force indicates lower coping skills. The healthiness of working wives is not reflected in health gains for their husbands. One may speculate that working wives cause additional stress for husbands in the form of less attention and more household obligations.

When both husband and wife are wage earners, the scarcest family resource is time. Role conflict and role allocation are almost inevitable in dual-career families, especially if there are children. When wives functioned only as homemakers, men who were good providers felt they discharged their obligations as husbands and fathers. As the primary wage earner and the only wage earner, the father felt entitled to consideration and usually got it. If promotion or advancement for father required relocating, mother and children put aside their own preferences and followed father. In families with two wage earners, however, the wife may be as committed to her job as her husband is to his. Therefore, difficult decisions must be made as to which career is more meaningful. The decision is often made on the basis of the husband's larger salary.

Inequities exist in the salaries paid to men and to women. Furthermore, women are more likely to leave the work force periodically to have children and to care for family members who are ill or incapacitated. When salary is the criterion, decisions to relocate are made by the husband even though most wives have some input. Even so, the wife who leaves a cherished job to accompany her husband does so reluctantly. Her feelings of self-sacrifice add to the stress of moving from one place to another.

The women's movement has removed some occupational barriers for women. Ambitious women are no longer limited to teaching and nursing but have entered male-dominated fields. Women acknowledge some gains, but some are beginning to wonder if the gains are worth the cost. Some working women contend that they have two full-time jobs, that of homemaker and that of paid employee. Husbands today perform more household tasks than their fathers did, but overall responsibility for housekeeping and child care remain with the wife. When the husband helps out, the wife is expected to be appreciative because his contribution is voluntary while hers is compulsory. Wives react to this predicament in idiosyncratic ways. Some refuse to be grateful and feel resentful instead. Others coax or cajole their husbands into helping, pretending a gratitude they may not feel.

The lesser earning power of women has enormous ramifications. The average female worker earns 70 cents for every dollar earned by a male worker. Equal pay for equal work is not the practice throughout the nation (Belkin, 1989). This inequity puts female heads of households at great disadvantage. There is general agreement that working women perform more homemaking and parenting tasks than their husbands (Cowan, 1989). This may be due to the lesser financial contribution made by working wives, as well as the entrenched belief that a woman's first duty is to husband, home, and children regardless of outside demands made on her. Figure 8.3 contrasts the median earnings of men and women over the last 20 years.

An insidious risk in dual-career families stems from opportunities available to husband and wife for meeting attractive members of the opposite sex. Such opportunities were always available to men, but less so for homebound wives. Successful men have always attracted women for whom wealth and power are aphrodisiacs. In recent years a pattern has become apparent among high-achieving men. Many of them, in late middle life, divorce the first wife and remarry, choosing a younger woman who is attractive and accomplished. The second wife is an adornment, attesting to their success as surely as an expensive car. When husband and wife are both successful, their achievements on the job may engender low tolerance for boredom or frustration at home.

Success in any job does not come without effort, and hard-working achievers expend the bulk of their energy on job-related activities. For a dual-career marriage to survive, the partners must make a commitment to the marriage at least equivalent to that given to their careers. In assessing the interactional patterns and sources of conflict in dual-career marriages, it is advisable to look for the following behavior patterns.

FIGURE 8.3. Median Earnings of
Women as a Percentage of Median
Earnings of Men

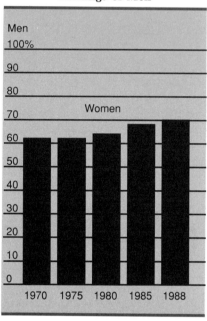

Source: U.S. Bureau of Labor Statistics.
Reported by Cowan (1989).

- Competition between husband and wife regarding advancement and promotions
- Counterdependent behavior by the wife as she tries to be superwoman
- Disagreement between the partners about whose job is more important
- Sacrifices made by one partner to advance the career of the other
- Resistance to role redistribution to accommodate tasks at home and work
- Extreme dedication by one or both partners to career or job

Clinical Vignette: Imbalance in a Dual-Career Family

Jason and Rachel are a young married couple without children. They married after graduating from college; both entered graduate school and were serious about their respective vocations. Rachel completed her architectural program easily and obtained a position with a firm where her talent was soon recognized. She was awarded a prestigious architectural prize a year after being hired and there was growing demand for her services. Jason's progress was less expeditious. He was enrolled in a doctoral program in clinical psychology and worked as a graduate assistant. After finishing his course work, Jason had difficulty writing a dissertation that met university standards.

As Rachel advanced in her career, Jason became sarcastic and critical. Nothing Rachel did seemed to please him. He began to spend more time on campus with other graduate students and resisted invitations by Rachel to do things together. As time passed, he began an affair with a fellow student, which ended when she moved away. Rachel suspected her husband's involvement but hesitated to confront him. When she tried to talk about their relationship, she was outmatched by Jason's sophistication and superior language skills.

Jason's attitude prevented Rachel from enjoying her own success. She knew Jason worried about his lack of progress and endeavored to be supportive. At first she felt guilty because her career was advancing so rapidly, but guilt turned to anger when her conciliatory overtures were rejected. She compensated for Jason's lack of interest by investing more energy in her work. At the same time she repeatedly suggested marital counseling. When Jason refused to consider this, she urged him to see a vocational counselor in order to resolve his inability to finish his dissertation. Rachel was supported in her efforts by Jason's parents, who were distressed by their son's unproductivity and failing marriage. They admired their bright daughter-in-law and wanted their son to be just as successful. Jason continued to resist any form of professional counseling.

Several factors precipitated the problems of Rachel and Jason. When they married, both were recent graduates facing bright futures. As Rachel finished her program and began to rise in her profession, the balance in the marriage shifted. Jason found his inferior position intolerable. It was probably a mistake for Rachel to involve Jason's parents. His father had always been demanding and perfectionistic with Jason. When Jason's father interfered, old wounds were reopened. Jason became more defensive and self-destructive, withdrawing from his parents, whom he now saw as Rachel's allies.

When Jason's coldness to her continued, Rachel accepted an assignment in another city. She and Jason discussed the move and agreed to a trial separation. During Rachel's absence, Jason made some progress on his dissertation. Feeling better about his work, he contacted Rachel and made overtures toward reconciliation. Through her work, however, Rachel had become involved with another man who was older and a prominent architect. Rachel enjoyed his company; they spoke the same language and the man appreciated her professional competence. She decided to remain where she was and a year later sought a divorce from Jason, who did not contest her action.

Jason was in fact relieved when the marriage ended. No longer measuring himself against a successful wife, he was able to finish his dissertation and earn his degree. Eventually he married a former student of his, whose ambitions lay in being a wife and homemaker. Rachel continued her career elsewhere. She enjoyed an active professional and social life but had no plans to remarry.

Many dual-career couples can sustain rewarding marriages, but the partners must be able to adapt to changing circumstances. When necessary, traditional role enactment must be modified to meet the needs of both partners and of any children. Competitiveness should remain outside the marriage and flexibility maintained within it. Rachel was single-minded in her career goals and gave less priority to her marriage until she saw the relationship deteriorating. In subtle ways she conveyed to Jason her impatience with his failure to progress. Impatience was a familiar experience for Jason, who had witnessed it often in his father. He refused counseling from fear of seeming weak and of being controlled by a strong wife and a strong father. Both partners acted as if their marriage was less important than their work. Rachel was driven by desire for success while Jason was driven by fear of failure. For both of them, autonomy was more desirable than interdependence. It was a relief for both that they had no children to hold them together and therefore could go their separate ways.

Parenthood

Transition from marriage to parenthood changes family organization from a dyad to a triangle, often a precarious structure. Parenthood is an event most persons approach ambivalently, even when the child is planned and consciously desired. The wife has been told that motherhood is a rewarding, even joyous, experience, but she has misgivings. She has heard over and over that the mother is the most significant person in a child's life, and that the quality of mothering a child receives determines his or her adjustment to life. So for her, fear and insecurity are part of the ambivalence. The husband may welcome his wife's pregnancy as testimony of his manhood, but he too has misgivings. His fears come from feelings of responsibility and of inadequacy.

Parenthood may occur early in a marriage, after a brief delay, or after a prolonged delay. Pregnancy that does not occur immediately but is briefly delayed is thought to be optimal. Here the couple have an interval to enjoy the romantic phase of their marriage, to establish a comfortable household, and to discover gratifying ways of being a couple. Today, many couples choose a long delay before having children, either to acquire a sound financial base or achieve dual career goals. Unfortunately, many couples who defer childbearing face the problem of decreased fertility when they do decide to have a child. Gutman (1985) observes that there are advantages and disadvantages to childbearing, whatever the timing. Couples who must deal with an immediate pregnancy report financial and relationship problems, especially if the first pregnancy is soon followed by a second. Child care obligations are often a problem when pregnancy occurs just before or after marriage. New mothers in this group report that husbands are little involved with child care, either because they are struggling to earn a living or because they want to go on being free and unburdened. Developmentally, new parents who are very young hesitate to move from adolescence into adulthood. When a couple are young and a child arrives soon after marriage, they face the task of forging a new identity as a spouse along with forging a new identity as a parent.

Late-timing couples report different problems after the birth of a child. Here, problems center on time management issues. The wife who was deeply invested in job or career must now rearrange her life to make room for motherhood. Some drop out of the work force for a few years, reentering when the children start school. Others try to juggle work, home, and motherhood. Usually these couples have sufficient financial resources, and the husband is more actively involved in parenting than are younger men whose children arrived early in the marriage (Daniels & Weingarten, 1982). Even so, both partners have feelings of stress and role confusion as they move from a relationship centered in each other to one that is family-centered (Cohler, 1984).

Many young women feel overwhelmed after the birth of a child. Some react by devoting all their energy to being the perfect mother; others react by performing their mothering tasks in a perfunctory way. Neither course of action is particularly adaptive. Concentrating all her attention on the child excludes the father. The effects of indifferent mothering on children are well documented. Even if there are no ill effects for the child, the indifferent mother is the target of criticism by others, which impairs her feelings of competence.

Besides changing the way a husband and wife relate to each other, parenthood changes relationships with the families of origin. Grandparents who had accepted the independence of their married children now want to be more involved. Their involvement may be perceived either as helpful or as intrusive by the new parents. Unresolved issues between the couple and their parents may resurface. If the couple decide to use different child-rearing tactics than their parents did, the grandparents may interpret this as a criticism. All this causes additional tension for new parents, most of whom want some help, but not too much, from their families of origin.

Parenthood in and of itself is no guarantee of marital happiness. Child-less women have been found to be happier than women with children under 6 years of age. The most adverse consequences to marital happiness occur when the couple has numerous small children (Cohler, 1984). It is suggested that the quality of married life is better in the preparental period and after the children are teenagers.

Society takes motherhood seriously, whether the mother is under 20 or over 40. This cannot be said of expectant or new fathers, who are regarded as buffoons rather than heroes of an epic experience. The chain-smoking male in the maternity waiting room who faints at the announcement of the birth, or the proud dad who makes silly faces at his newborn in the nursery, is a figure of fun to onlookers. This has been mitigated by dad's admission to childbirth education classes and his role as "coach" during labor and delivery. Still, he is mostly on the sidelines, giving cues to his wife who is the star of the performance.

The transition of men into the parent role receives scant attention even though more is expected of them in child care and parenting than in past years. Parenthood expects of men, as well as women, participation and role enactment that are multidimensional (Pruett, 1987). During the wife's pregnancy the husband may adopt any of three interactional styles (May, 1980). There is the observing husband who is somewhat uninvolved; the expressive husband who shares emotional responses; and the instrumental husband who busies himself in activities related to the pregnancy, the delivery, and child care.

Jordon (1990) writes that the essence of expectant and new fatherhood is the male's search for relevance. As his wife's pregnancy advances, he tries to incorporate fatherhood into his sense of self and expand his repertoire of roles. In a study of expectant and first-time fathers, Jordon identified three processes that make up the man's search for relevance. The processes, which are facilitated or impeded by actions of the wife and others throughout the pregnancy, are shown in Table 8.2.

The term *alliance of pregnancy* has been applied to the shared activities of the expectant couple (Deutscher, 1970). Sharing their feelings and their preparations for the child confers on father the needed sense of relevance. If the partners experience the pregnancy as a shared venture, their chances of establishing a parental alliance are strengthened. Exclusion of fathers from the pregnancy and birth experience is no longer total, but more could be done in this area. Women who want coparenting behaviors from their husbands might well begin by treating their pregnancy as a family affair. A

TABLE 8.2. **Processes Involved in the Father's Search for Relevance**

Process	Characteristics
Accepting the reality of the pregnancy and the child	This is a gradual process, slow in the early months of the pregnancy, accelerating as the child begins to move in utero and the pregnancy becomes obvious.
Obtaining recognition from others as a father	This is an intermittent process involving wife, family, friends, and society at large; recognition from others gives a sense of inclusion and meaning to the role of father.
Expanding role performance to include functions	This is a later process that involves tangible preparations for the birth such as making new financial arrangements or preparing a nursery.

parenting alliance is possible only if men can participate more fully. Jordon (1990, p. 14) records the words of one left-out husband:

> There is no validation of the feelings. There is no recognition. I don't feel like I should deny my feelings and deny what's going on for me. The message is clear . . . "You need to focus on her." I just haven't found anybody that is real understanding, like "What is the experience like for you?"

Extramarital Relationships

During the working phase of a marriage, the stresses of earning a living and raising children may alter a couple's commitment to each other. Boredom is another factor contributing to infidelity in marriage, as is the realization that time is passing and youth is fleeting. For various reasons some individuals find it hard to be monogamous even though they may not want their marriage to end. The solution for many partners is the extramarital affair or affairs. Nass, Libby, and Fisher (1981) report that 65 to 70 percent of married men have extramarital affairs, as do 45 to 64 percent of married women. Some but not all affairs are clandestine and secret. The affairs may be one-night stands or durable relationships with persons of the opposite sex. The secrecy in which most affairs begin heightens the excitement, but it also robs the legal marriage of time and energy. Openness between husband and wife is lost when one partner is involved in an affair. The involved spouse feels guilty and deals with this by dwelling on the deficiencies of the other spouse. This reduces guilt and justifies the actions of the unfaithful spouse, who feels that the partner does not deserve honesty or fidelity.

In some cases, an affair makes it impossible for the marriage to continue. In other cases existence of an extramarital relationship is known but not openly acknowledged by the husband and wife. In such instances the marriage may actually be preserved by the affair. If one partner has a stronger sex drive than the other, the affair provides an outlet for sexual needs. The disability of one partner may also be a factor leading to an extramarital affair that helps preserve the marriage.

It is extremely difficult to continue an affair and have it remain a secret. Unless the couple lead very separate lives, sooner or later the husband or wife begins to suspect. Suspicions, even if unconfirmed, impair the marital relationship. If secrecy continues, deceit and duplicity increase. If a full disclosure is made, anger and recriminations follow. Some motivated couples are able to strengthen their marriage in the aftermath of an affair. Discovery of an affair frequently injects strong emotions into an otherwise monotonous marriage. Faced with the prospect of breaking up, the couple may decide to deal with problems they have been avoiding. The discovery that one partner found the marriage deficient and looked elsewhere may induce a crisis that leads the couple to face and talk about failed hopes. Even when reconciliation proves impossible, the crisis may help the couple to learn something about themselves that will prove useful in subsequent relationships. In helping couples to deal with infidelity, the health care professional must be accepting and nonjudgmental. The success of counseling does not depend on salvaging the marriage. With the partners already blaming each other, the last thing they need is a moralistic counselor. Unless health care professionals can discard their own moral scruples, they should not continue working with these couples. Because emotions are apt to run high for the couple, a primary task of the counselor is to reduce emotionality and promote a climate where rational discussion is possible.

Companionship Phase: Winding Down

The later years of married life can be a time of contentment and comradeship. The hectic years of working and raising children are over, and for many couples this is a rewarding time. Couples once distracted by multiple obligations can renew their interest in each other. With children out of the home and a measure of financial security, the couple can take stock of their accomplishments and of what lies ahead (Guerin & Fay, 1982). Compatible couples move toward each other and attend to each other in a way that previously was impossible. Husband and wife start to recognize their mortality and to realize that life is finite. For some, these intimations of mortality are frightening; they dwell less on what they have done and more on what they have not done.

Retirement is an event that produces drastic changes in the interactions of any couple. Upon retiring, people lose meaningful associations and roles that enhanced their self-esteem. The world of the retired worker narrows. Husband and wife find themselves spending more time together through necessity, not choice. In traditional families where the husband was the only wage earner, he enters household territory presided over by his wife and often feels like a stranger in his own home. This is true even in dual-career families, for the home still is considered the wife's realm more than the husband's.

If both partners have been employed and retire together, they are more likely to plan for retirement and to anticipate future problems. Because wives are often younger than their husbands, the partners may not retire at the same time. A wife who has taken time out to raise children may not be ready to give up an enjoyable position. Lessened income is a frequent consequence of retiring, and this may persuade the wife to continue working. This situation may become problematic. With the husband at home and the wife working, she may expect more assistance from him. Already deprived by loss of the work role, the man may resist becoming a house husband, and arguments follow.

Couples who retire at the same time also face adjustments. They have more time to spend together, but this may not be equally agreeable to both partners. If one partner is more active socially than the other, the less outgoing partner may place limits on the other. Unless the couple can agree to balance independent and interdependent activities, the more outgoing partner will feel controlled while the less outgoing partner feels abandoned.

Clinical Example: Marital Dysfunction after Retirement

Just after his 60th birthday, Hugh Reynolds suffered a heart attack while working in the factory where he was plant foreman. Rushed to the hospital by ambulance, Hugh spent two weeks in intensive care. After another four weeks he was discharged with the provision that he return three times a week for cardiac rehabilitation. Hugh was a jovial, outgoing man who was confident that he could complete the rehabilitation program and return to work shortly. He followed his prescribed regimen faithfully and looked forward eagerly to working again. When Hugh filed a request to return to work, his application was rejected because his physician stipulated limited exertion. The family did not suffer financially. Hugh had thirty-five years of service with the same company, and the pension plan was generous. Marie, Hugh's wife, was an excellent musician who taught piano at home and was a paid organist and choir director in their church.

When he was told he could not return to work, Hugh was very upset. He appealed the decision, but without the endorsement of his physician he was powerless to change it. Without prior warning, Hugh found himself an unwilling retiree. Soon after his forced retirement, Hugh stopped attending the rehabilitation program. He began to stay out of the house and spend most of his time at a tavern. He became indifferent to his appearance and irritable with his wife. When he was at home, he complained about Marie's music lessons and ridiculed her pupils. Marie was patient for a while, but in a short time she rented a nearby studio and moved a piano there so she could give lessons without hearing complaints from Hugh. The couple settled into a routine in which Marie did housework in the morning and left for her studio about noon. Hugh spent his mornings in bed and his afternoons at the tavern. Communication between them was almost nonexistent.

The couple's oldest daughter came to visit and saw the angry truce between her parents. Distressed for them both, she insisted they see a marriage counselor. Their daughter made the appointment and drove them to their first visit. Hugh's attitude was that things were not likely to improve because Marie was now "king of the hill." Marie's response was that Hugh was a sick man and she would try to help him even if he had driven her and her pupils from the house.

Assessment

Hugh was frightened by his sudden illness and unprepared for retirement. He was proud of his independence and feared being dependent on anyone, but he denied these feelings. He masked his anxiety and depression by being angry and critical; Marie misinterpreted his actions and became angry and impatient. While Hugh struggled with loss of the work role, Marie moved further from the orbit of home. When she rented a studio, she did not consult Hugh or consider the effect of this action on his fragile self-esteem. Her impulsive move added to Hugh's feelings of loneliness.

Until Hugh's retirement the marriage was apparently harmonious, but the partners went their separate ways. For Hugh, his work associations were sufficient and all-important. He was accustomed to letting Marie make decisions about the house and the children without consulting him. Marie's competence and self-sufficiency threatened him only when he had no external sources of satisfaction. He felt he could not explain his feelings to Marie, and he behaved in ways that alienated her. This led Marie to withdraw further from Hugh and added to his loneliness. He hid his feelings behind a mask of irascibility and heavy drinking.

Planning

While Hugh was hospitalized, Marie was attentive and devoted. His inability to resume work shocked her, and his presence in the house upset her schedule. She was used to having the house to herself and resented interruptions to her lessons. In the marital sessions the counselor thought it imperative for the couple to talk about what Hugh's retirement meant to each of them so that they could negotiate some compromises. Throughout their married life, both had found friendships outside their relationship. Hugh had always spent time with pals from the factory, Marie with a group of women who shared her interests. Hugh bowled and enjoyed baseball games; Marie played bridge and went to concerts. For years they had accepted each other's differences until Hugh's retirement altered the balance. The isolation experienced by Hugh and his heavy drinking meant that the couple had to reconcile some of their divergent interests. Neither could be expected to give up accustomed pursuits altogether, but compromise was necessary for the sake of the marriage and Hugh's health.

Intervention

With the aid of the counselor, the couple identified activities they might continue to enjoy individually and activities they might share. A trade-off was recommended, with Hugh agreeing to learn bridge if Marie was willing to be introduced to bowling. Hugh's baseball games and Marie's concerts were designated as individual activities. Because Marie had already rented a studio, the couple decided to continue this arrangement. Marie expressed her concern about Hugh's drinking and the state of his health. Hugh seemed surprised at her solicitude and was able to tell Marie that he believed she no longer cared for him since his illness. A number of sessions were devoted to improving communication between the partners. The counselor recommended that the couple put aside time to have their evening meal together and exchange news of what each had done during the day. Hugh was encouraged to move out into the community in order to enlarge his circle of friends beyond the tavern. Marie suggested that he join the retirees' association of his company and join in their social and charitable activities. She assured Hugh that she would be willing to participate if he became active in the association.

Evaluation

The medical attention Hugh received was excellent, but his psychological needs were ignored, especially by his wife. When Hugh retired, Marie acted like a hostess with an unwelcome guest. She was insensitive to Hugh's feelings of loss; when he seemed angry, she reacted more angrily. Yet she was insightful enough to see, when it was pointed out to her, that she had more resources at her disposal than Hugh had. Self-engrossed and self-satisfied for many years, the couple now were called upon to give more to each other. Marie was encouraged to look beyond Hugh's blustering and understand his real emotions. Theirs was a marriage based on separateness, and the counselor respected the differences between them. However, sudden retirement demanded realignment of their relationship. Counseling neutralized their anger so that neither partner acted out conflicts but both verbalized what they wanted from the other.

Therapeutic Guidelines

When a couple seek professional help for their problems, they begin by describing their difficulties in broad, accusatory terms. Their initial statements are used not to provide information but to attack and blame each other. Without contradicting these sweeping generalizations, the counselor can ask for specific examples of situations when the husband was abusive, for example, or the wife was demanding. It is then possible to ask questions about what led up to the objectionable behavior and what followed it. Occasionally one partner comes to the first session armed with a written litany of grievances. The partner who has not compiled a written list is at a disadvantage, as is the counselor who is pushed into the position of judge. In these circumstances the counselor might comment that the sessions are obviously important to the partner with the list. Without reading the list, the counselor might ask the other partner to bring a similar list at the next session, adding that they can then discuss both lists at the same time.

When the counselor asks for specific information, a pattern emerges of how the couple interact. Does the husband habitually arrive home from work in a bitter, quarrelsome mood? Is he willing to explain the reasons for his negative state of mind, or does he expect his wife to understand without being told? When the wife is overwhelmed or exhausted by events of the day, how are her feelings expressed? Whom does she hold responsible when things go badly—herself, her husband, the children, or someone else?

Regardless of the phase of the marriage, reviewing premarital and post-marital history is valuable. This causes the couple to recall happier years and remember why they were attracted to each other. The marital history should include their early expectations of marriage and whether the expectations were met. Discrepancies in their expectations may reveal the source of current problems. The woman may have married with the hope of achieving status and affluence; the man may have married with little thought of rising in the world. If he has changed jobs frequently, the upward mobility so important to the wife may be elusive. He cannot understand her emphasis on money, and she cannot understand why he ignores prospects for promotion.

The way the couple interact in therapeutic sessions demonstrates some of their interactional patterns at home. The wife may look away or interrupt whenever her husband speaks. The husband may speak for his wife as well as for himself, telling her what she thinks and feels instead of listening. Besides being specific, couples must learn to speak only for themselves, not for each other. A bombastic or controlling partner may be disarmed by a counselor who insists that authoritative statements be prefaced by the phrase "It seems to me." Similarly, the less dominant partner can derive more authority by using the same phrase, which has an equalizing effect on the statements of both partners.

Communication patterns can be extremely complex, especially for less experienced health care professionals. Sholevar (1985) outlines various aspects of marital role enactment to be used in analyzing a couple's communication and interaction modes.

1. *Marital role:* Are the couple equipped by temperament and intellect to share companionship and understanding?
2. *Management role:* Are the couple fair and responsible in allocating and carrying out the daily tasks of family life?
3. *Parental role:* Are the couple able and willing to attend to the needs of the children?
4. *Sexual role:* Is the sexual relationship of the couple gratifying for both?
5. *Provider role:* Are material needs adequately met and family resources equitably distributed?
6. *Organizational role:* Are family boundaries clear and consistent; are subgroups defined by natural divisions of age, gender, and family position?
7. *Problem-solving role:* Do partners search for acceptable solutions; is decision making a shared process?
8. *Reciprocal role:* Is role enactment of the partners complementary or symmetrical; if complementary, is one partner dominated by the other; if symmetrical, do the partners compete for dominance or for dependency?

9. *Negotiating role:* Are statements of feelings or opinions presented as facts; are factual statements specific and explicit; are both positive and negative aspects of a situation acknowledged?
10. *Executive role:* Are decisions made in a rational, objective way; are managerial functions shared according to agreed-on rules?

Categorizing the couple's communication and interactional modes facilitates analysis of what needs to be changed and what the couple are likely to change. This analysis lends itself to specific interventions by the health care professional. Rules for more adaptive communication and interaction may be modeled by the health care professional in therapeutic sessions and taught to the couple. In trying to modify communication and interactional modes, four basic questions should be addressed. Is communication between husband and wife clearly expressed and transmitted by both partners? Are messages conveyed in words consistent with the mood of the interaction? Are messages validated by the partners so that there is little chance for misinterpretation or distortion? Is equal importance and equal weight given to the perceptions and views of each partner?

SUMMARY

This chapter discussed marital heterosexual relationships using a culturally oriented, life cycle model. Gender-related differences in the moral development of men and women are the focus of Carol Gilligan's work. These differences are culturally reinforced and exacerbate misunderstandings between husbands and wives. Most marriages in the United States begin with a romantic phase. At first newly married couples tend to idealize each other, but the romantic phase passes and is replaced by interactional patterns that are more mundane. The middle or productive years of marriage are characterized by multiple demands and responsibilities that accompany jobs and parenthood. This excessive busyness reduces the time and attention that husband and wife can give to each other; yet many marriages flourish because the couple have common goals and replace romantic love with conjugal commitment.

Extramarital affairs are frequent in contemporary marriages and do not always result in separation or divorce. As the more productive phase of marriage ends, new issues arise. Retirement is rarely an easy time for couples; problems surface both in traditional and in dual-career marriages as a consequence of retirement. There is more opportunity for intimacy and leisure pursuits, but loss of meaningful work roles requires adjustment, especially for the husband. The wife who has been a full-time homemaker considers the household her territory. Even when a wife has been employed full time, she is likely to see the home as her turf. Unless the couple can anticipate retirement problems and talk about arrangements, the retired husband may feel like a stranger in his own home.

In working with married couples, health care professionals should identify the phase of the marriage and observe how the couple handles phasic tasks. After the phase of the marriage is recognized, it is easier to assess idiosyncratic patterns that create problems. Most essential is the avoidance of blame or partisanship by the health care professional. Neutrality on the part of the counselor moderates the emotional climate so that the partners can move from bitter recrimination to rational problem solving. Preserving the marriage is not the major goal of counseling. A decision by the partners to end the marriage does not represent failure of the counseling process. Even when partners choose to divorce, effective intervention can do much to make a painful experience less intense.

REFERENCES

Barringer, F. (1989). "Doubt on Trial Marriage Raised by Divorce Rates." *New York Times*, June 9, p. A1.

Belkin, L. (1989). "Women's Lives: A Scorecard of Change," Part III. *New York Times*, August 23, p. A1.

Bjornsten, O. J., & Stewart, T. J. (1985). "Marital Status and Health." In O. J. Bjornsten (Ed.), *New Clinical Concepts in Marital Therapy*. Washington, DC: American Psychiatric Association.

Cohler, B. J. (1984). "Parenthood, Psychopathology, and Childcare." In R. S. Cohen, B. J. Cohler, & S. H. Weissman (Eds.), *Parenthood: A Psychodynamic Perspective*. New York: Adelford.

Cowan, A. L. (1989). "Women's Lives: A Scorecard of Change," Part I. *New York Times*, August 21, p. A1.

Daniels, D., & Weingarten, K. (1982). *Sooner or Later: The Timing of Parenthood in Adult Lives*. New York: Norton.

Deutscher, M. (1970). "Brief Family Therapy in the Course of First Pregnancy." *Contemporary Psychoanalysis*, 7(1): 21–35.

Dionne, E. J. (1989). "Women's Lives: A Scorecard for Change," Part II. *New York Times*, August 22, p. A1.

Friedan, B. (1986). *The Second Stage*. New York: Summit.

Gilligan, C. (1982a). *In a Different Voice*. Cambridge, MA: Harvard University Press.

Gilligan, C. (1982b). "New Maps of Development: New Visions of Maturity." *American Journal of Orthopsychiatry*, 52(2): 199–212.

Gilligan, C., Ward, J. V., & Taylor, J. M., with Bardige, B. (1989). *Mapping the Moral Domain*. Cambridge, MA: Harvard University Press.

Goleman, D. (1986). "Two Views of Marriage Explored: His and Hers." *New York Times*, April 1, p. C1.

Guerin, P. J., & Fay, L. F. (1982). "The Envelope of Marital Conflict: Social Context and Family Factors." *The Family*, 10(1): 3–14.

Gutman, M. A. (1985). "Infertility, Delayed Childbearing, and Voluntary Childlessness." In D. C. Goldberg (Ed.), *Contemporary Marriage: Special Issues in Couples Therapy*. Homewood, IL: Dorsey.

Jordan, P. L. (1990). "Laboring for Relevance: Expectant and New Fatherhood." *Nursing Research*, 39(1): 11–16.

Kohlberg, L. (1968). "Moral Development." In *International Encyclopedia of Social Science*. New York: Macmillan.

May, K. A. (1980). "Three Phases of Father Involvement in Pregnancy." In *Nursing Research*, 31(4): 337–342.

Nass, G. D., Libby, R. W., & Fisher, M. P. (1981). *Sexual Choices: An Introduction to Human Sexuality*. Belmont, CA: Wadsworth.

Prose, F. (1990). "Confident at Eleven: Confused at Sixteen." *New York Times Magazine*, January 7, pp. 23–25, 37–45.

Pruett, K. D. (1987). *The Nurturing Father*. New York: Warner.

Segraves, R. T. (1985). "Marital Status and Psychiatric Morbidity." In O. J. Bjornsten (Ed.), *New Clinical Concepts in Marital Therapy*. Washington, DC: American Psychiatric Association.

Sholevar, G. P. (1985). "Assessment of Marital Disorders." In D. C. Goldberg (Ed.), *Contemporary Marriage: Special Issues in Couples Therapy*. Homewood, IL: Dorsey.

Spanier, G. B., & Furstenberg, F. F. (1982). "Remarriage after Divorce: A Longitudinal Analysis of Wellbeing." *Journal of Marriage and the Family*, 44(3): 709–720.

CHAPTER NINE

Homosexual Families:
Patterns and Variations

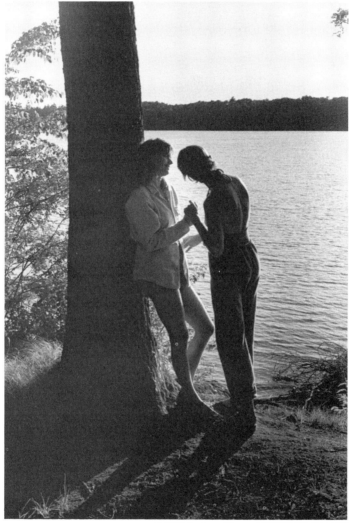

© 1990 by Jerry Howard/POSITIVE IMAGES

We prize individuality when it comes to the exercise of a man's aggressive spirit, but are inclined to despise it in the exercise of those aspects of his nature that are not perceived as conventionally masculine.

Richard A. Isay

This chapter reviews homosexual relationships of gay men and lesbians, their life patterns and variations. It begins with a look at homosexuality in a historical context: In ancient Greece, Rome, and Egypt, same-sex relationships were valued and condoned. Later, Western attitudes, largely influenced by Judeo-Christian beliefs, condemned homosexual behavior as immoral. Still later, the medical-psychoanalytic world labeled it as a sickness, a disease. Official psychoanalytic attitudes began to change in 1973 when, in the United States, the American Psychiatric Association changed its definition of homosexuality from a disease to a way of life. The chapter reviews several aspects of prejudice and discrimination and lists the most common myths about homosexuality.

The search for a sexual identity is discussed, along with the effects on the "coming out" process for gay men and lesbians of the women's liberation and the gay rights movements. The impact of the disclosure of a homosexual orientation on the gay man's or lesbian's family of origin is discussed. The similarities between the sexual behaviors of heterosexual and homosexual persons are revealed. The subject of gay men and lesbians as parents is explored, with motivations for parenthood reviewed. Guidelines for the disclosure of a parent's homosexuality to the children are presented. Issues for married gays and lesbians with nonhomosexual spouses are discussed, and special issues for aging gay men and lesbians are addressed. The impact of AIDS on homosexuals is acknowledged, and the emphasis on intensification of the public's homophobic attitudes is seen as a setback for the gay rights movement. In the last part of the chapter, therapeutic guidelines for working with homosexual persons are discussed, with some do's and don't's outlined for the health professional. A clinical example completes the chapter.

During the last two decades, as many homosexual persons pressed for social acceptance, professional groups and the general public became more aware of the prevalence of homosexuality. The term *homosexual* is usually applied to the sexual orientation of men and women who derive their primary emotional and sexual fulfillment from intimate relationships with persons of their own gender. Homosexuality, like heterosexuality, is only one aspect of human personality. Like heterosexuality, homosexuality is expressed in diverse ways. Identifying individuals solely through their choice of sexual partners ignores such diversity and demeans them by conveying the impression that persons with homosexual preferences are interested only in the sexual aspects of personal relationships. When the label *homosexual* is applied, other aspects of an individual's personality and character tend to be overlooked. Therefore, such labels should be used carefully and with the understanding that the only overriding difference between heterosexual and homosexual persons is in their choice of sexual partners.

In the ancient world, among Greeks, Romans, Egyptians, Etruscans, Carthaginians, Sumerians, and others, homosexual behaviors were accepted, even fostered. It was in countries bordering the Mediterranean Sea and the Euphrates and Nile Rivers that homosexuality received the most approval. In China and Japan homosexual activities were considered acceptable; during feudal times in those countries, homosexual attachments were thought to be more "manly" than heterosexual ones. Male geishas were common in Japan until the mid-1950s, when they were suppressed by the American Occupation Army. Among religious groups, homosexuality was deemed acceptable by Moslems and Buddhists and was even practiced among Buddhist priests and monks. In Hindu law, homosexual behavior is viewed as a minor offense (Gramick, 1983). The tolerance displayed in various countries at various times and among various religions is in marked contrast to prevailing Western attitudes of disapproval and negativism.

WESTERN ATTITUDES TOWARD HOMOSEXUALITY

Prior to 1973, traditional psychoanalytic theory attributed homosexuality to unresolved masochistic attachment to the preoedipal mother, a distant relationship with the father, defense against castration anxiety, and an immature ego (Bell & Weinberg, 1978; Carrera, 1981). One psychoanalyst (Bergler, 1956), referring to the Oedipal romance, described homosexuality as an "unfavorable unconscious solution of a conflict that faces every child" (p. 27). The general opinion was that homosexuality represented a neurotic condition or a mental disorder. As such, homosexuality was given a diagnostic label and included in the classification manual of the American Psychiatric Association. Bergler wrote that "regardless of level of intelligence, culture, background, or education, all homosexuals had a mixture of the following traits" (p. 27). These are listed in Table 9.1.

A significant change in the traditional approach to homosexuality took place in 1973, when the board of trustees of the American Psychiatric Association voted unanimously that homosexuality should no longer be

TABLE 9.1. Neurotic Traits Previously Attributed to Homosexuals
• Masochistic provocation and injustice collecting
• Defensive malice
• Flippancy concealing depression and guilt
• Hypernarcissism and hypersuperciliousness
• Refusal to acknowledge accepted standards in nonsexual matters
• Belief in their right to challenge moral standards because of their "suffering"
• General unreliability of a more or less psychopathic nature

Source: Adapted from Bergler (1956), p. 44.

classified as a mental disorder in the *Diagnostic and Statistical Manual of Mental Disorders*, which was then being revised. Protests against the Trustees' decision brought about a referendum in which a majority of American Psychiatric Association members supported the decision. These actions paved the way for homosexuality to be considered a way of life rather than a disease. The only reference to homosexuality in the current revision of the *Manual*, the DSM-III-R (1987) is under the heading "Sexual Disorder Not Otherwise Specified." It is specifically limited to persons evincing "persistent and marked distress" about their sexual orientation (p. 296).

Alfred Kinsey's studies in 1948 and 1953 demonstrated that millions of Americans had engaged in homosexual activities at one time or another. His surveys showed that 50 percent of American men and 28 percent of American women had some homosexual experience during their lives. The data made it clear that a person's sexual preference is rarely fixed but can be seen as subject to variation along a continuum. Kinsey developed a six-point scale rating people from "entirely heterosexual" to "entirely homosexual." In applying the scale, Kinsey found that nearly half of the subjects fell between the two endpoints. This indicated that there is a wide variation in forms of sexual expression among human beings.

Richard A. Isay (1989) is one of the first analytically oriented psychiatrists to discuss a normal route of psychological development for gay men. Isay has twenty years' experience in treating gay men and believes that there is no more psychopathology in homosexual men than in heterosexual men. He accepts the premise that there may be a constitutional or genetic factor involved in the etiology of homosexuality, but he also acknowledges that there is a complex set of environmental, social, and cultural elements that allow predisposition to homosexuality to express itself. He believes that there are two disabling obstructions to maintaining lasting and loving homosexual relationships. These are parental rejection and Western society's severe homophobia. Rejection, derogatory attitudes, and punitive measures undoubtedly have adverse effects on one's capacity for trust and intimacy.

According to census reports of 1988, fewer than 27 percent of the nation's 91 million households fit the traditional model of a family. The same reports showed that there were 1.6 million same-sex couples living together, an increase from 500,000 in 1970. Reasons for these changes included divorce, delayed marriage, and the strength of the gay liberation movement. Admittedly, the Census Bureau still excludes many nontraditional living arrangements from the definition of *family*. In the next few decades, the federal legal definition of family is likely to broaden, following the example of a number of states.

PREJUDICE AND DISCRIMINATION

Homophobia may be defined as a strong, irrational fear of homosexuals, sometimes exacerbated by the fear of homosexual urges within oneself. In Western culture there are well-entrenched attitudes about what is masculine and what is feminine. For example, aggressive characteristics are highly valued in men but denigrated in women. Gentler virtues of loving and caring are highly valued in women but undervalued in men. There are some theorists who believe that hostility and distrust of "feminine" characteristics in men may be the root of homophobia (Isay, 1989). Homophobia is so pervasive in our society that many homosexuals are physically assaulted by people who believe that homosexuals deserve mistreatment. Often they are regarded as safe targets by criminals who rely on homosexuals' reluctance to press charges lest this lead to unfavorable publicity. Bell and Weinberg (1978) reported that one-third of their homosexual subjects stated that they had been assaulted or robbed at least once as a consequence of their homosexuality. These researchers also noted that 25 percent of their homosexual men and women had been threatened with blackmail because of their sexual preference.

In our culture men appear to be more overtly homophobic than women, and male homosexuals seem to feel more threatened than their female counterparts. Behaviors that indicate homophobia include jokes about "queers" and "fags," ridiculing or disparaging homosexuals, and attacking homosexual persons verbally or physically. Most homophobic men seem to hold rigid gender role stereotypes and avoid role enactment that might be considered less than masculine. They tend not to choose female-oriented professions or occupations, avoid hugging friends and relatives of their own sex, and are uncomfortable with manual–genital contact even with partners of the opposite sex. Homophobia and general ignorance about homosexuality lead to the perpetuation of many myths, some of which are outlined in Table 9.2.

The Wolfenden Report, based on a ten-year study by the Committee on Homosexual Offenses and Prostitution in Great Britain, was made available in 1957. It proved to be a milestone in legalizing homosexual behaviors in

TABLE 9.2. Common Myths about Homosexuality
• If homosexuality is sanctioned, the world population would become extinct.
• It is possible to identify people's sexual orientation by looking at them.
• Homosexual persons are all very much alike.
• Homosexual persons have uncontrollable sexual drives.
• Homosexual persons are usually unstable emotionally.
• Homosexual persons can convert heterosexuals to homosexuality.
• Lesbian women cannot be good mothers; gay men cannot be good fathers.
• Homosexual persons are responsible for the majority of sexual violence.
• Homosexual teachers molest the children whom they teach.
• In homosexual relationships, one partner enacts the woman's role and the other enacts the man's role.

Britain and Europe. The report recommended that homosexual behavior between consenting adults in private no longer be considered a criminal offense. Following this recommendation, the laws were altered in a number of European countries, notably, France, Belgium, West Germany, and the Scandinavian countries (Katchadourian & Lunde, 1972). Although homosexual behavior has been decriminalized in many countries, the United States has lagged. Most states still have laws on the books regarding homosexual activities. In twenty-four states sodomy laws remain; sodomy legislation makes persons engaged in oral and anal sexual intercourse subject to arrest. To date, only two states, Wisconsin and Massachusetts, have passed laws banning discrimination against gays and lesbians. Homosexuals are often arrested for loitering to solicit and for disorderly conduct. Police officers have been found to use entrapment by posing as decoys soliciting sexual favors.

Homosexual persons who are open about their sexual orientation often are deprived of their civil rights in questions of housing and employment. Sometimes they suffer discrimination regarding credit, insurance coverage, and child custody or adoption proceedings. Because the safeguards of legal marriage are unavailable, they encounter difficulties with taxes, pensions, and property and inheritance rights.

Judeo-Christian positions on sex and morality are influential in many Western countries, and this has sustained the stigma attached to homosexuality. At present, religious groups struggle with homosexuality, not only among parishioners who have openly declared their homosexuality, but also among ministers, priests, and other religious figures who acknowledge a homosexual orientation as they continue to serve their church. Militant homosexual groups disrupt church services in their demands for acceptance and support; battles concerning the ordination of homosexual clergy continue in Catholic, Protestant, and Jewish congregations. Some aspects of homophobia are present in religious institutions. Clark, Brown, and Hochstein (1990) state that the Church's teachings force the gay person to choose between loyalty to the Church and loyalty to the homosexual person's true sense of self. The prejudicial attitude of the Church also has a negative impact on the family of the gay or lesbian person, because it teaches that homosexuality is deviant or immoral. Many families trying to come to terms with the homosexuality of a son or daughter need a place to take their disappointment, confusion, and sadness. For the most part, institutionalized religion has not provided a safe, nonjudgmental haven where families can deal with their distress. At present there is a growing trend among some religious groups to be more accepting and more liberal in their attitudes and actions toward persons who are homosexual. Neither Conservative nor Orthodox Jewish congregations accept homosexual rabbis, but Reform Jewish congregations and rabbis are more liberal, and the ordination of a homosexual rabbi in a Reform synagogue has been predicted (*Democrat and Chronicle*, Rochester, New York, June 1990). Unitarian congregations display the greatest tolerance, and Unitarian churches perform a number of ceremonies each year celebrating the unions of homosexual couples.

The Roman Catholic Church does not regard homosexual behavior as a morally acceptable option. The Episcopal Church, however, affirms the right of homosexual couples to a "covenant relationship," as set forth in a statement by the Episcopal dioceses of Rochester, New York (*Democrat and Chronicle*, June 1990, p. 4).

In summary, the statement from the Episcopal diocese supported significant same-gender committed relationships and stated that Christian tradition and biblical theology supported the basic need of all human beings to enjoy an intimately affectionate and long-term relationship with another person. It stressed that this reality goes far deeper than sexual orientation.

Despite opposition, liberalized attitudes toward homosexuality have begun to emerge. In 1972 the United Church of Christ became the first major denomination to ordain a homosexual clergyman. The Unitarian Universalists have warmly accepted the ordination of gay clergy. In San Francisco, the parishioners of a Lutheran church, half of whom are homosexual, voted in 1989 to accept a lesbian couple as assistant pastors. However, the Lutheran bishop of the area refused his approval because the lesbian couple did not commit themselves to sexual abstinence. As most homosexual persons believe, their progress toward acceptance seems to threaten traditional attitudes and values even in this secular age.

THE SEARCH FOR IDENTITY

The development of a sexual identity is a complex and not thoroughly understood process for men and women alike. Isay (1989) states that the development of a homosexual identity has its roots in early childhood, and in our culture is accompanied by guilt and self-loathing that inhibits stable personality integration. "Coming out," or declaring oneself a homosexual in the 1980s and 1990s, is very different from admitting one's homosexuality in earlier decades. There was such widespread intolerance of homosexuality during the 1930s, 1940s, 1950s, and even 1960s that it was very hard for anyone to feel good about being homosexual (Lewis, 1984). The decade of the 1960s brought the "sexual revolution," feminism, and the gay liberation movement. An obvious result was the raising of public consciousness and greater acceptance of alternative life-styles. When the American Psychiatric Association decided in the 1970s that homosexuality was not a disease but a way of life, homosexual pride and visibility increased. This does not mean that acknowledging one's homosexuality is ever an easy process. For health care professionals it is essential to examine the nature of the coming-out process and its implications for homosexuals and their families. Only then is it possible to formulate effective strategic interventions when homosexual persons seek professional assistance.

Disclosure of one's homosexuality to parents, relatives, and friends is often a risky and difficult undertaking even though secrecy creates a painful emotional distance between homosexuals and significant others. Disapproval and rejection may take the form of withdrawal of affection and friendship. Parents who had looked forward to welcoming grandchildren may be very disappointed. Stigma continues to be attached to homosexuality, in part because stigmatizing others allows some people to feel superior and to disown any homosexual feelings of their own (O'Donnell & Bernier, 1990). Fathers seem to have greater difficulty accepting homosexuality in a son than mothers do. Difficulties develop between parents of a homosexual when each expects the spouse to act and feel in similar ways. It is not uncommon for parents to become estranged from each other upon learning of their child's homosexual orientation. The problem becomes acute when one parent is more accepting than the other or wishes to express feelings to which the other parent does not want to listen. A proper therapeutic stance is to help these distraught parents realize that each one experiences stress in different ways and employs different coping mechanisms, but neither is alone in his or her distress. There are a number of community support groups to which relatives and friends may be referred. These include such groups as Parents and Friends of Lesbians and Gays, which may be reached through community agencies or local phone directories (O'Donnell & Bernier, 1990).

Secrecy concerning one's homosexuality is designated "being in the closet," in contrast to "coming out," the phrase applied to disclosure of one's homosexuality. McWhirter and Mattison (1984) identify five steps used by male homosexuals in their revelatory process, as shown in Table 9.3.

The steps in the disclosure process are not linear, and coming out is not a one-time-only event but a continuous one. In the first step of the process, a growing awareness of sexual feelings toward persons of the same sex may be accompanied by denial and the suppression of feelings or, at times, by fantasies. In this early stage, there may be a wide and varied range. For

TABLE 9.3. Steps in the Disclosure Process of Male Homosexuals
1. Self-recognition of oneself as gay
2. Selective disclosure to others
3. Socialization with other gay people
4. Positive self-identification
5. Integration and acceptance of oneself
Source: Adapted from McWhirter and Mattison (1984).

some, self-recognition is relatively easy, but for most it is accompanied by confusion and conflict. In the second step, the response of the person or persons to whom the disclosure is made is of crucial importance. Negative reactions will undoubtedly intensify conflicted feelings and delay the coming-out process, while acceptance and support will facilitate it. The third step, socialization with other gay persons, should produce positive experiences that dilute the loneliness and isolation often felt by the emerging homosexual. Positive relationships with other homosexual persons and with close heterosexual relatives and friends lead to a positive self-image. Even in stage four, the gay person may be partly hidden "in the closet." To reach the last stage of accepting and integrating one's homosexuality into the whole personality means that an open, nondefensive outlook on sexual orientation has been achieved. As with heterosexuals, homosexual persons vary in the coping methods they choose. Some become vocal advocates for changing public and legislative attitudes toward homosexuality. Others live quietly, acknowledging their sexual preferences but avoiding a militant lifestyle.

The coming-out process of lesbians is described by Lewis (1984) in stage-specific terms. Lewis emphasizes the adolescent girl's awareness of not "fitting in" and of feeling "dissonant" as she struggles with feelings of being sexually drawn to other adolescent girls or to older women. As the young girl grows older and her erotic attraction to other women continues, she resorts to denial accompanied by feelings of anxiety, shame, guilt, and ambivalence. Her dilemma about choosing a socially approved path leading to marriage and children or embarking on a socially stigmatized road is compounded by her wish to be true to her inner feelings, even if this means giving up her genuine wish to have children. Declaring one's lesbianism remains difficult despite greater acceptance of homosexuality in general, of feminism, and of the women's liberation movement. As with gay men, lesbian women find that disclosure is a difficult decision. Having decided to make an open declaration, the homosexual person must decide whom to tell first and what to say. Another consideration shared by gay men and lesbian women is the analysis of their motives for revealing their homosexuality at a particular time and to particular people. When deciding these matters, the homosexual person should determine whether the decision is made with a desire to improve communication and intimacy or with a hostile wish to punish or exact revenge (Shernoff, 1984).

Many gay men and lesbian women seek professional help at one point or another; in counseling them, it is advantageous to help them assess their own readiness to disclose their sexual preference and to balance the pros and cons of disclosure. Here an examination of their motives may be suggested, as well as an analysis of their relationship with significant family members. If the relationship between homosexuals and their parents is distant or troubled, an initial goal might be to improve communication with parents about other aspects of the homosexual person's life. Fostering rapport with parents and strengthening family relationships helps homosexuals decide when, how, and with whom to discuss the issue of sexual orientation. The gay or lesbian client will benefit from being prepared for possible reactions from parents and others. Many parents react with shock, anger, or dismay even when the disclosure is not altogether surprising to them. Some react with disbelief and try to send the gay or lesbian person to a psychiatrist to be "fixed" or cured of homosexuality (Shernoff, 1984).

The term *passing* is used to denote a male or female homosexual who chooses to remain silent about sexual orientation. At the present time, many gay men and lesbian women who came to terms with their homosexuality during the 1930s, 1940s, and 1950s have constructed happy, satisfying lives without making a public disclosure of their sexual preferences. They have decided on this course with or without a long-term partner.

From the family's point of view, knowledge of a child's homosexuality is usually traumatic, but there has been little substantive research in this area. Bozett and Sussman (1990) note that the pain and distress of family members is similar to that experienced by homosexual persons during the coming-out process. In this comparison may lie some direction in dealing with the discrimination attached to a homosexual identity (Strommen, 1990). Upon learning that a family member is homosexual, the family, especially parents, feel guilty, blame themselves, and wonder where they failed. These negative attitudes toward homosexuality are counterproductive, and the family must be encouraged to redefine its values and stereotypes. In all probability, the family holds traditional ideas of male and female role enactment, which have never been examined or questioned until now and which are not easily relinquished. This is especially true if family beliefs are reinforced by religious convictions.

Family therapy may be a useful approach in helping gay men and lesbian women communicate with their families of origin regarding the decision to "come out of the closet." Depending on the circumstances, all or some family members may be invited to participate. Such meetings demand great skill on the part of the health professional; they should be carefully timed and attempted only by experienced family therapists.

RELATIONSHIP PATTERNS

A sample group of 979 homosexual persons was matched to a control group of heterosexual persons for comparison purposes (Bell & Weinberg, 1978). Because the subjects were volunteers, they were expected to be more open about their sexual orientation than a random sample of homosexual subjects, although there has never been a true random sample of homosexual men and women in the United States because of inherent problems in obtaining such a sample. In their study, Bell and Weinberg reported the following data. Homosexual relationships are often thought to show rigid patterns, but this was not true of this homosexual sample. Their relationship patterns were as diverse as those of the heterosexual group, with the same joys, sorrows, commitments, and breakups. Five basic homosexual relationship styles are reported, to which 71 percent of the homosexual group belonged. These are described as follows.

1. *The closed-couple relationship*: The partners are closely bound and relate in a quasi-marital style. They report fewer sexual problems, have fewer partners than other homosexuals, and report little regret over their sexual orientation. They made up the happiest, most relaxed group. This group included 28 percent of the women and 10 percent of the men in the homosexual sample.
2. *The open-couple relationship*: These couples are also quasi-marital but tend to have more partners and to report more sexual problems. They participate in more "cruising," the activity of frequenting known gay establishments in the hope of finding new sexual partners. In this group were 17 percent of the women and 18 percent of the men in the homosexual sample.
3. *The functional homosexual relationship*: These are "single" persons who have a number of partners, a high level of sexual activity, little regret about their sexual orientation, and few acknowledged sexual problems. Ten percent of the homosexual women and 15 percent of the homosexual men in the sample were in this group.
4. *The dysfunctional homosexual relationship*: Persons in this group have the most troubled psychological adjustment pattern. They are not coupled, and have a number of different sexual partners and a high level of sexual activity, along with many sexual problems. Five percent of the homosexual women and 12 percent of the men were in this group.
5. *The asexual homosexual group*: These persons are more covert than members of the other groups. They are not coupled, have few partners, and describe themselves as lonely. They exhibit lower levels of sexual drive and sexual activity than persons in the other groups. Eleven percent of the homosexual women and 16 percent of the men were in this group.

Using a less stratified model, Isay (1989) describes three kinds of gay relationships: long-term relationships that last a year or longer; short-term relationships that last from a few nights up to a year; and anonymous sexual encounters in which affection may be briefly expressed but emotional bonding does not occur. These last forms of sexual encounter usually take place in public restrooms, gay movie houses, bathhouses, gay bookstores, and video shops where booths are available. These transitory encounters serve as sexual outlets for closeted gays and for bisexual men who dread discovery, perhaps because of heterosexual marriages or conventional religious affiliations. From outward appearances, these men conform and are accepted in the heterosexual community.

The extent of a gay man's sexual activity is influenced by biological factors such as the strength of the sex drive and by opportunity for sexual expression. It is generally believed that gay men tend to be more promiscuous than gay women. Isay (1989) attributes fears of intimacy in homosexual men to avoidance of the emotional pain they experienced earlier. Fear of emotional closeness stems from the rejection and left-over anger generated in the early father–son dyad.

SEXUAL BEHAVIORS

A common misperception is that certain sexual behaviors and practices are exclusively homosexual. The reality is that homosexual persons make love in much the same fashion as heterosexuals, except that they do not engage in penis–vaginal penetration. Homosexual couples kiss, caress, and stroke each other. In descending order of frequency, homosexual males use oral sex, hand–genital manipulation, and anal intercourse. Homosexual women use hand–genital stimulation most often, followed by oral sex, and by body rubbing. Contrary to popular belief, only 2 percent of homosexuals use dildos in their lovemaking. None of the foregoing practices is exclusive to the homosexual population (Bell & Weinberg, 1978; Crooks & Bauer, 1983).

GAY MEN AND LESBIANS IN FAMILIES

Gay Men and Lesbians as Parents

Parenthood and homosexuality constitute an enigma for heterosexual society. The terms *gay father* and *lesbian mother* are paradoxical and therefore puzzling. The words *gay* and *lesbian* denote homosexuality, while the words *mother* and *father* imply heterosexuality (Bigner & Bozett, 1990; Gottman, 1990). Why, then, do homosexual men and women want to be parents, and what is the impact of their sexual orientation on the children they raise? These are complex questions that deserve serious consideration.

Gay Fathers

Gay men who are fathers belong to two subcultures, homosexual and heterosexual, and perhaps are not fully accepted in either. The gay community is oriented toward a single person's life-style, where personal freedom and autonomy are of primary importance. In contrast, fatherhood requires a long-term commitment and financial obligations, in addition to expenditures of time and energy. The relationship between a gay father and children may threaten the partnership between the father and his lover unless the father and the lover share the parenting role. The gay father may have "come out of the closet" after a heterosexual marriage into which children were born. In another scenario, the gay person may wish to become a father regardless of his homosexual prediliction. Perhaps he experienced some dissatisfaction with his homosexual life-style and felt a need to father and raise children (Bigner & Bozett, 1990).

Little is known about the subjective experience of fatherhood for gay men or about the perceptions of children who have a gay father. Bigner and Bozett (1990) report the mixed reactions of such children and emphasize several aspects of the experience. Most children seem concerned about what their peers will think about a gay father and ask whether and how to tell their friends. They also wonder if they, too, will become gay because they have a gay parent. Some are embarrassed by the situation and reject the whole idea of homosexuality. Depending on the nature of their ties to the gay parent, they may or may not reject the parent as well. One interesting study of the role enactment of gay fathers found that they were less traditional in their overall approach to parenting. They stressed paternal nurturance and gave less attention to economic providing as the primary aspect of fatherhood (Scallen, 1981). The research of Turner, Scadden, and Harris (1983) indicates that (1) the father's sexual orientation is of little importance in the total parent–child relationship; (2) most gay fathers have positive relationships with their children; and (3) gay fathers try harder to create a stable home environment and foster positive relationships than would be expected among traditional heterosexual parents.

Bigner and Bozett (1990) identify disclosure of their homosexuality to significant others as the most crucial issue faced by gay fathers. Hiding one's sexual orientation means pretense and hypocrisy toward oneself and others. Revealing it risks the loss of social acceptance, economic security, and perhaps the custody of one's children. Bozett (1980, 1984) indicates that losing a marriage is less traumatic and upsetting for gay men than losing the love of their children. Although children of a gay father may not be happy with the knowledge, they rarely repudiate or disavow him. Some suggestions are available for gay fathers contemplating disclosure to their children (Bigner & Bozett, 1990). First, the gay father should have dealt with his own feelings about his homosexuality and be comfortable with his sexual orientation. Next, the disclosure should not be impulsive but carefully planned.

In making the disclosure, the gay father should *inform*, not *confess*, and disclosure to children should take place before children know or suspect. These researchers believe that children are never too young to be told and will absorb only as much information as they can understand. Age-appropriate language should be used, and, above all, children should be reassured that their relationship with father will not change as a result of the disclosure.

Lesbian Mothers

Research on gay and lesbian parenthood is deficient in several respects. Gottman (1990) points out some limitations, including the lack of control groups, unavailability of valid and reliable measurement tools, and relatively small sample sizes. Most of the studies focus on the adjustment of younger children, although the overall adjustment of children reared by homosexual parents can be evaluated only at later stages of development, from adolescence through adulthood. Gottman differentiates gender identity from gender role, stating that "gender identity refers to the individual's experience of self as basically male or female, while gender role refers to behaviors and attitudes that society positively sanctions for members of one sex and negatively sanctions for members of the opposite sex" (p. 180). On the basis of a literature review of relevant research, Gottman concludes that no study reported negative effects on children attributable to the parent's sexual orientation. The children studied showed no problems in gender identity, sexual orientation, or social adjustment. Problematic issues in the children's growth and development stemmed more from society's rejection of homosexuality than from dysfunctional parent–child relationships. No evidence was found suggesting that daughters of lesbian mothers became homosexual themselves.

A number of legal issues have arisen concerning parenting activities of gay fathers and of lesbian mothers (Bigner & Bozett, 1990; Gottman, 1990). Often the judicial system holds that a parent's homosexuality may prove harmful to a child. Consequently, the courts have tended to deny custody to a gay father or lesbian mother. This speaks to the influence of homophobic reactions in society, which maintain that a homosexual parent is apt to molest a child sexually, that his or her partner may do so, and that a child raised in such an environment is likely to become homosexual. Bigner, Bozett, and Gottman all emphasize that homosexuality does not in itself imply pathology in the child or family, and that there is no relationship between sexual orientation and the ability to be a good parent. Rather than invoke parental sexual orientation as the primary standard in custody proceedings, courts should consider a parent's relationship with a child, the quality of home life that is provided, the ethical values that are maintained, and the child-rearing tactics that are employed.

Some lesbian women want to raise children without biologically bearing them, while others view pregnancy as a fulfillment of their identity as women. A number of options are open to lesbian women who wish to be parents. Many of them adopt children; others avail themselves of artificial insemination techniques. Frequently, a woman will marry and bear children before recognizing her homosexual orientation. When such women eventually seek divorce from a heterosexual mate, they may try to hide their sexual orientation lest disclosure jeopardize their chance of obtaining custody of children.

Gay Men and Lesbians with Heterosexual Spouses

Many gay men and lesbian women who enter heterosexual marriages are unaware of their sexual preferences at the time of the marriage. Others who are aware of their homosexual leanings may not reveal this to the prospective spouse before marriage (Bozett, 1982; Wyers, 1987). Although marriages between a heterosexual and a homosexual partner usually culminate in divorce, Auerback and Moser (1987) note that group treatment for the wives of gay or bisexual men helps the women work through the issues of a failed marriage and make some constructive changes in their own lives. Reporting on a group program for 50 women in the San Francisco area, these investigators found that none showed signs of major mental illness or of drug or alcohol abuse. The anxiety and depression displayed by the women appeared appropriate to the life stress they were experiencing. Themes dealt with in the group were anger, hurt, betrayal, homophobia, children, sexuality, and the need to receive the support of peers. The emotional climate of the group was accepting and nonjudgmental rather than blaming. Factual information was used by the leaders to reduce homophobic thinking and to resolve misconceptions. A number of wives in the study chose to remain in their marriages. Of the wives who wanted to make their marriages work, they recognized that they could not accomplish this alone, without the motivation and involvement of the husband. Those who were unwilling to continue in marriage reported that the group helped prepare them for marital separation and possible divorce.

AGING GAYS AND LESBIANS

Often overlooked is the population of aging gay men and lesbian women in society. Studies of aging and elderly people neglect this group; consequently, research studies are rare. One problem is that researchers probably find it hard to locate this group. Many of them live quietly, choose their friends carefully, and do not congregate in bars or actively participate in the gay community. Berger (1982) describes some of the problems faced by older homosexuals and offers suggestions about providing services to them. Here the focus is mostly on older male homosexuals, about whom information seems more readily available. The aging male homosexual in his sixties grew up during World War II and the McCarthy years, when sexual deviance and corruption were closely associated in the public mind. With memories of epithets like "pervert" and "sexual deviate," many older homosexual persons feel threatened by younger homosexuals who publicize their sexual orientation and make demands on society. It is not easy for older homosexual people to throw aside the deeply rooted fears that resulted from constant and burdensome psychological pressure for so many years. Berger writes, "The elderly male homosexual has always been a pathetic figure, both in the professional literature and in the popular media" (Berger, 1982, p. 237).

The older lesbian woman is often equally unhappy and lonely. Like the male homosexual, the lesbian woman is unattractive to younger persons who might become partners. In addition, the older homosexual man or woman often has lost or never developed the ability to enter or establish a supportive social group. Saghir and Robins (1973) note some differences between older gay men and lesbian women. They indicate that a youthful appearance and sexual activity are less important to homosexual women than to men. Lesbian women are therefore less concerned about aging and are more likely to continue with a partner.

On a more positive note, Berger emphasizes some strengths of older gay men who have survived in a hostile society by finding sources of mutual comfort and understanding. Many, but not all, older homosexual persons have achieved an integrated identity and a satisfying way of life despite the barriers imposed by society. They bring their coping strategies with them into old age in a society that devalues aging as well as homosexuality. Berger reports that gay men and lesbian women have less trouble dealing with the physical changes of aging because their self-concepts are less dependent on stereotypes of what is feminine and what is masculine. He further suggests that health professionals should include the following areas when working with homosexual clients: emotional needs, institutional issues (religious, occupational, political), legal issues, and medical problems. To be helpful to older homosexual clients, health professionals should become familiar with the diverse life-styles among them, the effects of discrimination on the homosexual community, the nature of identity concealment, and the extent of the client's commitment to homosexuality.

Many institutions such as hospitals and nursing homes unwittingly create problems for elderly homosexual persons. Visiting and decision making may be limited to close relatives. In such situations, a partner of many years may have no legal standing and therefore have no voice in crucial life-and-death issues. The legal system is largely designed for the heterosexual majority, although legally binding "relationship contracts" are increasingly used by homosexual couples, as are joint wills and property ownership. Sexual dysfunction is not uncommon among aging homosexuals, and counseling services need to be developed in this area. Among any sexually active group, the risk of AIDS exists, along with other sexually transmitted diseases. (Because AIDS is not restricted to homosexual persons, it is discussed in greater detail in Chapter 10, which deals with the effects of physical illness on families.) Some sex-related medical problems of gay men are pharyngeal and anal gonorrhea and anal fissures resulting from rectal penetration. The older gay man may be unaware of available procedures to diagnose and treat these conditions, or may be too embarrassed to inquire. In these instances, health care professionals need to be knowledgeable and sensitive in overcoming psychological obstacles that prevent older homosexuals from accepting methods and procedures that maintain or restore physical health.

HOMOSEXUALITY AND AIDS

Although AIDS is not confined to homosexual persons, it has far-reaching and tragic consequences in the homosexual community. Chapter 10, which deals with the effects of physical illness on families, presents demographic data on the extent of this disease among homosexual persons. As Fineberg (1988) noted:

> The AIDS epidemic exposes hidden vulnerabilities in the human condition that are both biological and social. The epidemic has touched almost all aspects of society — extends to every social institution from families, schools, and communities, to businesses, courts of law, the military, and the Federal, State, and local governments. It also has had a profound impact on the ways science, medicine, and public health are practiced in the world. (p. 128)

The prevalence of AIDS among homosexual persons has changed the tenor and direction of the gay rights movement. The loss of so many of their number to AIDS has increased the militancy of the movement. The homosexual community accuses public officials of providing too little in prevention and treatment programs. Officialdom is also accused of allocating insufficient funds for research and for withholding drugs that might help AIDS sufferers. Unjustly, AIDS has been called the "gay disease," and its presence has intensified discrimination against homosexual persons. Some opponents of homosexuality go so far as to assert that AIDS is God's punishment for an unnatural and sinful way of life. Despite increased prejudice, gay and lesbian groups have refused to abandon the political arena. Their response to the AIDS epidemic and their demands for governmental help have overshadowed other issues with which gay and lesbian persons are concerned. Such issues include legal recognition of long-term partnerships, Social Security and medical benefits, child custody, and homosexual marriages.

The crisis of AIDS has produced profound emotional and social consequences for healthy gay men. Sexual encounters for many gay men are fraught with anxiety for themselves and their partners. Although some healthy young gay men perceive themselves as potential carriers of death, others have become extremely anxious about contracting the disease (Isay, 1989). Many watch helplessly as cherished friends and lovers succumb to AIDS, and must grieve for them in a homophobic social world. As Chapter 10 indicates, the families of homosexual persons find that the threat or presence of AIDS in a loved one adds another dimension to the difficulty of acceptance and reconciliation.

Shilts (1987) cites the recommendations of former Surgeon General Koop that schoolchildren should be educated about AIDS and that the use of condoms should be advocated for sexually active persons. Koop indicates that widespread testing is impractical *unless* job protection and medical coverage can be guaranteed. According to Shilts, these recommendations have not been implemented by governmental, educational, or health care institutions.

The AIDS epidemic has contributed to division and controversy within the gay liberation movement itself. The more militant organization within the movement is the AIDS Coalition to Unleash Power (ACT-UP). A more restrained faction exists that seeks political change but decries extreme methods that may antagonize political forces that have the power to facilitate change.

When a homosexual person is diagnosed with AIDS, there follows a realization that the disease is a terminal illness. The nature of this realization is largely determined by the relationship between the ill person and the family that existed previously. When families were previously unaware of the infected person's sexual orientation, there is an additional burden of distress. Some family members may abandon the sick person, while others put their own feelings aside and are able to offer comfort as the condition of the patient declines. Another aspect of this confusing situation is the grief of other homosexuals who must witness the approaching death and see in it a reflection of their own future. A sequential model of grief resolution is offered by Lovejoy (1990), who describes four phases families experience upon learning that a member has AIDS.

- *Crisis phase*: This initial or impact phase is induced by feelings of shock, anxiety, and denial.
- *Transitional phase*: This phase occurs as families experience extreme, exaggerated fears of HIV (human immunodeficiency virus) transmission or infection, mingled with feelings of anger, depression, and guilt. In this phase, families tend to seek information and social supports. In some instances, family role enactment may be altered to meet new demands.
- *Acceptance/adjustment phase*: In this phase, families try to cope with limitations caused by the illness. Care for the person with AIDS is a

primary focus, along with planning for the future. The setting of concrete, realistic goals helps immeasureably in this phase.

- *Anticipatory mourning and bereavement*: During this final phase, the ill person and the family prepare themselves for eventual loss through death. This is the period during which unfinished emotional issues are addressed. The ill person approaching death may express desires surrounding his care and the disposition of possessions. For surviving family members and friends, the grieving process may continue for many months, even years.*

THERAPEUTIC GUIDELINES

Homophobia is widespread in Western society, and much of it is unconscious. Therefore, an early task of a health professional working with gay and lesbian clients is to examine his or her own attitudes and biases in this emotionally charged area. It is essential for health professionals to communicate that being homosexual is acceptable. Many gay and lesbian persons are not themselves accepting of their own sexual orientation and are very conflicted. Not only do they feel that something is wrong with them, but they feel alienated and different from most other people. The question is often asked by homosexual and by heterosexual persons alike as to whether a nonhomosexual therapist can work effectively with gay or lesbian clients. In the NASW *Practice Digest* (1984), a known practicing lesbian therapist working in a homosexual counseling program, says that heterosexual therapists who have worked through their feelings about homosexuality can be helpful to homosexual clients dealing with generic or family issues. If a homosexual client wants help with sexual issues or with the decision to "come out," a gay or lesbian therapist is more likely to be helpful. Moreover, health professionals who work with homosexual clients should become acquainted with the gay and lesbian culture and resources in general and in the specific locality. By learning about available resources, the health professional can refer homosexual clients to nonjudgmental priests, ministers, and rabbis, as well as to physicians and lawyers who are sympathetic and supportive (NASW *Practice Digest*, 1984).

A valuable set of rules for health professionals working with homosexual clients is provided in the *Practice Digest* by Whiting who also decries the lack of homosexual support groups and organizations in small towns or rural areas.

Source: Adapted from "AIDS: Impact on Gay Men's Homosexual and Heterosexual Families" by Nancy C. Lovejoy, in *Homosexuality and Family Relations*, edited by Frederick W. Bozett and Marvin B. Sussman, pages 285–316, copyright © 1990 by The Haworth Press, New York.

RULES FOR WORKING WITH HOMOSEXUAL CLIENTS*

1. If you are uncomfortable working with homosexual clients, do not work with them. Sometimes the best thing to do for a client is to make a referral to another therapist. Then examine and, if necessary, seek help in dealing with your own feelings of discomfort. Develop awareness of homophobic reactions or stereotyped views that you may have. Develop awareness and comfortable acceptance of any homosexual feelings you may have that you may not recognize as sexual in nature.

2. Never establish a contract with a person who wants you to change his or her sexual orientation. Research shows that this goal is rarely achieved. Work instead to change the client's attitude about being homosexual. Ask clients what exactly they don't like about being gay. More often than not, clients are distressed not so much by their homosexuality per se as by the obligation to conceal their sexual preference.

3. Help clients recognize the actual prejudice and biases that exist, especially in nonmetropolitan areas. Homosexual persons do suffer threats of job loss and housing discrimination and must not be considered paranoid if they are fearful and suspicious.

4. Recognize the great stress homosexual persons experience beyond the usual life pressures of heterosexuals. Regardless of the circumstances, homosexual persons must constantly monitor themselves, change pronouns when alluding to their private lives, make choices about whom to trust and whom to distrust. They repeatedly ask themselves what will happen if this person or that person guesses the undisclosed secret. These concerns affect all homosexual persons to some extent, but are especially trying for those who live in inhospitable surroundings.

5. Discuss the stereotypes, misconceptions, and negative images that homosexual clients have concerning their own sexual orientation. Help clients discover the source of these negative images and correct them.

6. Be aware that many homosexual persons may be depressed. They expend a great deal of energy just to survive. In trying to shut off painful feelings, they shut off joyful feelings as well. They need encouragement in recognizing and expressing feelings of joy and happiness, and of pain and anger as well.

7. Become familiar with sources of assistance at the local, state, and national levels. The National Gay Task Force (NGTF) is a rich resource of information, distributing guidelines for starting self-help groups, news items, and a directory of services available in towns and cities throughout the United States. Included in the directory are counseling agencies, bookstores, coffeehouses, and religious organizations. Write to NGTF, 80 Fifth Avenue, New York, NY 10003, or call (212) 741–5800.

*Source: Adapted from NASW Practice Digest (1984).

Families are usually distressed upon learning of a friend's or relative's homosexuality, and this is heightened by their ignorance about what it means to be homosexual. Two helpful books are *Now That You Know: What Every Parent Should Know about Homosexuality* (Fairchild & Hayward, 1979), and *A Family Matter: A Parent's Guide to Homosexuality* (Silverstein, 1978). Finally, education of the public at large about homosexuality merits ongoing attention. Customs and beliefs about sexuality and sexual activity change at different rates in different places, and the extent of change varies from one family to another. Legislation can protect some of the civil and political rights of homosexual persons, but attitudes cannot be changed by legislative decree. Only an informed, more openminded society can lighten the onus felt by so many gay men and lesbian women. In this effort, health professionals can play a significant role.

CLINICAL EXAMPLE

Assessment

Jon was a 28–year-old gay man who requested professional help from an urban mental health center because of depression. In the course of the initial interviews, he revealed that he was gay and really wanted help with how to tell his family. There were a lot of social and family pressures for him to marry and "settle down," and he felt they "had to know sooner or later." Jon had been aware of his erotic feelings for other males since age 14 or 15, when he was in high school, and he had been very upset about them, thinking there was "something basically wrong with me." He had participated in some mutual masturbatory behavior with other adolescent boys but had never told anyone. He had thought this was "normal" behavior. He had allowed himself to be persuaded to have anal intercourse by an older college student when he was 18, and then he was sure he was "abnormal." His sexual daydreams and fantasies about other men persisted, as did his wish for sexual activity with other men. While in college, he had had a series of sexual encounters with men but never developed a lasting relationship. He became more and more ashamed and guilty. He began to participate in body-building exercises, weight lifting, so he could become strong and muscular, in the hope that then "no one would even know." He had dated a few girls, but as soon as they "got romantic," he broke it off. One of the girls to whom he had become somewhat close had accused him of "being a queer" and had recently stopped seeing him. After this, he became quite depressed, had difficulty sleeping and eating, and was filled with self-loathing and remorse. The girlfriend's comment was actually the precipitating event for the call for help.

Jon came from a middle-class family in a small midwestern town. His family subsequently moved to a suburb of the large northeastern city where he now lived. He attended college in an eastern city and graduated with a B.A. degree in French language and literature. He was slight in stature, quite shy, and made few friends. He held a job as a translator for a small publishing company. He had spent two summers in France while in college, working as a cook and kitchen helper in a small hotel in the Loire Valley. In his family of origin, Jon was the third of four children; he had an older brother and sister and a younger sister. All had college educations, and all were married but Jon and the younger sister, who had recently become engaged. His father was a bank vice-president, and his mother taught math in a suburban high school. Jon described his parents as "strict but generous," and said his family were "fairly close but didn't talk much together." His best relationship was with his older sister. He felt closer to his mother than to his father, but he knew his father "respected" his language skills. As a child he had been close to his father until his younger sister was born when he was four. He recalled how he felt abandoned by his father at that time, since the father devoted all his time to his younger sister. His mother kept asking him whether he had a steady girl and just shook her head when he kept saying "no." He hated to go home because his mother would invite various young daughters (his age) of family friends over for dinner, which made him quite uncomfortable. He liked to go on fishing trips with his dad, and the last time they went together, he had almost broached the subject of his being gay, but "just couldn't get it out."

Planning

The mental health professional assigned to work with Jon was an older male social worker who was not gay, but who had taken workshops on working with gay men. He and Jon established good rapport. Jon's mood lifted somewhat after talking with a nonjudgmental person about his homosexuality, and he commented how relieved he felt about being open and honest for the first time about his true feelings. He was, however, quite anxious about disapproval and rejection of others, and in general he felt sad about his life. He was very concerned about hurting or disappointing his parents. Because of his persistent depressive affect, he was seen by a psychiatrist to evaluate whether antidepressant medication was indicated. It was agreed that it was not indicated for now, since Jon was eating and sleeping better, did not show any negative signs of a more serious depression, and had responded so well to the initial therapeutic encounter. After the initial assessment was completed, it was recommended that Jon and the individual therapist continue to meet weekly, with the possibility of a family meeting at a future date, should Jon wish this. Should Jon and the family be seen together, it could then be evaluated whether further family therapy sessions would be useful. Depending on how the family responded, a referral to a supportive or educational group for them could be considered.

Implementation

As Jon felt more comfortable in the individual therapy, he brought up the subject of approaching his family, and the therapist made it clear this was Jon's decision only when he was ready. Jon decided he was not ready and wanted to focus more on establishing better communication with his parents. He had thought he might tell his older sister first about his homosexuality, so that perhaps she could help when he told his parents and other siblings. Family meetings were offered to aid in this process, when Jon felt ready. He did want the individual sessions to continue.

In six months, through his therapy sessions and with an expanded social life, Jon's option of eventually "coming out" to other gay men had given him a greater sense of self-worth, and his self-esteem increased. Eight months after he first entered the mental health clinic, Jon had developed an intimate relationship with another gay man about his age, who had majored in Spanish studies in college and had lived in Spain. They shared many interests and decided to move in together. It was at this point Jon felt strong enough to share with his family information about his new life-style. He had already talked with his older sister, who was neither shocked nor surprised and who proved to be supportive. He felt on a more comfortable footing with his parents after he had initiated a discussion with them about his career goal of working at the United Nations as an interpreter/translator. They had been enthusiastic and supportive. Jon admitted he was "too scared" to take the "big step" alone and disclose to his parents that he was gay. Therefore, he asked his therapist to meet with him, his older sister, and his parents. He felt more comfortable breaking the news in this setting, where he knew both he and his parents could get some support. He was sure they would ask a lot of questions he would not be able to answer, such as, "What causes a person to be homosexual?" "How is it cured?" "How should they (his parents and family) treat him?" Most of all, Jon feared his parents would blame themselves and feel they had failed. His mother would probably cry, and his father would be very intellectual and would probably say Jon "would get over it with some treatment with a good psychiatrist."

The day of the conjoint appointment found the therapist anxious also — about what would happen and whether he would be able to help the parents hear Jon's desperate need for their acceptance and affection. The goals for the family meeting were to identify conflicting feelings of Jon and of his parents and to clarify that Jon's sexual preference was not attributed to any parental failure or deficiency, nor was it a rejection of the heterosexual relationship of his parents.

In spite of some initial anxiety and stiffness at the beginning of the interview with Jon, his sister, and his parents, the session, which lasted for two hours, went well. Jon was near tears as he spoke of his sadness and his wish not to disappoint or hurt his parents. The sister sat by Jon and touched his arm on several occasions. The therapist encouraged them to talk to each other and was sensitive to the father's early discomfort. He asked the father about his interest in fishing, commenting Jon had told him how much he had enjoyed their fishing trips as a child. After this discussion, the father became noticeably more comfortable. Neither of the parents was shocked at the information about Jon's homosexuality; the mother said she had "suspected" it for some time. True to Jon's prediction, the parents tended to blame themselves and asked where they had "gone wrong." In contrast to Jon's fears, the mother did not cry, and the father did not become overly intellectual. The father did appear to be visibly upset and disappointed and said that he "hoped Jon would get over this phase and marry and have children someday." He did seem open to learning more about homosexuality, and both parents readily accepted a referral to a support group for families and friends. The sister proved to be a major support and a strong link between Jon and the parents. She said she and her husband had gay male friends with whom they were close, and she expressed her concern for the pain Jon had "silently" suffered through the years. As they left, the mother reached out to Jon with affection. She invited him and his live-in friend for dinner the following week. The father looked sad and withdrawn. He hesitantly shook the therapist's hand at the door of the office. Another family meeting was planned for a month later, to which the father responded, "I'm glad we're going to meet again." Clearly, the family meeting had a strong impact on the participants, and the father (if not all) had become aware that there were many more feelings to express and ideas and questions to discuss.

Evaluation

Jon established a strong therapeutic alliance with his therapist, and this, plus his motivation to make some changes in his life, helped him in his painful psychological work over many months. Not all persons so distressed work as hard as he did, and not all families are so caring and open to help. Jon was able to become more comfortable himself with being gay and to have some relationships with other gay men. Although it was stressful, the initial family interview and those that followed opened new doors in Jon's relationship with his parents and, later, with his other siblings. He was unwilling or unable to break ties with his parents, and it was hoped that the positive aspects of their relationship could be reinforced as time progressed. There were other crossroads to meet and other hard decisions to make, and Jon knew he could not depend on therapists forever. His newly gained self-confidence helped him to feel he would not need therapy forever.

The therapist recognized the disquieting nature of a father's distress at having a son who does not choose to follow his father's masculine identity and role. The therapist also was sensitive to the guilt and painful feelings of all parents who visit a mental health professional's office about problems with their child—problems that they cannot identify easily, understand, or rectify. It was important, therefore, for the therapist to reach out to the parents and particularly to the father early on, to demonstrate that he (the therapist) was not there to judge or condemn. The therapist also gave Jon plenty of time to decide about having the family meeting. To push prematurely for such a conjoint family session might have been disastrous, and Jon might have fled treatment. The therapist knew as well that deeply felt emotions were only partially expressed in the first meeting and that further work with the family was needed.

In conclusion, the more Jon could experience that he is a likable and lovable human being, the more able he could be to risk letting other people see him and know him as a whole person. The sexual orientation is only one part of the whole person, and Jon, like all homosexuals, needs to be accepted as a *whole* human being.

SUMMARY

This chapter has reviewed homosexuality, its patterns, and its variations. It has described attitudes toward same-sex behavior, beginning with the countries in the ancient world (Greece, Egypt, Rome, etc.) where it was accepted and fostered. In the modern Western world, homosexuality was banned and viewed as a mental illness, although Alfred Kinsey's research in 1948 and 1953 showed that millions of Americans (both men and women) had engaged in homosexual activities at one time or another. In this country, prejudice and discrimination against homosexual persons has developed to an alarming degree, and is called homophobia. It is defined as a strong, irrational fear of homosexuality and is felt to be exacerbated by the fear of homosexual urges within oneself. In our culture, men appear to be more overtly homophobic than women and seem to hold to more rigid gender role stereotypes and to avoid role enactment that might be considered less than masculine. Myths about homosexuality are plentiful, and ten of these are mentioned.

The Wolfenden Report in the 1950s in Great Britain proved to be a milestone in promoting a more liberal attitude and legalizing homosexual behaviors in Britain and some European countries. Today in the United States discrimination continues, and homosexual persons are deprived of their civil rights in issues of housing and employment, credit, insurance coverage, child custody, and adoption. Some aspects of homophobia are present in religious institutions as well, and many families of homosexual persons who struggle with their disappointment and confusion are not able to find understanding and comfort in their church. Unitarians show the greatest tolerance for homosexual behavior, as do the United Church of

Christ, some branches of the Episcopalian denomination, and some congregations of the Reform Jewish faith.

The search for a sexual identity is a complex and not thoroughly understood process. *Coming out* is the process of declaring oneself a homosexual, and this disclosure is seen as often a painful process because of the homosexual person's fear of prejudice and discrimination. *Passing* means that a homosexual person's sexual orientation is kept "in the closet."

Relationship patterns of homosexuals are described from two points of view: 1) five basic styles, described by Bell and Weinberg's study in 1978, and 2) Isay's description in 1989 of a less stratified model, which includes three kinds of gay relationships. A certain misperception is that certain sexual behaviors and practices are exclusively homosexual, but studies have shown that no sexual practice or behavior is exclusive to the homosexual population.

Gay men and lesbians in families are discussed, with the focus on gays and lesbians as parents, and on those with heterosexual spouses. Parenthood and homosexuality are an enigma for heterosexual society. Homosexual persons are in parental roles either because they have been in a marriage that produced children or because they have been able to adopt children. Little is known about the subjective experience of parenthood for either gay men or lesbians, or about the perceptions of children who have a homosexual parent. Some research shows that although children of a gay father may not be happy with that knowledge, they rarely repudiate or reject him. The studies of Bigner and Bozett (1990) reveal that disclosure to children of a parent's homosexual identity should be carefully planned and viewed as an informing process rather than a confession. It should take place only when the homosexual parent is comfortable with his or her homosexual orientation. More research needs to be done in the area of homosexuals as parents.

The aging gay and lesbian population is often overlooked, and research studies here are few, as well. Many older homosexuals, who grew up in the 1940s through the 1960s when sexual deviance and corruption were closely associated in the public mind, feel threatened by younger homosexuals who publicize their sexual orientation and make demands on society. Some research with older homosexuals reveals some differences between older gay men and lesbians. A youthful appearance and sexual activity are less important to homosexual women than to men, and they are more likely to continue with a partner.

The occurrence of AIDS, which has reached epidemic proportions, has far-reaching and tragic consequences for homosexuals. Prejudice and discrimination have intensified. The prevalence of AIDS has changed the tenor and direction of the gay rights movement; some homosexuals have become more militant, demanding more governmental support for AIDS research. The crisis of AIDS has produced profound emotional and social consequences for healthy gay men. The crisis has also stirred the public to press for education in the schools about AIDS and sexual behavior.

REFERENCES

American Psychiatric Association. (1987). *Diagnostic and Statistical Manual of Mental Disorders*, 3rd edition, revised. Washington, DC: Author.

Auerback, S., & Moser, C. (1987). "Groups for the Wives of Gay and Bisexual Men." *Social Work*, 32(4): 321–325.

Bell, A., & Weinberg, M. (1978). *Homosexualities*. New York: Simon and Schuster.

Berger, R. M. (1982). "The Unseen Minority: Older Gays and Lesbians." *Social Work*, 27(3): 236–242.

Bergler, E. (1956). *Homosexuality: Disease or Way of Life?* New York: Collier Books.

Bigner, J. J., & Bozett, F. W. (1990). "Parenting by Gay Fathers." In F. W. Bozett & M. B. Sussman (Eds.), *Homosexuality and Family Relations*. New York: Haworth Press.

Bozett, F. W. (1989). "Gay Fathers: How and Why They Disclose Their Homosexuality to Their Children." *Family Relations*, 29: 173–179.

Bozett, F. W. (1982). "Heterogenous Couples in Heterosexual Marriages: Gay Men and Straight Women." *Journal of Marital and Family Therapy*, 8(1): 81–89.

Bozett, F. W. (1984). "Parenting Concerns of Gay Fathers." *Topics in Clinical Nursing*, 6: 60–71.

Bozett, F. W., & Sussman, M. B. (Eds.). (1990). *Homosexuality and Family Relations*. New York: Haworth Press.

Carrera, M. (1981). *Sex*. New York: Crown Publishers.

Clark, J. M., Brown, J. C., & Hochstein, L. M. (1990). "Institutional Religion and Gay/Lesbian Oppression." In F. W. Bozett & M.B. Sussman (Eds.), *Homosexuality and Family Relations* (pp. 265–284). New York: Haworth Press.

Crooks, R., & Bauer, K. (1983). *Our Sexuality*. Menlo Park, CA: Benjamin/Cummings.

"Reform Jews Expected to Ordain Gay Rabbis." (1990). *Democrat and Chronicle*, Rochester, New York, June 25.

Fairchild, B., & Hayward, N. (1979). *Now That You Know: What Every Parent Should Know about Homosexuality*. New York: Harcourt Brace Jovanovich.

Fineberg, H. V. (1988). "The Social Dimensions of AIDS." *Scientific American*, October.

Gottman, J. S. (1990). "Children of Gay and Lesbian Parents." In F. W. Bozett & M. B. Sussman (Eds.), *Homosexuality and Family Relations*. New York: Haworth Press.

Gramick, J. (1983). "Homophobia: A New Challenge." *Social Work*, 28(2): 137–141.

Isay, R. A. (1989). *Being Homosexual: Gay Men and Their Development*. New York: Farrar, Straus, & Giroux.

Katchadourian, H. A., & Lunde, D. T. (1972). *Fundamentals of Human Sexuality*. New York: Holt, Rinehart and Winston.

Kinsey, A., et al. (1948). *Sexual Behavior in the Human Male*. Philadelphia: W. B. Saunders.

Kinsey, A., et al. (1953). *Sexual Behavior in the Human Female*. Philadelphia: W. B. Saunders.

Lewis, L. A. (1984). "The Coming-Out Process for Lesbians: Integrating a Stable Identity." *Social Work*, 29(5): 464–469.

Lovejoy, N. C. (1990). "AIDS: Impact on Gay Men's Homosexual and Heterosexual Families." In F. W. Bozett & M. B. Sussman (Eds.), *Homosexuality and Family Relations* (pp. 285–316). New York: Haworth Press.

McWhirter, D. P., & Mattison, A. M. (1984). *The Male Couple: How Relationships Develop*. Englewood Cliffs, NJ: Prentice-Hall.

Mead, M. (1973). "Bisexuality: What's It All About?" *Redbook Magazine*, January 1.

NASW *Practice Digest*. (1984). "Working with Gay and Lesbian Clients," 7(1).

O'Donnell, T. G., & Bernier, S. L. (1990). "Parents as Caregivers: When a Son Has AIDS." *Journal of Psychosocial Nursing and Mental Health*, 28(6): 14–17.

Saghir, M. T., & Robins, E. (1973). *Male and Female Homosexuality: A Comprehensive Investigation*. Baltimore, MD: Williams & Wilkins.

Scallen, R. M. (1981). "An Investigation of Paternal Attitudes and Behaviors in Homosexual and Heterosexual Fathers." *Dissertation Abstracts International*, 42, 3809-B.

Shernoff, M. J. (1984). "Family Therapy for Gay and Lesbian Clients." *Social Work*, 29(4): 393–396.

Shilts, R. (1987). *And the Band Played On: Politics, People and the AIDS Epidemic*. New York: Viking Penguin.

Silverstein, C. (1978). *A Family Matter: A Parent's Guide to Homosexuality*. New York: McGraw-Hill.

Strommen, E. F. (1990). "Hidden Branches and Growing Pains: Homosexuality and the Family Tree." In F.W. Bozett & M.B. Sussman (Eds.), *Homosexuality and Family Relations* (pp. 9–34). New York: Haworth Press.

"The 21st Century Family." (1990). *Newsweek Magazine*, Special Edition, Winter–Spring.

Turner, P. H., Scadden, L., & Harris, M. B. (1983). "Parenting in Gay and Lesbian Families." Paper presented at the Future of Parenting Symposium, Chicago.

Wyers, N. L. (1987). "Homosexuality in the Family: Lesbian and Gay Spouses." *Social Work*, 32(2): 143–148.

PART
FIVE

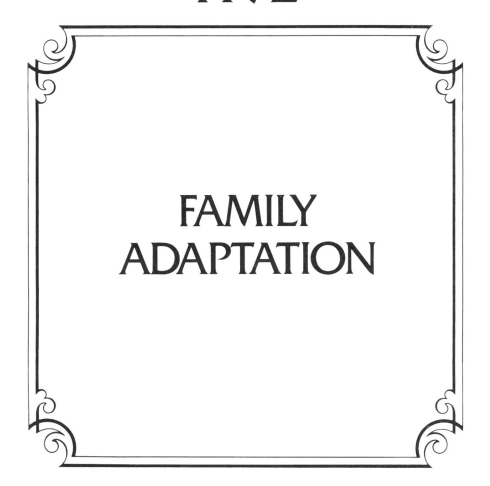

FAMILY ADAPTATION

CHAPTER TEN

Physical Illness in the Family

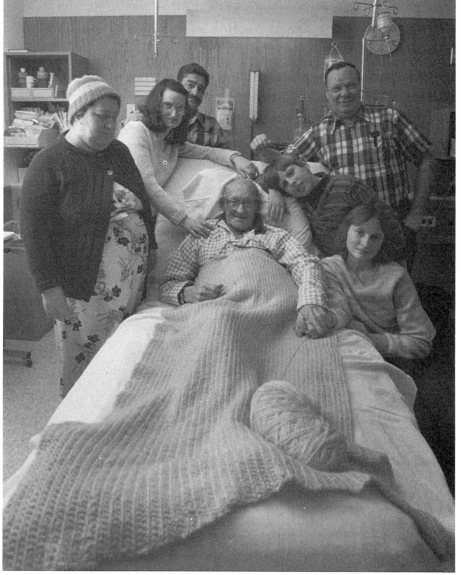

© Frank Siteman MCMLXXXIII

All any of us can do, my friend, whether we're sick or well, is to live one day at a time.

Claire Safran

The customary behavior patterns of families are drastically changed, permanently or temporarily, by the illness of any member. Because families are interdependent systems, changes introduced by illness are reflected in the role performance not only of the person who is ill but of those who are well. Every family deals with illness in a special way, revealing its strengths and weaknesses and employing its own methods of coping with new demands. The effectiveness of family responses to illness depends largely on habits and attitudes already present, on socioeconomic circumstances, on psychological resources, and on cultural attitudes toward health and illness. Family coping is also influenced by the identity of the member who is ill and by the life stages of the family and its members. The prognosis of the illness and its likely duration and course are other factors affecting a family's response to illness.

Ours is an age that searches for connections between cause and effect. In part this is due to our desire to control a world that is often inexplicable and unmanageable. We look for answers that help us understand the mystery of who gets sick, and why or when. There is nothing intrinsically wrong in this, but definitive answers are elusive. It is true that our wish to understand and control what happens to us may persuade us to adopt wholesome health practices. The other side of the coin is that when good health is lost, there may follow the suggestion that the person is responsible for the impairment. Many, perhaps most, illnesses have a psychological component. There are persons who claim that virtually all ailments can be averted through a wholesome life-style and that illness, when it occurs, can be influenced constructively through self-directed psychological channels. Without evaluating the validity of such beliefs, it may be said that total reliance on them can add to the suffering of ill persons and further complicate conflicted family feelings. Thus, it is dysfunctional for health professionals to add to the concern of family members and of the patient by suggesting in any way that they somehow caused the illness.

Early in our lives we learn to feel responsible for getting sick or causing someone else to get sick. There are few adults who cannot recall being told by mother that they wouldn't have caught cold if they had come home earlier, worn overshoes, or whatever. So the habit of attributing illness to certain behaviors is fostered quite early. Of course, many forms of behavior do contribute to ailments and illness. Smoking, alcohol abuse, and intravenous drug use are among the undisputed contributors to illness. But the time to call attention to unhealthy and self-destructive actions is *when* the behavior is manifested, not *after* painful symptoms arrive. Once illness occurs, regardless of its origin, blaming the patient or the family is counterproductive. The patient does not need the additional burden of self-recrimination, and families are less able to cope if energies are dissipated by feeling guilty. Cognitive acknowledgment of contributing causes is permissible but should be promptly put aside in dealing with the current situation (Lerner, 1985; Wechsler, 1990).

LEVELS OF PHYSICAL ILLNESS

Based on duration, course, and prognosis, there are three general levels of illness: acute, chronic, and terminal. Within these levels are overlapping and transitional phases, for many illnesses exist at different levels at different times. Depending on their nature, illnesses may be characterized by recovery, remission, stabilization, crisis, recurrence, and deterioration, and sometimes death. Acute illness is apt to be sudden in onset and to impair individuals for a while, after which they usually recover their previous functioning. Chronic illness tends to be less predictable. There may be times of recovery or remission followed by relapse, so that the person suffers or is incapacitated for many years. Some chronic illnesses such as diabetes can be stabilized; others, such as rheumatoid arthritis, tend to be progressively debilitating. There is no fixed progression from one level of illness to another, nor are the levels impassible frontiers. An acute illness may become chronic or terminal; a chronic illness may enter an acute phase, improve, or reach a terminal state. As the levels of an illness change, the behavior and attitudes of patient and family alter responsively.

The value of delineating three levels of illness is in assisting assessments made by health care professionals. The outcome of an acute illness depends chiefly on the medical treatment that is instituted. The outcome of a chronic illness depends more on combined measures undertaken by the patient, the family, health professionals, and the community. Chronic illness requires sound medical treatment, but ongoing responsibility for nursing, nutrition, and maintenance falls heavily on the patient and the family. When chronic illness deteriorates into terminal illness, the family may be somewhat prepared, having already learned to deal with chronicity.

Frequently, however, a chronic condition that becomes terminal may have already depleted family energy and resources. Such exhaustion is experienced by many families dealing with the chronic illness of a loved one for many years before the onset of terminal conditions. Acute illness mobilizes many families in a positive way, especially if a favorable outcome is expected, but chronic and terminal illnesses are another matter.

It was Talcott Parsons (1951) who clearly described the privileges and obligations that accompany the "sick role." Whenever a person becomes ill, that individual is exempt from certain responsibilities. Sick people have the right to receive care, but they also have an obligation to accept help, to cooperate, and to try to recover. Persons with disorders such as alcoholism may be rejected by the family because they do not accept the sick role obligation of accepting help and trying to recover. There are several psychiatric conditions in which the identified patient seems to defy the obligation to get help and follow a recommended treatment plan. Parsons also states that the sick role imposes some passivity on the patient because freedom from responsibilities may lead to less autonomy and decision-making power. The concept of the sick role illuminates some differences between acute and chronic illness. In acute illness followed by recovery, the sick role is enacted for a while but eventually discarded. Victims of chronic illness can seldom relinquish the sick role completely, and this necessitates permanent shifts and realignments in family life.

Family Consequences of Acute Illness

How an illness is discovered or recognized influences the way it is handled by the family. When an illness comes without warning, changing an apparently healthy person into a sick one, most families rise to the occasion. Sudden, serious illness cannot be easily denied or ignored. The urgency of the situation establishes priorities: (1) Obtain medical care immediately; (2) reassign family functions in order to carry out essential tasks; and (3) reassure, support, and assist the sick person. Most of the practical problems attending acute illness are solved within a few days. Transportation, housekeeping, and other responsibilities are delegated to family members or helpful friends. When the patient is out of danger and beginning to convalesce, family members and health care professionals may become cheerleaders, telling the patient how lucky he is to be getting better and how grateful he should be. The convalescent patient may not feel lucky at all. Even with recovery in the offing, acute illness gives patients a wrenching sense of how fragile life is. Norris (1990) describes the bewilderment felt by recovering patients who ask, "Why did I survive when other people die from this disease? What was I saved for? What can I do to pay back the debt of life? . . . Why did this happen to me? What did I do to deserve it? What is the meaning of illness? What purpose does it serve?" (p. 47).

For various reasons, patients are being discharged early from hospitals and sent home to recover. This means that families who have never witnessed a convalescence are now being asked to participate. Most of them need help in caring for someone who is getting stronger physically but seems to be experiencing emotional turmoil. The physical and psychological effects of acute illness are likely to cause patients to react strongly to minor disappointments and mishaps. The health professional involved in the situation should discourage a family's unrealistic expectation that the recovering patient will be happy and appreciative. Often the convalescent period ushers in an existential crisis for the patient, to which the family should be sensitive. Families feel relieved when a patient is mending and may become intolerant of moodiness and irritability. They need to know that in addition to physical restoration, convalescence is used by many patients to (1) allow time to redefine the meaning of life, (2) provide opportunity to reassess lifetime goals, and (3) discover more satisfying paths to fulfillment and self-actualization (Norris, 1990). The mood swings, anger, and restlessness of convalescing patients take a toll on family members. In an early article, Van Kaam (1959) describes the in-between, hovering state of mind in which many convalescents find themselves. Sick people confined to their room listen to household noises as family members come and go, and they see themselves as outsiders, exiles, with no part to play in everyday life. They feel a great distance between themselves and the life going on outside their room. Even their well-meaning visitors who bring news of the outside world merely accentuate their feelings of isolation.

There is a great deal that health professionals can do for families during the recovery period. First, they can interpret the behaviors of the patient and of family members in ways that defuse the tensions between them. It is helpful to guide patient and family members to a cognitive, rational understanding of events that have occurred and of what may be expected in the future. Families need to know that it may not always be possible for them to keep the patient cheerful and contented no matter how hard they try. Fostering open communication between the patient and family members can be done by modeling active listening and by indicating that convalescence is a complex process made easier if patient and family members try to share their viewpoints with each other.

An illness that previously existed but gradually becomes acute presents different problems. If the illness was present for weeks, months, or years before becoming acute, strong feelings of regret or anger may surface. Family members who believe they could have done more feel guilty; their anger or bitterness may be directed at the patient or other family members for not taking more steps to avoid deterioration. Thus, many forms of acute illness are exacerbated by feelings derived from earlier, chronic phases. A wife may feel that her husband knew he had a chronic condition but did not have enough regard for his family to take care of himself. An ill husband may justify failure to take care of himself by citing family responsibilities or his wife's indifference to his health. Each spouse may blame the other for the worsening illness, or they may blame themselves. In some respects this is a control measure. Feeling powerless at present, they comfort themselves by insisting that somehow conditions were preventable. Meanwhile, the children react with fear and confusion to changes in the family and the realization that their parents are mortal.

Family Consequences of Chronic Illness

Chronic illness includes all conditions that necessitate prolonged treatment, supervision, observation, or care. In chronic illness the sick role is more or less permanent, and the illness is marked by residual disability and pathological change. Constant, ongoing adjustment is demanded of the person who is chronically ill. Neither acutely sick nor completely well, the chronically ill person lives with uncertainty and ambiguity. Griffin (1980) enumerates some of the problems accompanying chronic illness. These include (1) avoiding medical crises and dealing with them when they occur, (2) controlling symptoms and preserving the quality of life, (3) arranging and coordinating treatment modes, and (4) coping with recurrent patterns and developments of the illness.

Like all levels of illness, chronic illness requires sacrifices from the family on behalf of the patient. When illness is chronic, the sacrifices are not temporary but become a family way of life. One or more family members frequently become expert on the particular illness affecting one of their number, and their expertise provides reliable data for health care professionals in attendance.

During the acute stage of an illness, the patient tends to be preoccupied with life-and-death issues. This preoccupation lessens as conditions become chronic. After patients realize that they will probably survive, they take notice of the damage that has been done. Most persons with progressive disorders or impairment of a body part have great difficulty reconciling themselves to changes in body image. At times the family is more accepting of the altered soma than the patient is, and this is beneficial even though the patient continues to express self-loathing. In other instances family members are more shocked and unaccepting than the patient. This is difficult for the patient and poses a serious challenge for health professionals striving to alleviate the family's dismay while strengthening the patient's shattered self-image. The woman who has a colostomy, for example, must come to terms with a greatly altered body image. First comes the knowledge that cancer cells have invaded her body, with terrible results. Then comes the unending job of handling an abdominal orifice from which odorous fecal material seeps. In the hospital the woman was probably aided by matter-of-fact nurses who were competent and gentle in their ministrations. Only after the patient goes home does the enormity of her situation intrude. If family members have participated in teaching sessions and prepared for what is needed, the patient is less likely to feel that she is repulsive. But even with family involvement, negative feelings may prevail. Norris (1990) notes that many spouses of colostomy patients never see the stoma, and some who do react initially by showing signs of disgust that may include fainting or vomiting.

As early hospital discharges continue, many families are being expected to offer assistance in the home. Even when family members are willing to participate in home care, sick people dread being a burden or arousing disgust in others. Dreading rejection, they may appear to reject those who love them. This apparent rejection distances family members and may be self-perpetuating. To alter mutual withdrawal, individual counseling for the patient, family meetings, and support group referrals may be indicated. Home care for chronically ill persons is a formidable endeavor, and families require practical and emotional help. Chronic patients must cope with their own distressing reactions; it is too much to expect them to reach out for acceptance. And it is too much to expect families to respond positively to illness and abnormality unless they are prepared for the responsibility they must assume and have access to support services.

There are time limits to both acute illness and terminal illness, but this is less true of chronic ailments. Management of chronic illness should be shared among family members, with the patient participating as much as possible. Dependent patients with little control of their own lives may be easier to care for in some ways, but families pay a price when they take complete charge of persons who are capable of some autonomy. The ill person should do as much self-care as possible, and families should be encouraged to set reasonable limits on their own performance. This ultimately benefits everyone, for relatives who are not worn out are less apt to grow resentful. Respite for primary caretakers is essential, and conscientious family members need not feel guilty for taking care of themselves. When they take time away from the patient, they may feel like deserters, and the patient may sometimes complain of being abandoned. An appropriate response is for the family members to acknowledge the reactions of the patient, but not to the extent of giving up their own plans. Rest and diversion for the caretakers should be included as a matter of course in long-range plans for home care.

Family Consequences of Terminal Illness

Terminal illness is defined by its resolution, namely the death of the person who is ill. As with most levels of illness, the onset of terminal illness may be abrupt or gradual. Realization of terminal illness arrives when denial is no longer possible and the truth must be faced. The impact of this realization is so great that the family reacts with shock and cannot deal with practical matters until their shock lessens. The essential element that affects everyone involved is that regardless of the efforts being made, the patient will not recover. In terminal illness, emotional support extended to family members may be the most crucial factor of all.

Some theorists believe that terminally ill people pass through a sequence of stages before accepting the inevitable. The most well known model is that of Kübler-Ross (1969), who believes that the diagnosis of terminal illness is initially denied by the patient. Later, as the implications of the diagnosis are realized, the patient becomes angry. Anger is directed at God or destiny for permitting the illness. There is anger toward health professionals who cannot produce a cure, and even toward family members because they are not sick. At such times family members need help in responding to the patient's anger, and health professionals who are targets may need help as well. As anger subsides, the patient begins to bargain for an extension of life. Promises are made to God, to favorite saints, and to family members in exchange for a few more years of life. When bargaining proves fruitless, despair follows. This may take the form of depression or detachment from family members. The patient may express a desire for death and an end to suffering. Finally, for some but not all patients, acceptance is reached. Sometimes patients consciously choose to make the most of whatever time is left, and draw closer to loved ones. Some terminally ill people, frail and in pain, nevertheless have the spiritual and emotional strength to make what our grandparents called a "good" death. After accepting the inevitability of death, some patients enter a period of withdrawal and remoteness that families find hard to bear. This may stem from failing strength, but it may also represent an effort by patients to prepare themselves and their families for their departure. Withdrawal by the patient may cause family members to draw closer to one another and to look for comfort within the family system. In such instances the dying person may be offering one final gift.

Families of terminally ill people may undergo stages similar to those of the patient. After experiencing shock and denial, they may begin to hope that the patient will die so that the ordeal will be over. They may have fantasies of dying with the patient rather than suffer separation, and they may feel anger for being abandoned. These confusing reactions add to the family's grief and inhibit their ability to help the patient. A therapeutic intervention is to assure family members that they are not unique, evil, or self-serving and that their feelings are normal in the circumstances.

During the last days or weeks of a terminal illness, health professionals can act as linkages between family and patient, explaining, interpreting, and comforting. Activities of the family should be directed not toward cure but toward easing the patient's discomfort. If the patient's suffering is alleviated, the pain of the family also lessens. Even terminally ill patients give indications as to what they want from the family and other caregivers. As far as possible, cues given by the patient should be respected. Any messages or requests should be granted, if possible. One dying, elderly man from another culture asked his nurses to remove his mattress from the bed and place it on the floor. With proper regard for cleanliness, this was done, whereupon family members quietly squatted on the floor around the dying patriarch. A few members of the hospital staff were offended, but the contentment on the face of the old man showed how much it meant to him to die not in a bed but on a pallet with the faces of his loved ones close by, just as his forefathers had done.

Implicit in the emphasis on comfort rather than recovery is realization by health professionals and by families of the dying that death is not unnatural but part of the human condition. Eakes (1990) cautions health professionals to structure relationships with families of the dying to avoid being overinvolved and "consumed" by the situation. Health professionals who become too involved lose their objectivity and encourage dependence on themselves rather than interdependence among family members. When they do too much for families, they may enjoy gratifying expressions of appreciation, but they impair a family's capacity to function. Families that become very dependent avoid accomplishing tasks of which they are capable. After the death they may blame themselves for relying on others instead of taking a more active role. From the first therapeutic encounter, a partnership should be established that gives family members as much responsibility as they can manage. Involving them is one way to guide them from futile curative measures to comfort-increasing measures on behalf of the patient. When families make this transition, they find solace in realizing what they can do for their loved one as death nears (Rando, 1984; Weizman & Kaam, 1985). In addition, activity at this time often reduces the anxiety. Another reason for encouraging participation and independence in these families is that the professional relationship is time-limited, since it generally ends soon after the death occurs. If the health care professional has become indispensible during the dying process, it is more difficult for the family to resume taking charge. Family members who have been making decisions and participating all along are less likely to be distracted and overwhelmed at the end. Health care professionals can make themselves available and give necessary help, while trying to promote self-sufficiency in family members. Always there are some members so distraught that they are almost useless. Even so, there are usually one or two members self-possessed enough to take charge for a while and function as family executives.

Witnessing terminal illness at close range makes enormous demands, as many health workers can attest. Very few of us can confront death and remain untouched. The imminent death of another human being brings us face to face with our own mortality. Sontag (1978) states that "Death is the obscene mystery, the ultimate affront, the thing that cannot be controlled" (p. 55). Death evokes dark images of dissolution, decay, and finality to which people react in strange, unexpected ways. Small wonder, then, that the approaching death of a family member brings out the best and the worst in us.

CLINICAL VIGNETTE: RESPONSES TO ACUTE ILLNESS IN A CHILD-REARING FAMILY

Stuart Mills, married and the father of three school-age children suffered a heart attack while watching television in his own home. He was rushed to a hospital and admitted to the intensive care unit. The reaction of Lou, his 34-year-old wife, and his children was shock and disbelief. In many ways, the family's reaction paralleled that of Stuart. Because the family had ample insurance and Stuart had job security, money worries did not intrude. The initial phase of Stuart's illness focused on his medical treatment. Drugs, monitoring, and good nursing care stabilized his condition. After a few worried days, it became evident that Stuart would recover. Lou and the children became more cheerful, but Stuart continued to be anxious and depressed even after being transferred from intensive care. Because the heart may recover more rapidly than the psyche of patients suffering a heart attack, the predictability of this reaction was explained to Stuart and his wife. This eased the tension that had arisen between the two, but the unit social worker arranged several counseling sessions for the couple.

In the sessions Lou was encouraged to listen as Stuart tried to express his feelings about getting sick and his fears for the future. Accustomed to discharging the role of family provider and primary decision maker, Stuart keenly felt the loss of autonomy and executive functions. He was concerned about returning to work and very apprehensive about having a second heart attack. He felt that his wife was overreacting to his illness and resented her constant surveillance and attention. The hospital staff had already observed Lou's excessive involvement in her husband's care and her tendency to treat him like a child. During the sessions and on the hospital unit Lou was encouraged to give Stuart more independence. Efforts were made to keep Lou informed of his progress but a clear message was relayed that compliance was Stuart's responsibility and that most decisions about his care could be left to him. With role modeling and suggestions from the health care professionals, Lou was able to find a balance between solicitude for her husband and dominating him. Their three children were invited to attend one family session, which was used to help them reach a better understanding of recent events, explain their parents' distress, and reassure them about the immediate future.

Two themes emerged in the counseling sessions and became the basis of certain goals that the couple accepted. One theme was that Stuart, despite his illness, was a rational, competent man with the capacity to direct his own recovery; a goal was established that Lou would recognize this and restore her husband's autonomy. The second theme was that Stuart's illness had introduced a new dimension into family life that could not be denied; a goal was established that Stuart would permit himself a certain amount of dependency and would accept some assistance from his wife and children, who wanted so much to help. The protective actions of his family were interpreted to Stuart as signs of their affection, not as threats to his autonomy or masculinity. The onset of his illness threatened Stuart's self-image. When his wife and children rose to the occasion, Stuart perceived this as an additional threat. In counseling sessions, Lou was able to express her love and gratitude to her husband who had provided so well for his family "in sickness and in health." Her acknowledgment reinforced the strength of the family system and reduced Stuart's feelings of being diminished. Lou began to understand her husband's reaction to role shifts in the family and was actually relieved when Stuart reasserted himself and resumed his accustomed performance in the marital/parental dyad. Predischarge counseling lowered tension levels in the family and enabled Stuart to get on with the work of recovery and resumption of a relatively normal life.

THE AIDS PATIENT AND FAMILY ISSUES

The AIDS epidemic is a challenge for the health care system and a greater challenge for friends and relatives who must stand by and watch the inroads of the illness. AIDS, regardless of other considerations such as sexual preferences or transmission modes, is probably the most urgent public health problem today. Projections are that by the end of 1992 more than 365,000 Americans will be diagnosed with AIDS, and the annual death toll will exceed 170,000. With about 1.5 million Americans affected with the human immunodeficiency virus (HIV) that causes AIDS, the Public Health Service predicts that 20 to 30 percent of these people will contract the disease within five years (Leukefeld, 1989). In the absence of effective medical treatment for AIDS, psychosocial and family interventions are extremely important. The disease is one that encompasses acute episodes, chronicity, and deterioration leading to untimely death. Prospects for AIDS patients are not hopeful at present, and as their condition deteriorates they are overwhelmed by pain and fear. For the homosexual person afflicted with AIDS, suffering is intensified by social and emotional issues involving families and lovers that have not been fully resolved.

The most effective weapon against AIDS at the present time is prevention. Most persons who are HIV-positive are apparently well and do not know they are infected. Health professionals should be familiar with the following recommendations and impress them upon clients who are at risk (U.S. Public Health Reports, 1988).

- Individuals should not have sexual relations with persons having AIDS or belonging to any group at risk for contracting AIDS.
- Individuals should not have sex with multiple partners or with anyone who has multiple partners.
- Individuals with AIDS or at risk for contracting AIDS should not give blood.

- Extreme care should be exercised by health workers handling or disposing of hypodermic needles and syringes.
- Individuals should not use intravenous drugs. If they persist in intravenous drug use, needles and syringes should not be shared.
- Women who use intravenous drugs or have sexual relations with a partner belonging to a high-risk group should avoid pregnancy because of transmission of AIDS to the unborn.

Persons suffering from AIDS, their families and their loved ones, need a wide range of services, not all of which are available across the country (Chaches, 1987).

- *Housing:* Misconceptions about contagion and transmission modes make it difficult for persons with AIDS to obtain adequate housing.
- *Finances:* Costs of treatment for AIDS are staggering. Jobs are lost; insurance benefits are exhausted; impoverishment is added to the indignities of the disease.
- *Home care:* Persons with advanced AIDS are likely to be hospitalized three or more times within the space of a year. Between hospitalizations home care services are essential, especially if no hospice or voluntary caretaker is available.
- *Child care and foster care:* Mothers with AIDS and mothers of children with AIDS need child care in order to obtain treatment. Temporary foster care may be needed when the mother is hospitalized; permanent foster care may be needed when the mother dies.
- *Legal advice:* Decisions about child custody, power of attorney, and wills are expedited through legal assistance.
- *Medical care:* Different treatments are needed at different points in the illness. Coordinating treatment plans is necessary. A health care professional coordinating treatment should also take responsibility for explaining and humanizing procedures as much as possible.
- *Public education:* The person with AIDS, friends and relatives, and the general public deserve accurate information about AIDS with emphasis on prevention measures.

AIDS is no respecter of persons; it afflicts men, women, and children, heterosexuals, bisexuals, and homosexuals. It is the homosexual person with AIDS, however, who seems the victim of a special kind of torment. Even when the family of a homosexual person has become reconciled to the sexual orientation, the diagnosis of AIDS seems to open old scars. In addition, there is the widespread stigma engendered by the behaviors of certain high-risk groups, such as drug addiction, promiscuity, and prostitution (Newman & Taylor, 1987). Wallach (1989) reports that physicians and nurses are not immune to anxieties about homosexuality, and that these anxieties are exacerbated by the AIDS epidemic. AIDS at present is an incurable disease that primarily attacks young people. The age of the patients operates to break down the psychological defenses of health professionals who are not able to prevent death. Fear of contagion adds to their anxiety, causing some of them to avoid or neglect these patients. Wallach notes that minority health care providers seem more troubled about the contagiousness of AIDS, more distrustful about information on risk and safety, and more uneasy when dealing with homosexual patients. The data suggest a need for educational programs designed for health care professionals educated abroad and now practicing in the United States.

The deterioration, physical and emotional, produced by AIDS leads to regression in the patient and in family members as well. One consequence of AIDS is the reemergence of parents as caregivers to their adult child who is so gravely ill. In their dilemma, parents look for someone or something to blame. They may blame themselves in some way for being poor parents who caused the life-style that led to the illness. At the same time they may blame the patient for putting himself in danger. AIDS differs from other disorders in that it brings into the open actions that parents may want to keep secret. O'Donnell and Bernier (1990) explain that relationships between homosexuals and their parents may have been troubled for years before the onset of AIDS. Even when parents tried to be understanding, there may have been little contact between them and their homosexual son or daughter. The diagnosis of AIDS is sometimes a catalyst that does not greatly change parental attitudes but may change parental behavior. For example, a son who has become accustomed to his parents' remoteness may find them overly solicitous as they try to compensate for previous behavior. This naturally requires readjustment on the part of the ill person and any partner with whom he is involved.

The homosexual person with AIDS must deal with the reality of a fatal illness. Parents must deal with the reality of AIDS in their son, but also with a resurgence of feelings about his homosexuality. Parents of a homosexual child with AIDS may find it hard to tell others of the diagnosis. Some parents continue to be ashamed and angry, even when others are sympathetic and accepting. Even with these negative feelings, parents may become very protective of their son and defiant toward society. If they have avoided meeting any of their son's companions until now, they may have to encounter their son's lover for the first time. Occasionally the mother of the person with AIDS and the son's lover see each other as rivals for the affection of the patient, replicating the competing posture of a parent and a son- or daughter-in-law. Fathers are less likely than mothers to become involved in giving direct care, but they too are beset with grief and ambivalence. In the natural order of things parents do not expect their children to die first, and the early death of a child is terrible to contemplate. Ideally, parents will rally and join with their son's lover in caring for the patient. When parents permit the lover to share their grief and their decisions, their own isolation is reduced. As they come to accept and respect their son's lover, they gain more respect for their dying son and for the meaningful relationships in his life (Newman & Taylor, 1987).

Parental reactions to a son with AIDS are varied. Kübler-Ross (1987) writes that between 1984 and 1986 about half the mothers of AIDS-stricken sons actively cared for them and a third of the fathers in her sample were also involved. In many cases the mothers relocated to distant cities to be more available. Because AIDS is progressively debilitating, patients become increasingly helpless. However, steps should be taken to give patients whatever decision-making and self-care activities they can handle. Family conferences that include parents, the daughter or son's partner, the patient, and other supportive companions should take place at frequent intervals. The objective of meetings need not be specific, but they should offer opportunities to share concerns and promote problem solving. A health care professional who is coordinating the patient's care may be the person best suited to arrange these meetings and introduce supportive and networking groups to assist the patient, parents, and the primary partner through this tumultuous time.

Not every health professional is capable of giving AIDS patients the compassion they so much need. If health professionals are to make valid contributions to the care of AIDS patients and their families, they must recognize in themselves any limitations and negativism that are detrimental. Leukefeld (1989) lists a number of useful considerations for practitioners:

- It is possible to establish rewarding and mutually beneficial relationships with persons who have AIDS.
- Working with an AIDS patient is very demanding, and burnout is a constant threat. Access to professional reference groups, support groups, and AIDS network groups can be a sustaining force.
- Practitioners should avoid excessive self-sacrifice and martyrdom. They should take care of their own needs and maintain interests in activities and diversions unconnected with their professional life.
- Practitioners should examine their feelings about AIDS and death and familiarize themselves with literature on AIDS and on death and dying. They should expect to experience feelings of despair and futility at times, even as they try to maintain a balanced sense of reality.
- Practitioners should not become the sole care providers of a person with AIDS. They should share responsibilities with others in order to avoid feelings of isolation and engulfment.
- Practitioners should take an active part in reducing prejudice and ignorance about AIDS. They should try to eradicate boundaries and limits regarding the allocation and distribution of services to persons with AIDS.

CLINICAL VIGNETTE: HIGH-RISK BEHAVIORS
IN AN HIV-POSITIVE MALE

Clinical and legal experts face problems in the management of HIV-positive persons who continue to engage in high-risk activities. Some states have passed *noncompliant carrier statutes* aimed at protecting the public. Unlike other statutes that mandate reporting of activities such as child abuse, these regulations make reporting discretionary. As a result, a clinical and legal impasse exists (Carlson, Greeman & McClellan, 1989).

Tyler Green, a 25-year-old drug user, was found to be HIV-positive. He learned this from a community-based program that guaranteed anonymity but offered no posttest counseling for those with positive results. Two of Tyler's close friends had recently died of AIDS, and he was very upset by the test results. Following a serious suicide attempt, he was admitted to the psychiatric wing of a midwestern urban hospital. His presenting symptoms were drug addiction, depression related to his HIV-positive status, and the suicide attempt. Other issues related to his life-style as a prostitute, his sexual liaisons with two partners who had died of AIDS, and his belief that he, too, would soon get sick. He also admitted a pattern of deliberately trying to infect other people to get back at whoever had passed the infection to him. He was unwilling to remain long in the hospital or to accept residential care. A hospital psychiatrist sought legal advice from local officials but was told there were insufficient grounds for involuntary commitment. Authorities did advise hospital staff to make reasonable efforts to notify persons at risk in the community.

Efforts were made to discharge Tyler to a halfway house where he would receive some supervision and his behavior would be monitored. No suitable facility in the area was willing to accept him because hospital staff could not guarantee that Tyler would remain drug-free and sexually inactive after leaving the hospital. He had a sister living in the neighborhood who had visited him a few times while he was hospitalized. Family meetings were arranged with the hope that Tyler could live with his sister and her husband. At first she was willing, but when she learned that Tyler was HIV-positive she reported that her husband and mother-in-law would not let her take Tyler in, and insisted that she not see her brother again.

Failing to find a place for Tyler with relatives or in a halfway house, hospital staff tried to persuade him to enter an inpatient drug dependency program. They hoped that treatment for his drug addiction would lead to his giving up the prostitution he engaged in to support his habit. Before arrangements were concluded, Tyler signed himself out of the hospital to live with a male friend who was a known drug user. Tyler and his friend had previously attended an outpatient drug program where they were known to share syringes and needles. Following the state regulation concerning HIV-positive status, hospital personnel notified the health department. Public health officials tried unsuccessfully to discover where Tyler was living. Neither he nor his roommate was enrolled in any drug program, and there was concern that Tyler would continue his drug abuse and sexual prostitution. Some eight months after Tyler's disappearance, he was brought by police to the emergency department of a city hospital. It was determined by clinical staff that he had died of an intentional or unintentional drug overdose.

The case of Tyler exemplifies the multiple problems connected to his care. Aftercare programs considered him unsuitable because he was HIV-positive and an unrehabilitated prostitute and drug user. Staff members at community programs felt compelled to protect their own somewhat vulnerable clientele. The regulation in force recommended reporting his HIV status but did not contain measures to enforce compliance on Tyler. It is also possible that personnel of aftercare programs feared contagion for themselves as well as their clients. Clearly, state regulations and community resources were inadequate in this situation.

ROLE FACTORS IN ILLNESS

When a parent becomes ill, there are two overriding considerations that are interdependent. One consideration is role performance; the second relates to the life stage of the family and of the person who is ill. Many present-day families depend on the earnings of both parents in order to make ends meet, and the illness of either causes financial problems. Still, in most families it is the husband and father who is the primary provider. Therefore, it is father's illness that is apt to have the most pronounced financial effects. If he is incapacitated for a lengthy period, will the family be able to live on a reduced income? If so, for how long? What can be expected in the form of insurance or unemployment compensation? What effect will a prolonged illness have on savings? On outlays for a new car or vacation? What will happen to teenagers' plans for college? If it is a nonworking mother who gets sick, the financial strains may be less, but arrangements must be made to take care of her and the children so that the father can continue to work. There may be less financial pressure when mother is the patient, but her illness deprives the family of a source of nurture and care. When mother is ill, members of the extended family may join the household to "help out," and this in itself may cause contention in the family. It can safely be said that father's illness leads to financial disorganization and mother's to emotional disorganization.

Every aspect of family life undergoes change when a parent falls ill. To make up for the lost income of an ill husband, a wife may have to find employment outside the home or work longer hours if she is already employed. Children find themselves giving up free time because they are expected to do more at home. Older sons may perform home maintenance tasks once done by father. If mother is working long hours or attending to father, children are assigned jobs as house cleaners, cooks, and babysitters, with different jobs apportioned among them. The same reorganization of family tasks takes place when mother is the patient and father must depend on the children to keep the household functioning. Leventhal, Leventhal, and Van Nguyen (1985) warn that role confusion may follow the redistribution of family assignments, when this is carried to extreme lengths. The danger is not in the delegation of chores but in the new patterns of emotional responses that may result. By trying to shield the patient from the stressful details of everyday life, the well parent and the children may unknowingly exclude the patient from meaningful aspects of family life. For many parents, accustomed to being at the hub of the household, this exclusion further erodes their lowered self-esteem and aggravates their feelings of uselessness. Some patients react by becoming depressed, by disengaging from family life, while others antagonize hard-working family members by trying to reassert their authority. None of these reactions contributes to harmonious family life.

When the patient begins to recover, the return to prior role performance may prove neither easy nor simple. During the illness of a husband and father, other family members may have moved in the direction of freedom and autonomy that they are reluctant to give up later on. Without an able-bodied husband to lean on, mother may have become a more active disciplinarian and household manager. Children who have been performing more tasks in the household may now be less docile and tractable. As a result, the recovering patient may believe that his importance to the family has diminished, and feel more disappointed than grateful that the family has gotten along so well without him. Concepts that may aid the family at this point include role realignment, role competence, and role ambiguity. At the onset of illness in a parent, it was necessary for the family to engage in role realignment to take care of family tasks usually done by the patient. Role realignment proceeded because family members extended themselves and became more or less competent in performing new tasks. With the patient improving, role ambiguity develops. Every family member, especially the patient, has memories of previous role performance in the family when everyone was well. These memories, combined with recognition of roles as they are now performed, creates uncertainty and unclear expectations in the family. It is unrealistic for family members to pretend that role shifts have not taken place, but these should be labeled contributions made by the family on behalf of someone they loved. Role changes were motivated not by a desire to usurp the functions of the person who was ill, but by a wish to speed the recovery process. At first, the patient can be told in all honesty that the role competence shown by family members is a sign of regard for the patient, and that any role ambiguity that continues to distress the patient can be negotiated after recovery is complete. Sharing rather than shielding a recovering patient from routine household matters can be therapeutic.

If an illness is followed by full recovery, role shifts are rarely a serious problem. When recovery is incomplete, when illness becomes chronic, or when there is a possibility of recurrence, it may not be possible to return to former role organization. Uncertainty about the future may cause a wife to continue her dominance in the family, a husband to tolerate role ambiguity, and children to act in ways that are not age-appropriate. Unhappily, the illness of a parent makes many families think in all-or-nothing terms. The patient is thought to be either wholly sick or wholly well. The illness is not perceived as a process on a continuum. Such absolutism perpetuates role ambiguity and impedes patients' attempts to rejoin family life. Illness and wellness are better viewed as gradations or matters of degree. It is not easy for families to accept additional duties, but they may deny feeling tired. Sometimes, reluctance to restore role functions to a recovering parent is a way to deny feelings of exhaustion. During the early phase of a parent's illness it may not have been possible to reorder roles in a sensible, equitable way. Desire of all family members to perform well may sustain a family for a while but be impractical on a permanent basis. When family circumstances are less critical, members can give time to resolving role conflicts. Families that respond well to the illness of a parent have shown themselves capable of role flexibility and role realignment when necessary.

LIFE STAGE FACTORS IN ILLNESS

In family illness there are a number of chronological or temporal considerations arising from life stage factors. Family obligations change over the years; young families in the child-rearing or launching stages have different reactions from those of older families when illness strikes. The life stage of the family and of the person who is ill affect the perceptions of various members regarding the implications of the illness. Leventhal, Leventhal, and Van Nguyen (1985) compare family reactions to cancer in an 80-year-old woman and family reactions to cancer in the mother of young children. Although the older woman may be well loved and her illness may distress her family, the quality of grief will be different from that felt for a young woman whose husband and children are dependent on her. The middle-aged children of the older woman will grieve, but they probably have attachments to their own children that will mitigate their sorrow to some extent. If the mother of the stricken young woman is alive and well, she will question the meaning of her daughter's untimely fate. In the early childbearing and child-rearing stages of family life, parents are immersed in responsibility. During the launching stage, the physical demands on parents may be less but financial and career challenges continue. Thus, illness that develops in relatively young parents can be particularly disruptive to the family system. Illness never comes at a convenient time, and the impact on older families can also be heavy. Because life stage issues are crucial in family assessment and planning, they offer a focus for health professionals trying to lighten the worries of patients and their relatives.

Burish and Bradley (1983) indicate that illness that is untimely, in the sense of being unusual at a particular life stage, tends to generate great anger in patients and family members. Emotional distress and bitterness are more common among younger patients with serious illness than among older ones. They believe that becoming ill is unfair, and their feelings of injustice are generalized to the people around them, including caretakers and the health care system. Frequently they expect others to share their anger, and are disappointed by responses that are reasonable rather than emotional. When anger and resentment are discharged to family members or to health professionals, the target persons may protect themselves by disengaging to avoid confrontation (Leventhal, Leventhal, & Nguyen, 1985). A more therapeutic strategy is not to become defensive of either oneself or the health care system, but to respond to understandable anger and discouragement. Expressing acceptance and understanding of negative feelings can be done without taking sides and does not negate the client's right to feel as he or she does.

In contrast to younger people who fall ill, older patients try to monitor the intensity of their reactions. This sometimes causes them to avoid being rebellious and to substitute a narrow range of feelings, such as resignation or passivity. The emotions felt by older patients may be intense, but they are sustained by a sense of completion of the life cycle. Emotional responses to illness displayed by families at a later life stage usually revolve around different issues. Adult children contemplating the approaching death of a parent may have strong feelings about who is the favorite child and who is the outcast. Sibling animosity may surface, and left-over feelings from childhood may be dredged up again. If there is an estate to be disposed of, an adult child who has devoted years to a patient's care may fear being replaced by a less responsible but charming sibling (Silverstone & Hyman, 1982).

ETHICAL ISSUES IN ILLNESS

When a person is terminally ill or so impaired that the quality of life is doubtful, some hard decisions must be made. If the ill person has previously written his preferences regarding heroic measures, these will be honored. If there is no record of the patient's preferences about life-sustaining measures but he remains capable of making decisions for himself, his expressed wishes will be honored. Sometimes, however, there is no way of knowing a patient's wishes because the ability to make decisions has been eroded by illness or accident. Ascertaining a patient's decision-making ability should be neither capricious or unilateral but should follow the outlined policy of the care facility.

Depending on the physical condition and the age of the patient, family members may want to withhold or terminate heroic treatment, including life support systems. Often the question of treatment is decided by the family in collaboration with the primary professional care provider. Usually the primary care provider is a physician, but input from other professionals working with the patient is part of the decision-making process. When health care professionals believe that legal repercussions may follow the withholding or termination of treatment, the decision may be left to the courts. Even when there is no fear of legal consequences, health care professionals may regard failure to offer treatment or termination of treatment as betrayal of their professional or personal code of ethics.

The Supreme Court ruling that states could compel hospitals to sustain life in a comatose person against the family's expressed desire has activated ethics committees of hospitals throughout the nation. Hospitals are becoming more aggressive in arranging for patients to sign "living wills," which are advance directives to be used if a patient becomes irreversibly ill and is unable to express a treatment preference (Lewin, 1990). Living wills are also useful for persons who wish all possible forms of medical treatment to be used to prolong their lives, even if an irreversible condition is present. An alternative to the living will is the appointment of a trusted friend or relative who may act as a proxy or surrogate in making treatment decisions when the patient is no longer able to do so. In some states a friend or relative to whom power of attorney has been delegated is permitted to make treatment decisions. The Patient Self-Determination Act passed by Congress requires hospitals and nursing homes to ask whether patients have a living will or a health care surrogate. The legislation was effective December 1991.

Lewin (1990) reports the findings of a study concerning patients' right to die that reveal considerable gender bias. The sample consists of 22 cases involving patients who were mentally competent before an illness but had no written instructions regarding treatment. In such instances courts of law try to construe the patient's preferences by means of values and sentiments previously manifested in their lives. In cases involving women, the courts said they were unable to construe the patient's preferences on life support measures in 12 out of 14 cases. In cases involving male patients, the courts refused to construe the patient's preferences in only 2 out of 8 cases. Throughout the court reports, female patients are referred to by their first name and male patients by their last name. Also, the comments of a 31-year-old woman on life support measures are characterized as "offhand remarks made by a patient when young." The comments of a 33-year-old man on life support are described as "deeply held" and "showing solemn, intelligent determination" (p. A-13).

Health care professionals, lawyers, and ethicists discuss the relative usefulness of a living will and the appointment of surrogates, with many of them recommending both. A living will does not help a patient who cannot instruct caregivers on the whereabouts of such a document and is no longer able to make a competent judgment. A previously appointed surrogate would know the location of the living will and presumably be cognizant of the patient's wishes in the matter. In the absence of a living will or a surrogate, certain considerations should prevail. The first is the patient's well-being, meaning the probable benefits of the treatment to the patient. Unless the treatment is likely to produce physiological benefits, there is no obligation to undertake it unless psychological benefits are likely to ensue. The second consideration is the patient's right to make decisions on her own behalf. Some but not all patients are capable of this. For those who lack this capacity, the health care professional who is functioning as the primary care provider may name a surrogate. The surrogate may be one person or several relatives and friends. If only one surrogate is named, that person should not be an isolate but someone willing to consult with other friends and relatives. If this proves difficult because of family disagreements, a surrogate may be appointed by the courts.

When decisions on life-sustaining treatments are being made, more than the surrogate and health care professionals are likely to be involved. An institutional review should precede implementation of life-and-death decisions. A consensus exists that it is ethically better to provide treatment and withdraw it if it fails, rather than not initiate it at all. If health care professionals who are not the primary care providers object to treatment decisions made by the patient and/or the surrogate for reasons of conscience, they are not obligated to implement the treatment. These health care professionals should ask to withdraw from the case, and the request should be granted. If the objector is the primary care provider, he or she should inform the patient or surrogate of the reasons for objecting and discuss any viable options. If a compromise cannot be reached, or an alternative care provider or facility cannot be found, an institutional or judicial review may be necessary.

Conditions where patients can no longer make their own decisions are extreme, but they do happen. Judicial reviews should be a last resort because they take matters out of the hands of families and the health care professions, and the judgments may not be in the best interests of everyone concerned. A great amount of distress can be avoided if adults in good health record in writing their treatment preferences. In the absence of the so-called living wills, the next recourse is the appointment of a surrogate or group of surrogates to make life-and-death decisions with the advice and consent of the health care professionals who are involved.

FAMILY CONSEQUENCES OF A CHILD'S ILLNESS

Advances in medical science have lowered the incidence of acute illnesses in children, and transformed some terminal disorders into chronic ones. Before insulin was discovered in 1922, diabetic children had an ominous future. Until antibiotics were developed, children with cystic fibrosis lived only a very few years. Despite progress, the number of serious illnesses still affecting children is overwhelming. Johnson (1985) reports that 7 to 10 percent of children in the United States have a serious disorder, and this group constitutes 50 percent of pediatric practice. The following partial list of long-term childhood disorders is a solemn reminder of progress not yet made.

- Disorders due to chromosomal defects: Downs' syndrome, Klinefelter's syndrome, Turner's syndrome
- Disorders due to hereditary factors: sickle cell anemia, hemophilia, cystic fibrosis, muscular dystrophy, diabetes mellitus; congenital malformations such as club foot, spina bifida, cleft palate, deafness, blindness
- Disorders due to unfavorable uterine factors: congenital syphilis, rubella; damage from radiation, various drugs, prenatal hypoxia, and blood incompatibilities
- Disorders due to traumatic perinatal events: neurological and motor damage
- Disorders caused by infections, trauma, and neoplasms during the postnatal period or childhood: meningitis, encephalitis, tuberculosis, rheumatic fever, renal disease, leukemia, convulsive disorders, mental illness or mental retardation of organic origin

Chronic childhood disorders take a toll on the child, the parents, and siblings as well. Although some generalizations are made in this chapter, chronic illness is by no means a single entity, as the foregoing list indicates. The chronicity of these illnesses is the common feature that makes generalization possible. It should be kept in mind, however, that different illnesses make different demands on the family, and that families find their own ways of responding.

Consequences to the Child

First of all, no child can manage a serious illness without family and professional assistance. Parents often receive glib advice about involving the child in managing the illness, without understanding how much involvement a child can accept and at what age. LaGreca, Follansbee, and Skyler (1982) stress the value of matching responsibility to a child's capacity, and report that among diabetic children disease stabilization was related to high levels of maternal knowledge. Among preadolescent children greater management responsibility of the child was associated with poor control. The implication here is that responsibility may be inadvisable for young children, and that self-injection and urine testing should be goals for late childhood and adolescence. Naturally, the cognitive and emotional abilities of children improve over time. Therefore, parents should be encouraged to relinquish management tasks gradually unless the severity of the illness and the status of the child preclude this. Even after a child's self-management skills improve, parents should be prepared to observe and monitor progress regularly.

Children with a chronic disorder have lives quite different from those of their peers. If they can attend school, they are frequently absent. If they require frequent hospitalizations, they endure separations from home and family. Often their disability is so severe that they cannot attend the same school as their brothers and sisters. When they attend a special school or are tutored at home, they are left out of neighborhood activities. Most of them are very lonely, and the normal developmental tasks of childhood and adolescence are especially hard to achieve. They see other children enjoying friendships and an active social life, while their world is more restricted. Usually the relationship between mother and the sick child is very intense, and this also may become conflict-ridden as the two struggle with dependency and separation issues.

Children with chronic illness are often ambivalent about their own health. They yearn to be like other children, but the solicitude and attention they receive may compensate for other losses. Matus (1981) suggests that some asthmatic children may deliberately forget to take medication or choose an activity that brings on an attack. They may use their illness to get things they want, and come to rely on being the center of family attention. Parental attitudes toward the child and the illness may have reciprocal elements. For example, the overly concerned, overly protective mother may relay her fears to the child through words and actions. Johnson (1985) reports that diabetic children whose mothers are rigid and authoritarian in connection with the illness replicate these maternal attitudes. Johnson further notes that marital discord, overprotective or overcontrolling parents, low parental self-esteem, and high parental anxiety all contribute to the poor adjustment of children with chronic illness. Many parents of impaired children adopt an active directing manner to stimulate the responses of the child. This excessive parental directiveness may be ultimately unproductive because it reinforces passivity and inattentiveness in the children, perhaps reducing their willingness to initiate interaction.

In some families, the needs and limitations of the sick child rule the household and take precedence over the needs of other family members. Preoccupation with the impaired child may represent parents' attempts to compensate for the child's deficiencies, but it is likely to inhibit the child's mental and emotional growth. Some parents are so intent on making up for the child's handicap that they see only the deficits and ignore the potential. Grey, Genel, and Taborlane (1980) report that parents of children with stabilized diabetes engaged in the following behaviors:

- They encouraged independence in their children.
- They encouraged free expression of feelings in the family.

- They maintained low levels of conflict in the environment.
- They showed cohesiveness in family transactions.

In an investigation of the coping responses of disabled children, Zeitlin and Williamson (1990) find a wide range of coping styles, ranging from consistently effective to consistently ineffective. For the most part the coping strategies of disabled children were determined by the immediate situation. The children seldom generalized effective behavior and applied it to future situations. Their coping behaviors were erratic, inflexible, and restricted. The directiveness used by many parents of disabled children may be due in part to the children's failure to adapt coping measures from one situation to another. The reluctance of many disabled children to engage in spontaneous, self-directed interaction may reflect their limitations but also may be a function of structured, parent-directed interactions (Dunst, Cushing, & Vance, 1985).

Consequences to Parents

The birth of a child is usually a happy event even when the parents were not overjoyed at the prospect. This is not the case when a flawed child is born, for bringing an ill, handicapped, or disabled child into the world is one of the most heartbreaking events parents ever face. Because the situation is so frightening, many parents at first cannot accept the diagnosis. Even when they have been told the facts, they hold on to the hope that things are not as bad as they seem. Depending on the reactions of the parents, planning sessions should begin immediately at which feelings can be expressed and the search for solutions can begin. Moos (1977) suggests that the baby be brought in the room as parents are first told, and held or touched by the health professionals who are present. This gives parents the message that their child needs and deserves human contact. Often parents do not know what to tell their relatives or children at home and will need help with this. The focus of health professionals should be on the family as well as the child, since the problem is a family one. As the meaning of the diagnosis is realized, parents and child embark on a medical odyssey that is often doomed to failure. They go from one treatment center to another looking for a miracle. When the miracle is withheld, they return home again and again with their sick child, having spent time and money that they could not afford.

When a child has multiple problems or when treatment can only prolong the child's suffering, parents and health professionals face the legal and ethical dilemma of deciding to withhold or institute heroic measures. The 1984 Child Abuse and Neglect Prevention and Treatment Act provides some guidelines. The act states that withholding "medically indicated" procedures from a child is a form of abuse and neglect. Exceptions are made for (1) infants who are irreversibly comatose, (2) infants for whom treatment would merely prolong dying without correcting the life-threatening conditions or ensuring the infant's survival, and (3) infants for whom treatment is futile and providing it would be "inhumane" (Cohen, Levin, & Powderly, 1987). The Act is helpful to a degree, but infants are a special group because they cannot make their wishes known. Dormire (1989) questions whether parents alone can make the wisest decisions about treatment. They may love their child deeply but lack sufficient information on which to base a judgment. This causes them at times to insist on overtreatment or undertreatment of the child. Physicians and nurses are legally bound to act in the best interests of the child, and they are likely to have information that parents may not know. Dormire warns against relying too much on statistical probability when weighing possible outcomes of treating a child. For example, statistical norms might recommend not treating newborns who weigh less than 500 grams. It is true that intervention for a very tiny infant may preserve the life of a severely impaired baby. On the other hand, providing treatment to very small babies also means that some will live normal lives who might otherwise have died. The recommended approach is to individualize decision making. This means that treatment is instituted for every infant; meanwhile, data are collected concerning the infant's status at present and the implications for the future. In addition to utilizing all available medical information, this approach explores the parents' feelings, answers their questions, and fosters a sound relationship between the parents and the professionals caring for the child. A panel of experts in the child's disorder would be consulted, as would members of the hospital's ethics committee. Through collaborative decision making, the interests of the child and of the parents are protected. This approach does not eliminate all possibility of making unwise decisions, but does safeguard families and health professionals from unwarranted courses of action that parents may later regret or that may have legal consequences for health care professionals.

The financial burden of a chronically ill child falls most heavily on middle-class families. Wealthy families have sufficient means to defray costs. Poor families have access to public funds such as Medicaid. Palfrey et al. (1989) finds that educational level and socioeconomic factors have significant effects on parental stress. Among parents of disabled children, 16 percent of those without a high school education reported stress, as compared to 42 percent of those with post–high school educations. Among parents of children with multiple problems, 51 percent of parents without a high school education reported stress, as compared to 79 percent of those with post high school educations. Black parents of children with multiple physical problems, sensory deficits, and emotional difficulties were less likely to report stress than were white or Hispanic families. The impact of mental retardation was greatest among the most affluent families.

It is possible to hypothesize that better educated, more affluent parents may see disabling illness as stressful because they can identify its presence as a negative factor among many positive ones. Less well educated and less affluent families may be conscious of the effects of many negative factors, such as poverty and unemployment, and may not attribute stress specifically to the child's disability. Better educated and more affluent parents may find the child's limitations more upsetting because they place a high value on success and achievement. The lack of distress reported by less educated and less affluent families correlates with their relative uninvolvement in special education programs designed for their disabled children. In many localities, Individualized Educational Plans (IEPs) have been made available to disabled children; greater parent participation is desirable for the parents regardless of educational or economic status. The increased participation of better educated and more affluent families is probably due to their feelings of empowerment and their desire to obtain from the educational system whatever their child needs. It is foolish to assume that the educated parents who participate in IEPs have solved most of their problems. The high distress levels reported by these families indicate that these parents may need help in accepting the child as he or she is and in adapting their aspirations to the child's abilities.

Only 15 percent of parents whose children had multiple physical problems report that the child's condition adversely affects the marriage (Palfrey et al., 1989). More distressing was the difficulty of obtaining child care; this was a problem for 38 percent of parents whose children had multiple physical problems. Job constraints were a problem for 31 percent of the parents of these children. Not only did they look for work in areas where there were services for the disabled, but they also had to devote considerable time to administering care. The same percentage reported constraints on choosing a house or community in which to live.

Relatives may disappoint parents by their reactions to the child. Grandparents may blame the disability on in-laws, or they may blame themselves for carrying defective genes. Aunts and uncles of the child may be worried by the possibility that they might give birth to a child with similar problems, and may choose not to become involved. Featherstone (1980) mentions the tendency of friends and neighbors to help when the child is born or during periods of crisis but adds that they are inclined to forget to offer help at ordinary times. Palfrey et al. (1989) elaborates this point: "Somehow extraordinary help is easier to give than ordinary help; thus getting equipment is much easier than getting the few moments of good supportive listening and conversation which may lend the confidence to carry on" (p. 102). Because parents of a seriously disabled child find it almost impossible to get away, a contribution can be made through the years by persons who offer respite or child care services.

Even though families appear to be coping, there should be periodic assessment of role performance. In the first months after the diagnosis, mother may gradually find herself situated in a daily routine that includes only herself and the child. She feels overwhelmed, although much of the situation may be of her own making. Father is deeply upset by conditions at home, but his life is less child-centered. As his wife devotes most of her time to the sick child, he and the other children feel neglected. They envy the close relationship between mother and the sick child while the mother envies them their freedom and outside interests. The needs of the sick child take precedence. Mother and father have differentiated their roles so completely that companionship between them has vanished.

A chronically ill child can simplify interactions between parents who subordinate the marital relationship to parenthood. As parents struggle to care for the child and preserve a semblance of family life, they are applauded by outsiders for their courage and resourcefulness. Mother especially may derive satisfaction from her accomplishments. After learning to care for their own ill child, many mothers become specialists or advocates for other children with the same disorder. Not a few of them return to school for professional education. Professionalization of the mother is constructive if it enriches her life and allows her to pay adequate attention to all family members. It is less constructive if it preserves mother's excessive involvement with the sick or disabled child at the expense of other family members and other interests.

The longevity of many children with chronic disorders has improved in recent decades, but there are some progressive diseases that culminate in the decline and death of the young child. In some communities there are established groups and networks of parents whose children suffer the same disability. These organizations help families by offering practical advice, answering questions, and providing emotional support. Not every parent is willing or able to participate in this fashion, but for many parents a group can be very therapeutic. Groups offer living proof that parents can face similar problems and survive. Support groups may be independent or affiliated with national organizations devoted to education or research for a particular disorder. Many associations publish newsletters that inform parents of relevant new developments. A prototype of a fatal disorder for which an association and network have been organized is Tay-Sachs disease, which is transmitted from an asymptomatic parent to the affected child.

Children with Tay-Sachs disease appear normal at birth but develop symptoms in their first year. As the disease progresses, they become blind, lose muscle control, and suffer seizures and respiratory problems. In past years these children were often institutionalized, but increasingly they are being cared for at home. Parents know that this child will soon die. If they want to have other children, they face ethical problems about reproduction, prenatal testing, and abortion.

The National Tay-Sachs and Allied Disease Association (NTSAD) holds yearly conferences and operates a national network for parents. Parents are encouraged to participate in self-help groups to share experiences and help one another. In an account of one such group, Mack and Berman (1988) report on themes that emerged in the meetings:

- Need was expressed for better medical care, for expanded home services, and for better support systems overall.
- Desire was expressed for more sensitivity from physicians, and a wish that they would make greater emotional investment in the child.
- Appreciation was expressed for those nurses who provided home care, valued the child, and shared parental concerns.
- Regret was expressed for the lack of privacy imposed by home care.
- Complaints were expressed for inadequate insurance coverage and community resources.
- Divergent opinions were expressed on prenatal testing, pregnancy, abortion, artificial insemination, and adoption.

The most intimate exchanges between group members took place just before and after a child's death. Before death parents were afraid that they might not be with a child at the end, especially if the child was hospitalized. One father and mother in the group described the home death of their little girl (Mack & Berman, 1988):

> *Mother:* It was hard . . . but it was the best it could be . . . I didn't hand her to anybody. I had her with me, on my lap . . . I took two hours . . . just the two of us . . . And then, I took her downstairs and held her on my lap for another 45 minutes. And that was helpful because she went from being warm to being cold. And then, when we were ready to have her go . . . she also stayed in my arms . . . I didn't let them take my baby when she was alive—she was dead. And she felt dead compared to how she had been feeling. I still had her in my arms when they came and brought a stretcher in. And I took her and wrapped her up again in a blanket . . . and I put her on the stretcher . . . and took a sheet . . . and covered her face. (p. 401)
>
> *Father:* And kissed her . . .
>
> *Mother:* And I kissed her and touched her head one more time.

These poignant descriptions underscore the positive effects of sharing and of mutual support. The group follows the NTSAD model, where families interact at different stages of their child's illness. Parents of children who have just been diagnosed may join, and parents of children who have died are permitted to continue for a time, until they feel themselves ready to leave. Although some parents become apprehensive as they hear accounts of what lies ahead, the group gives them an outlet and a place to work on their problems. As the group progresses, members are able to discuss with increasing ease subjects that were once unmentionable and that cannot be talked about outside the group.

The social work leaders of the group used a flexible, responsible style and became less active as members became more comfortable. They worked to create a safe climate in the group and to counter judgmental attitudes.

Because the group was open-ended, with members joining and leaving at different times, the leaders were available outside the sessions. They were involved in practical matters, contacting referral sources, acting as liaison between members and community programs, and facilitating contacts among members between meetings. The success of this and similar groups is undoubtedly related to the ongoing problems of the members, who found understanding and empathy they could not obtain elsewhere. Referrals to support groups are an excellent way for health professionals to assist families in coping. Many of these groups are not led by a professionally trained leader, but they are usually led by a dedicated person with personal knowledge of the disorder for which the group is organized. Generally, there is an educational component to group proceedings, as well as a psychosocial one. They can be a valuable adjunct to the health care plan.

Effects on Siblings

The adjustment of parents to the illness of a child receives more attention than the adjustment of siblings. In a study of sibling responses to the chronic illness of a brother or sister, Tritt and Esses (1988) report that 89 percent of the siblings had some knowledge of the disorder and of the ill child's condition. The extent and accuracy of their knowledge varied but did not correlate with the age of the respondent. Some siblings of an ill child tried to accumulate as much information as possible, while others were satisfied with only superficial knowledge. In some families there seemed to be a family rule about not asking questions or talking much about the illness. Two-thirds of the siblings believed that illness had changed their brother and sister in both positive and negative ways. Some commented on the irritability and temper tantrums of the ill child, while others mentioned improvement in the ill child's behavior and disposition. Most of the siblings reported that the first year of the illness was the worst and that family life improved afterwards. A large majority (92 percent) were aware of parental stresses and worries. More than half believed that the relatives paid more attention to the ill child, parents and grandparents included. Siblings complained of extra jobs they were given, saw themselves as somewhat unhappy, and expressed feelings of being excluded. When asked what advice they had for other children with a seriously ill brother or sister, they suggested that the ill child not be allowed to take advantage of family members. At the same time they stated that siblings should try to help their parents and the ill child. Obviously, the data point to the ambivalence and confusion these siblings experience.

Special problems may develop when the disability of a child is apparent at birth or shortly thereafter. Any long-term illness in a family member, child or adult, imposes hardship. When the ill person has been part of the family for years and has been integrated into family life, role shifts and adjustments may be easier to make. The child who comes into the family with a disability enters as a stranger, especially to siblings. The arrival of an imperfect child is an unknown element to which brothers and sisters, in addition to parents, must adjust. Healthy children in the family recognize the difficulties their parents face in caring for the sick child. They become hesitant about making requests that add to their parents' burden and simultaneously resent the circumstances in which they must live.

As a general rule, families try to attend to the sick child while disrupting family life as little as possible. Their efforts to maintain normality may take the form of "scapegoating" or blaming the child who is ill. When this happens, parents and siblings attribute all adversity and disappointment in family life to the presence of a child who is ill. Because the child is unlikely to recover, decisions can be delayed and conflict avoided. This pattern removes pressure on family members to improve communication and settle differences. The family accommodates to the child's illness in ways that avoid meeting the genuine needs of the parents and of their healthy children. Griffin (1980) describes this as the most pervasive distortion in families with a chronically ill child, regardless of whether a mother–child coalition controls the family.

THERAPEUTIC GUIDELINES

Acute Illness

When acute illness strikes a family member, with or without warning, a critical situation exists. Health professionals are called upon to assess the immediate dimensions of the problem and plan responsive actions to be taken by themselves or by family members. Practical decisions about medical treatment, jobs, child care, and household arrangements must be made promptly. Emotions are apt to be high, and family members are likely to be upset. Some of them are unable to function without direction and require active guidance in making decisions, but more self-possessed members may be able to fill the gap. Families that are mobile may have community links that are weak or nonexistent. If this is the case, health professionals may have to be more active. There are advantages to encouraging families to look for their own solutions to problems so that feelings of family competence and cohesion are enhanced. Because of the relatively brief duration of acute illness and the recovery that usually follows, the family may be strengthened by their experiences, with increased appreciation for the person who was ill and for the proven resourcefulness of family members.

Chronic Illness

When people do not recover fully from their illness but must be cared for at home for long periods of time, caring for the patient may become a permanent obligation for the family. During periods of hospitalization for a chronic illness, family members should be included in teaching sessions so that they are prepared for some responsibilities. If an individual has undergone surgical procedures or an illness that causes body changes, such as those that follow a colostomy or mastectomy, family members must be advised of major changes they will witness. If they are not prepared, their reactions may add to the patient's distress. Chronic illnesses and the aftermath of radical surgery vary greatly, as do the responses of different family members. In meeting family needs, the health professional should anticipate the demands imposed by a particular illness or disability, and move toward helping the family meet these demands. Among the demands made on families by the presence of chronic illness are the following:

• Dealing with pain and loss resulting from the illness or disability
• Dealing with health care personnel involved with the patient and family
• Dealing with present and future obligations related to the illness or disability
• Maintaining family functions and family equilibrium in the presence of illness or disability
• Safeguarding family relationships despite the illness or disability
• Responding to present and preparing for future contingencies

Health professionals involved with the families of chronically ill or disabled persons must recognize the fact that anger and frustration exhibited by the patient or the family are not personal attacks. They need to know that there are various emotional stages experienced by patients and families, and that the stages are not always fixed or sequential. It is enough to realize that the person with a chronic illness and the family may display a broad range of emotion, and that strong emotion in difficult situations is not pathological and may even be therapeutic. When emotions are high, explanations from health professionals should be cognitive, especially if those involved seek information. Requests of the patient and the family for participation should not be construed as interference or intrusion but encouraged.

Instrumental or practical support for families is best provided by persons with weaker ties to patient and family. Expressive or emotional support is best provided by persons with strong ties to patient and family, or by persons who have had similar experiences. This implies that spouses or partners, friends, colleagues, and support groups are appropriate sources of emotional support. Although professionals tend to be better sources of cognitive and practical assistance, many are able to build a therapeutic relationship strong enough for them to become sources of emotional support (Woods, Yates, & Primona, 1989).

Another function of health care professionals is linking families with formal and informal support groups in the community. The nature of family support services, whether instrumental or expressive, is determined by the needs that are being experienced. When the illness causes pain or physical discomfort, instrumental measures such as medication or hands-on care are more effective than expressive measures. A person dealing with problems related to self-image is helped more by expressive or emotional support. Deciding the type of assistance that is called for is a first step in formulating interventions.

Terminal Illness

In terminal illness, where there is no hope of recovery, families must be persuaded to turn from curative measures toward measures that increase the patient's comfort. This reduces their feelings of powerlessness and helplessness. Dying persons indicate as best they can how they want to be cared for, and health professionals can interpret to families what the patient seems to want. They can also avoid defensive reactions to criticisms of the care the patient is receiving. When the dying person is an infant or a young child, it is very hard for parents to say goodbye. They may need time to relinquish the body of their child, and exceptions should be made to accommodate their wishes, regardless of where the death occurred.

When a person is stricken with AIDS, social issues intrude that heighten distress. Any health care professional working with an AIDS patient must first deal with personal attitudes toward the patient and the illness. Not everyone is capable of working with AIDS patients, but everyone has a responsibility to learn about the disease and to disseminate accurate information. There is a great deal of hysteria about AIDS, and awareness of transmission modes and preventive actions is essential. In the absence of a cure for this illness, prevention is the best tool available. This is a worldwide public health problem as well as an individual and family problem.

Regardless of the level of illness, it is not helpful for the ill person or the illness to dominate family life. Siblings have legitimate claims on parents, who need to hear that family horizons should expand beyond the sickroom. This is also true for parents whose marital relationship has been overlooked in their zeal to help the sick child. Chronic illness in a loved one narrows the perspective of family members, especially the parents. Total family health can be achieved only by encouraging outside interests, arranging respite periods, and considering the needs of every family member.

Communication is an aspect of family life that is seldom improved by illness. Sometimes the ill person is close in age to a spouse or to siblings, but often there is a generation gap between the ill person and other family members. Meyerowitz, Heinrich, and Schag (1983) report that 72 percent of the patients in their study reported problems communicating with health professionals, and 86 percent reported problems communicating with family members. Communication problems may be specific, such as obtaining information about one's illness, or they may be general problems stemming from reticence, fear of asking too much, or protectiveness toward one's family. One problem is that family members may not know what to say to the patient, either because their own information is inadequate or because the situation has made them unsure. Adult children who find themselves enacting a parental role with an ill mother or father have a sense of incongruity that is hard to dispel. Similarly, a parent who is ill may have trouble asking or even accepting help from the children they raised. Illness tends to make patients feel constitutionally inferior, and families can exacerbate these feelings by their communication patterns. Even when they say the right things, their nonverbal behavior may contradict their words.

Communication can be aided by family meetings where messages between family members can be conveyed directly, and not mediated by a member or a health professional who has somehow become the switchboard or relayer of messages. Family meetings may be used to clarify what is happening to the patient, and to open communication channels so that all members have the same understanding of events. Discussing the life stage of the family and the patient helps determine what functions must be delegated and to whom. Patients need to be assured that their family duties are being carried out but reassured that they are not being replaced. The life stage perspective helps members see the illness as a family problem where everyone participates in finding a solution. Examining life stage issues can be a mnemonic technique for assessing needs and planning actions to mobilize family strengths. In the early phase of illness it may be necessary to devote greater attention to patient needs and less to family functions. Nevertheless, the mother who knows her children are receiving care, the father whose financial worries are dispelled, the elderly person whose spouse and children offer assistance find that the consequences of any illness, acute, chronic, or terminal, are less frightening.

CLINICAL EXAMPLE: FAMILY DYSFUNCTION IN CARING FOR A DISABLED CHILD

Paula and Stanley Essex are the parents of two children, a 6-year-old daughter, Susan, and a 4-year-old son, Johnny. Susan is a bright, winning child who is her father's comfort and joy. Johnny was born with spina bifida and cerebral palsy. His speech is incomprehensible to everyone but his mother. He is unable to walk, is incontinent, and has required constant attention and care since birth. Most of the burden has fallen on Paula, who accepts it without complaint because she is the parent who insists on home care for Johnny. Her husband helps with cooking and housework but not with the physical care of his son. Stanley spends a few minutes with Johnny every evening, but this usually follows a suggestion from Paula. Father and daughter have a very close relationship. Each evening Stanley spends several hours with Susan, reading to her or playing games with her. Susan has just entered first grade. An older child living across the street accompanies Susan to and from school.

Assessment

The physiotherapist who visits the family three times a week became aware of Paula's deepening depression. She noticed that Susan sometimes played at the home of classmates but that no children ever visited her. It was the physiotherapist who suggested that the couple consult a counselor at a local mental health center. Stanley was reluctant to do so but consented when Paula reported that the physiotherapist thought that Susan felt lonely. During the initial interview the counselor observed that although the family seemed to be coping, the distance between the spouses was very wide. They seemed to have no common interests except for their two children. Here their interests also diverged. Paula was extremely involved with her son, while Stanley's main concern was his daughter. Although she tried not to complain, Paula was very resentful toward her husband because of his indifference to Johnny. Stanley was repelled by the services his son needed and could not bear to observe the boy closely. Although it had never been discussed, Paula recognized these feelings in Stanley and was reluctant to ask him for help in caring for Johnny even though she often wanted to do so. She also felt excluded from the happy times that Stanley and Susan shared in the evenings. Because they never asked her to join, she felt that they considered both her and Johnny to be rejects.

Planning

It was apparent to the counselor that this family was a closed system in which all four members were socially isolated. Each parent interacted with only one of the children. The result was that Susan and Johnny each had only one parent. Because Paula's responsibilities were so heavy, the counselor suggested that a community health nurse come into the home regularly to help with Johnny's care. The possibility of using a home health aide was considered so that Paula would have a few hours to herself each week. Although the counselor was aware of problems within the marital relationship, a decision was made to approach this problem by addressing the children's needs. In many ways this was not a two-parent family, and a primary goal was to modify dysfunctional parenting patterns. It seemed necessary to reduce the excessive involvement of Paula and Johnny and to increase Stanley's participation. The exclusion of Paula from the father–daughter relationship was another pattern that required modification. Through these modifications the counselor hoped to lighten the load Paula was carrying and encourage a family reorganization that did not fragment parent–child relationships.

Implementation

The counselor formulated three major objectives in working with this family: to reduce Paula's obsessive attention to Johnny and simplify his care; to expand the relationship between Stanley and Susan to include Paula and, to some extent, to include Johnny as well; and to strengthen the marital relationship by improving communication between the parents. The presence of a community health nurse at times gave Paula access to expert advice on feeding Johnny, keeping him clean, and increasing his mobility. The nurse arranged to make some evening visits, ostensibly to observe the evening care of Johnny but also to involve Stanley and solicit his help.

The counselor noted Paula's need for companionship and suggested that the couple plan some recreational activities together. She gave them a list of qualified babysitters endorsed by the local cerebral palsy chapter. A suggestion was made for the couple to join a support group for parents of disabled children. Because Stanley resisted this idea and apparently needed more time to deal with his feelings, Paula followed through on her own. Even though Stanley did not accompany her, the group provided Paula with an opportunity to meet and interact with other adults. She was able to share with Stanley some of the things she had learned in the group. Thus, the sense of isolation was reduced for both parents.

Evaluation

Because Johnny's disability is permanent, the family will require help over the years. Neither Stanley nor Paula wants the problem of Johnny's care to fall upon Susan after they are gone, and they undoubtedly will need advice on this matter. Helping Stanley adjust to his son's illness is likely to be a lengthy process that may never be fully successful. Some of the major objectives have been accomplished already. Johnny's care has been simplified as much as possible. Arrangements have been made to give Paula some time to herself, and she has learned that it is possible to ask Stanley for help now and then. With more time at her disposal, Paula is able to pay attention to her daughter. The closeness between father and daughter continue, but Paula is now invited to join them.

At the suggestion of the counselor, Stanley has begun to spend more time in the evenings with his son. Surprisingly, Susan often wants to be included and has begun to read to Johnny on her own. Stanley is still unwilling to undertake much physical care of his son, but he does stay with both children when Paula attends group meetings. The evenings when Stanley and Paula go out together remind Stanley that she is a wife and companion rather than a harassed caregiver. Other people may see the family as still restricted and isolated, but considerable reorganization has taken place.

SUMMARY

This chapter differentiated three levels of illness: acute, chronic, and terminal. It compared the behavior patterns adopted by families in response to these levels of illness and suggests appropriate therapeutic strategies. Acute illness may have a sudden or gradual onset but constitutes a crisis that mobilizes most families. The short-term nature of acute illness may cause temporary role shifts but enables families to return to normal life after the patient recovers, although the convalescent period may be a difficult time for all concerned.

Chronic illness is more demanding for the patient and the family. Recovery from chronic illness is rarely complete or permanent, although there may be periods of remission or relative health. The strain on the family is severe, and some of the coping responses are maladaptive. Often the marital relationship suffers as a result of mother's excessive preoccupation with the sick child. Siblings report ambivalence and feelings of resentment toward parents and the ill child. In families that revolve around the sick child, the child may be the center of attention but may be blamed or scapegoated in subtle ways. Decisions in the family are deferred, and areas of disagreement expand because they are never discussed or resolved. Family unhappiness and disappointment are blamed on the ill child, and the real causes of family discontent are ignored.

Terminal illness brings its own distinctive features to family life. Reactions to terminal illness vary, but approaching death is always an ordeal for families. AIDS is a terminal illness that brings special difficulties for patients, partners, and family members. Although the prognosis is grim for AIDS patients, the diagnosis sometimes compels family members to overcome their prejudices, and may bring about reconciliation with a son or daughter who may have been estranged for years.

One consequence of terminal illness and of chronic illness as well is the social restriction it imposes on families. Involvement with networks and with support groups organized around a disorder can help patients and families avoid social isolation. Another sustaining influence for them is a good relationship with competent, caring health care professionals.

REFERENCES

Burish, T. G., & Bradley, L. A. (1983). *Coping with Chronic Disease*. New York: Academic Press.

Carlson, G. A., Greeman, M., & McClelland, T. A. (1989). "Management of HIV Positive Psychiatric Patients who Fail to Reduce High Risk Behavior." *Journal of Hospital and Community Psychiatry*, 40(5): 511–514.

Chaches, E. (1987). "Women and Children with AIDS." In C. G. Leukefeld & M. Fimbres (Eds.), *Responding to AIDS: Psychosocial Initiatives*. Silver Springs, MD: National Association of Social Workers.

Cohen, C. B., Levin, B., & Powderly, K. (1987). "A History of Neonatal Care and Decision Making." Washington, DC: *Hastings Center Report*, 17(6): 22–25.

Dormire, S. L. (1989). "Models for Moral Response in the Care of Seriously Ill Children." *Image*, 21(2): 81–84.

Dunst, C. J., Cushing, P. J., & Vance, S. D. (1985). "Response Contingent Learning in Profoundly Handicapped Infants: A Social Systems Perspective." *Analysis and Intervention in Developmental Disabilities*, 5(1): 33–47.

Eakes, G. G. (1990). "Grief Resolution in Hospice Nurses: An Exploration of Effective Methods." *Nursing and Health Care*, 11(5): 242–248.

Featherstone, H. (1980). *A Difference in the Family*. New York: Basic Books.

Grey, M., Genel, M., & Taborlane, W. (1980). "Psychosocial Adjustment of Latency Aged Diabetics: Determinants and Relationships to Control." *Pediatrics*, 65(1): 69–73.

Griffin, J. Q. (1980). "Physical Illness in the Family." In J. R. Miller & E. H. Janosik (Eds.), *Family-Focused Care*. New York: McGraw-Hill.

Johnson, S. B. (1985). "The Family and the Child with Chronic Illness." In D. C. Turk & R. D. Kerns (Eds.), *Health, Illness, and Families: A Life Span Perspective*. New York: Wiley.

Kübler-Ross, E. (1969). *On Death and Dying*. New York: Macmillan.

Kübler-Ross, E. (1987). *AIDS: The Ultimate Challenge*. New York: Macmillan.

LaGreca, A. M., Follansbee, D., & Skyler, J. (1982). "Behavioral Aspects of Diabetes Management in Children and Adolescents." Paper presented at the Annual Conference of the American Psychological Association.

Lerner, H. G. (1985). *The Dance of Anger*. New York: Harper & Row.

Leukefeld, C. G. (1989). "Psychosocial Issues in Dealing with AIDS." *Hospital and Community Psychiatry*, 40(5): 454–455.

Leventhal, H., Leventhal, E. A., & Van Nguyen, T. (1985). "Reactions of Families to Illness: Theoretical Models and Perspectives." In D. C. Turks & P. D. Kerns, (Eds.), *Human Illness and Families: A Life Span Perspective*. New York: Wiley.

Lewin, T. (1990). "With Court Leading the Way, Living Will Gaining New Life." *New York Times*, July 23, pp. A-1, A-13.

Mack, S. A., & Berman, L. B. (1988). "A Group for Parents of Children with Fatal Genetic Illnesses." *American Journal of Orthopsychiatry*, 58(3): 397–404.

Matus, I. (1981). "Assessing the Nature and Clinical Significance of Psychological Contributions to Childhood Asthma." *American Journal of Orthopsychiatry*, 51(3): 327–351.

Meyerowitz, B. E., Henrich, R. L., & Schag, C. C. (1983). "A Competency-Based Approach to Coping with Cancer." In T. G. Beirich & L. A. Bradley (Eds.), *Coping with Chronic Disorder*. New York: Academic Press.

Moos, R. H. (1977). *Coping with Physical Illness*. New York: Plenum.

Newman, B. A., & Taylor, E. H. (1987). "The Family and AIDS." In C. G. Leukefeld & M. Fimbres (Eds.), *Responding to AIDS: Psychosocial Initiatives*. Silver Springs, MD: National Association of Social Workers.

Norris, C. M. (1990). "The Work of Getting Well." *American Journal of Nursing*, 90(7): 47–50.

O'Donnell, T. G., & Bernier, S. L. (1990). "Parents as Caregivers: When a Son Has AIDS." *Journal of Psychosocial Nursing*, 28(6): 14–17.

Palfrey, J. S., Walker, D. K., Butler, J. A., & Singer, J. D. (1989). "Patterns of Response in Families of Chronically Disabled Children: An Assessment in Five Metropolitan School Districts." *American Journal of Orthopsychiatry*, 59(1): 94–104.

Parsons, T. (1951). *The Social System*. New York: Free Press.

Public Health Report No. 103: Supplement 1, Vol. 3. Washington, DC: NIH.

Rando, T. A. (1984). *Grief, Dying, and Death: Clinical Interventions for Caregivers*. Champaign, IL: Research Press.

Silverstone, B., & Hyman, H. K. (1982). *You and Your Aging Parent*. Mt. Vernon, NY: Consumers Union Press.

Sontag, S. (1978). *Illness as Metaphor*. New York: Farrar, Straus, & Giroux.

Tritt, S. G., & Esses, L. E. (1988). "Psychosocial Adaptation of Children with Medical Disorders." *American Journal of Orthopsychiatry*, 58(2): 211–220.

Van Kamm, A. L. (1959). "The Nurse in the Patient's World." *American Journal of Nursing*, 59(12): 1708–1710.

Wallach, J. J. (1989). "AIDS Anxiety among Health Care Professionals." *Hospital and Community Psychiatry*, 40(5): 507–510.

Wechsler, H. J. (1990). *What's So Bad about Guilt*. New York: Simon and Schuster.

Weizman, S. G., & Kamm, P. (1985). *About Mourning: Support and Guidance for the Bereaved*. New York: Human Sciences.

Woods, N. F., Yates, B. C., & Primona, J. (1989). "Supporting Families During Chronic Illness." *Image*, 21(1): 46–50.

Zeitlin, S., & Williamson, G. G. (1990). "Coping Characteristics of Disabled and Non-disabled Children." *American Journal of Orthopsychiatry*, 60(3): 404–411.

Psychiatric Illness in the Family

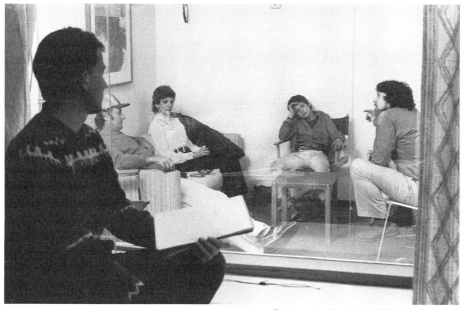

Knowledge of what is possible is the beginning of happiness.

Santayana

Although it is rarely classified as trauma, psychiatric illness in any form is a traumatic experience for everyone concerned. In particular, a psychiatric illness in which an individual seriously distorts reality is traumatic for the collective family as well as the individual. By its very nature, the course of a psychiatric illness tends to be lengthy, so that the individual and the family must live under trying circumstances for considerable periods of time. Under the best circumstances, psychiatric illness may be controlled or alleviated so that the family can reorganize itself in an adaptive manner. Under less than ideal circumstances, the trauma of psychiatric illness goes on, and family life continues to be disrupted.

In a psychiatric context, *trauma* may be defined as any overwhelming, uncontrollable experience that causes psychological vulnerability of long or short duration. This definition contains the idea that families as well as individuals are traumatized by psychiatric illness. Traumatic experiences provoke a variety of reactions such as self-concept deficits, self-destructiveness, and antisocial behaviors. James (1988) describes connections between the experience of psychological trauma and the subsequent appearance of psychiatric symptoms. It follows, then, that psychiatric illness in a family member produces profound disturbance within the family system. This is an important point to remember when dealing with such families. Disturbed family interactions may be the result as well as the forerunner of psychiatric illness. All that is known with certainty is that psychiatric illness itself is a trauma, exacerbating the suffering of the individual and the family.

Work with individuals who have endured the trauma of war, imprisonment, or disaster demonstrates to clinicians the impact that extraordinary events have on an individual's adjustment. The syndrome known as post-traumatic stress disorder demonstrates how traumatic events are relived in the form of intrusive thoughts and subjective perceptions. In psychiatric illness the individual often suffers from discrepancy between what is actually happening around him and what he thinks is happening. Everyone possesses certain beliefs, assumptions, and inferences that are more or less shared and understood by others. When an individual suffers a psychiatric illness, his beliefs, assumptions, and inferences are not validated by other people. The disparity between the individual's experience and that of others is frustrating and alarming for him and for the family. The individual who is ill often has a lowered threshold of arousal. His reactions to stimuli are different from those of other people, and he realizes that this is likely to be misunderstood. This frequently causes him to create a new version of events that confirms his false impressions. As a result he avoids interpersonal encounters that threaten his misinterpretations. The fearfulness, withdrawal, and psychic numbing seen in the person who is ill may also be replicated by the family members in their dealings with the ill person and with others in their social milieu. For the ill person and the family, these are self-protective maneuvers.

During a psychiatric illness the individual undergoes an extraordinary experience that few can imagine. Persons in the grip of a severe psychiatric illness abandon logic, order, and rationality. Unable to trust or understand what they alone think or believe, they experience anxiety approaching panic. Disorder and confusion prevail as they enter a world no longer ruled by reason or consensual validation. Anyone who has witnessed an acute psychotic episode can attest to the intense nature of the experience for the individual and for onlookers as well. Given the unpredictable nature of some forms of psychiatric illness, the psychotic process may abate or may persist for years. In some instances, extraordinary events preceding the onset of psychiatric illness actually happened in the external environment of the individual, and are discernible. In other instances there may be no recognizable precipitating events except those that are subjectively generated and exist only in the mind of the individual who is ill.

On the basis of the nature and extent of precipitating events, many forms of psychiatric illness can be seen as stress reactions. Included among these stress responses are guilt, anger, depression, suspiciousness, anxiety, hostility, and even violence. Clinical manifestations of psychiatric disorders include thought disruption, mood disturbance, and eating disorders. Somatic complaints are frequently part of the clinical picture and require investigation. Drug and alcohol abuse are common behavioral manifestations; delusions and hallucinations are idiosyncratic phenomena indicating that the individual has lost touch with reality.

Conceptualization of psychiatric symptoms as stress reactions has clinical value because it implies that dysfunctional symptoms may be moderated by stress-reducing interventions. This statement applies to the family as well as the client. The immediate social field with which care providers are concerned should encompass the biological, psychological, and environmental forces surrounding the individual client and the family.

Connections between individuals suffering a psychiatric disorder and their families are so entangled that it is hard to imagine any circumstance affecting the client that does not also affect the family.

By its very nature psychiatric illness, regardless of the form it takes, is rarely a short-term experience. Invariably it disrupts family life significantly. In the best circumstances the illness is controlled or alleviated so that the family eventually regroups itself and adapts. In less than ideal circumstances the family does not reorganize itself, and disruption caused by the illness persists for years.

This chapter describes mental illness in light of its effect on family life. It endorses the notion of mental illness as a severe form of trauma to which all family members must adapt. Three distinct manifestations of psychiatric illness are presented in the chapter: disorders of thought, of mood, and of eating. These disorders are selected because of their prevalence and their implications for the family. Therapeutic guidelines appropriate for each form of disorder are included. The guidelines vary in certain respects, but all emphasize the need to include the family as well as the identified patient, because all share the ongoing trauma of mental illness.

SPECIAL PROBLEMS OF PSYCHIATRIC ILLNESS

The ability of families to cope with the trauma of mental illness is largely dependent on three factors: (1) the personal factor, meaning the psychological strengths and weaknesses of the client and the family; (2) the nature of the psychiatric illness; and (3) the social context in which the illness manifests itself. Most people embark on marriage and parenthood with hopes and dreams that are tinged with some apprehension. On the whole, however, couples expect to be equal to the demands that will be made upon them. They believe that they, like most people, will be rewarded by producing children who will become useful citizens, of whom they can be proud. They anticipate changes as they grow older, but each partner expects the other to contribute to the smooth operation of family life; each thinks that losses and serious illness are possibilities more likely to happen to other people than to the founders of their new family. They trust that their marriage will last, that their children will prosper, and that they will grow old together surrounded by children and grandchildren. Usually they are optimistic about the future, considering the world to be a fairly orderly place in which hard work, commitment, and virtue are usually rewarded. This is not an altogether unrealistic set of beliefs, and it is fulfilled in the lives of many families.

For all too many families, however, the dream is unfulfilled. Despite the good intentions of family members, hopes are shattered by the serious psychiatric illness of any member. Someone in the family begins to act in strange, inexplicable ways, and the catchall term *nervous breakdown* is used to describe these worrisome behaviors. Before long the family becomes an autocracy ruled by the deviant member. When this happens, family life changes, depending on the form of the illness, on who is afflicted, and when the illness occurs in the family and individual life cycles (Romano, 1979). Within the limits of their ability, family members adapt as best they can (the personal factor). The range of psychiatric symptoms varies greatly. Some symptoms are extreme enough to terrify family members; others may be equally severe but constitute only a source of great anger or embarrassment (the nature of the illness). Finally, depending on support granted or withheld by friends, community, and professionals, the family is helped or hindered in its attempts to adapt (the context factor).

Unpredictability

The prognosis for most major psychiatric disorders is unpredictable. Asking an experienced clinician if a particular client is likely to recover or suffer future relapses rarely brings a definitive answer. Ask if the client will regain her premorbid personality and powers without residual impairment, and again the clinician is unwilling to give an unqualified answer. Such equivocation is due not to resistance on the part of the clinician but to uncertainty regarding the prognosis for most psychiatric disorders. The ambiguity is further compounded by the caution and concern the clinician already feels on behalf of the troubled family. With the prognosis so uncertain, it is not surprising that bewilderment about the client's illness is a common occurrence in families (Faloon et al., 1984). Some clinicians fear that describing the likely course of the illness to the family may become a self-fulfilling prophecy, leading to pessimism that opposes the client's recovery. Unfortunately, this reticence can produce unreasonable expectations and, ultimately, lead to bitter disappointment when expectations are not met. A basic principle in working with a psychiatrically disabled client is to explain to the family what is happening and what is likely to follow to the extent that this is possible.

Recurrence and Chronicity

Most major psychiatric illnesses are not a single event but a long, disabling process. Therefore, families need guidance in understanding and responding to recurring crises characterized by extreme dysfunction, followed by convalescence or remission (Seeman, 1986). Depending on the nature of the illness, lasting cure is sometimes possible but cannot be guaranteed. In thought disorders the most common course is one of acute relapses with some stabilization between episodes. When a family member is impaired by the thought disorder known as schizophrenia, the rest of the family needs to learn that periodic relapses are generally followed by the client's inability to return to previous functioning even when the most severe symptoms are controlled. The picture is less bleak for other psychiatric disorders in that residual deficits are not cumulative, but even here recurrence is possible. Although openness is the best policy, the health care professional must decide how and when to describe to the family what lies ahead. Indeed, it is not enough to "tell" the family in a hurried meeting what they should reasonably expect. Families deserve an ongoing period of psychoeducation to help them deal with the client and their own doubts and questions.

Stigma

Society is somewhat more enlightened about mental illness today than it was some decades ago. Mental health issues are better understood by the professional community and the general public, but much progress remains to be made. Families with a member who is mentally ill feel stigmatized for several reasons. First, there are unpleasant aspects to mental illness, such as unpredictability and chronicity. Second, families have sometimes been considered the cause of mental illness. Not long ago, theories of the etiology of schizophrenia centered on the idea of the schizophrenogenic mother who victimized her children (Fromm-Reichmann, 1948), faulty family communication patterns (Bateson et al., 1956), dysfunctional marital interactions (Lidz et al., 1965), and other phenomena that attributed schizophrenia to identified family patterns. Although the etiological pendulum has moved from unidimensional positions to multifactorial explanations, old beliefs and assumptions die hard, even though prevailing family emotions of anger, confusion, and uncertainty are now seen as reactions to rather than causes of mental illness (Abramowitz & Coursey, 1989). Still, there are some clinicians and theorists who continue to interpret such emotional reactions as indicators of family pathology. These interpretations persist even though research shows that global dysfunction in the realm of communication and interaction is not limited to families with a schizophrenic member.

In discussing the rigors of working with mentally ill clients, Romano (1979) notes that emotional maturity is needed to care for these persons, not only for those who remain disabled but also for those who recover slowly and minimally over time. Demands on health care professionals are great, but they are relative strangers to the client and are generally able to maintain professional objectivity. A great deal more is exacted from the client's family, who must face the unpredictability and chronicity of the client on a daily and nightly basis. They become preoccupied with "managing" the client's illness to the extent of neglecting family needs. This unending burden requires a reshuffling of priorities in the family, and frequently leads to fragmentation of family structure and function. The financial burden of psychiatric illness adds another dimension to the family's plight (Lefley, 1987). Instead of working together, the family is so overwhelmed that relationships may splinter; each member tries individually to endure and is preoccupied with self-preserving tactics. Thus, the family has come a long way from that eager and hopeful young couple described earlier in the chapter.

The stigma that continues to be associated with psychiatric illness is generalized to the family. Families withdraw from their accustomed social relationships; more often than not the withdrawal is reciprocal as other people distance themselves from what they do not understand. Social isolation becomes a way of life for the client and the family, each preferring privacy for different reasons. Families tend to avoid exposing themselves to questions from the curious, especially if the client engages in strange actions. Families wish to avoid further humiliation; friends and associates wish to avoid embarrassment. This results in a pattern of mutual withdrawal.

Blaming

When something goes wrong in the life of a loved one, people search for explanations. In the absence of sound explanations, they may begin to look at their own part in creating the dilemma. Family members who live intimately with the client may blame themselves to some extent for the client's illness. Unhappily, self-recrimination is often reinforced by health care professionals in subtle ways. Under the guise of client confidentiality, family members may be kept totally in the dark regarding the nature of the disorder. The exclusion of family members from useful cognitive information may be interpreted by them as an indictment of their part in causing the illness. They tend to assume they are being locked out by professionals because they are perceived as part of the problem. It is not necessary to relay confidential information to the family, but it is important to explain general ramifications of the disorder. No health professional overtly blames a family for the client's illness, but sometimes the message is implicitly sent by ignoring or excluding the worried family.

THOUGHT DISORDERS AND THE FAMILY

Schizophrenia is a major disorder of thought and perception. Contact with reality is broken and personality disorganization is shown in how the client thinks, feels, and acts. Initial onset generally occurs in adolescence or early adulthood. Three sequential stages are apparent in the disorder. The initial or prodromal stage is marked by unusual behavior which causes the individual to be seen by others as eccentric or different. Functioning in one or more areas of the individual's life becomes deficient. Usually this is followed by an acute psychotic episode. The more sudden the onset of acute psychosis, the more optimistic is the prognosis. A history of good premorbid adjustment is another hopeful sign. If the prodromal stage appears early in life and worsens gradually over the years, the prognosis is more pessimistic. Stage two of schizophrenia is the acute stage, marked by heightened emotionality, hallucinations and/or delusions, and strange thought patterns. The acute stage may or may not be a response to identifiable stressors. It is this stage that brings the client to the attention of mental health care professionals. Stage three is the residual stage. The storm of the acute stage subsides, but thinking continues to be strange. Behavior may be bizarre; emotions may be inappropriate and relationships impaired. Although hallucinations and delusions may continue, they have lost their disruptive force. The client has not become her premorbid self, but neither is she acutely disturbed. Overall functioning continues to be deteriorated and premorbid skills have not been regained.

The so-called positive symptoms of schizophrenia, such as hallucinations, delusions, and bizarre behaviors characteristic of the acute stage, are amenable to neuroleptic drugs. The so-called negative symptoms such as withdrawal, isolation, and apathy are not (West et al., 1985). For the individual client, recommended treatment combines psychopharmacological, psychological, and social interventions designed to meet specific needs. Interventions that utilize stress reduction and problem-solving techniques to help the client handle present circumstances are usually more beneficial than many sophisticated, dynamic approaches. Some clients can function with little or no medication; others may need it indefinitely. Whatever combination of treatments prevents relapse or promotes functioning is certainly the recommended route.

Terkelson (1987) and Lefley (1987) examine effects of schizophrenic illness on the family, based on the identity of the person stricken. The schizophrenic illness of a child is extremely painful, but it does allow the parents to continue in their nurturing roles. The issue of blame and responsibility for the illness is one that parents of any age will face. The older the parents are at the time of onset of schizophrenia in a child, the less threatened is their sense of identity and self-esteem. Younger parents seem more threatened by the schizophrenic illness of a child. Many undergo an identity crisis of their own upon learning the diagnosis and adopt a very dark view of the future.

Schizophrenic illness in a husband and father may have devastating financial as well as emotional consequences. Because father is the symbolic, if not the actual, head of the household, there is extraordinary role shifting within the family when he becomes ill. The wife generally becomes primary provider and decision maker, as well as nurturer and caregiver.

Perhaps the most extreme family adjustment follows the schizophrenic illness of the wife and mother. For a time the husband and children may cope successfully, but as time passes management problems usually become more complicated. Older children in the family strive to take mother's place to some extent. Like their younger siblings, they find themselves inhabiting an ominous world. Regardless of their respective ages, the children experience some developmental problems with identity formation, and with issues of trust and stability. In some cases children and adolescents may seek the constancy and balance lacking at home by looking outside the family household for companionship and support.

Regardless of who is afflicted, the primary caregiver is engulfed by manifestations of the illness. If other family members build barriers between themselves and the ill family member, by association the primary caregiver is very likely to be placed with the client on the far side of the barriers. Attempts on the part of the primary caregiver to involve other family members in the care of the client are usually unsuccessful, and result in stronger and higher barriers being erected. The only weapons available to the primary caregiver are guilt and persuasion. The effect of these on family members is not likely to produce desirable results, unless the primary caregiver is allied with another family member or assisted by a concerned clinician.

Therapeutic Guidelines

The vast majority of clients with chronic schizophrenia live at home with their parents, with spouses, or with other relatives. About 25 percent live in structured residential settings. Even those clients who leave their families and live on their own continue to be seen as a responsibility. In large part this is due to the deterioration that is so much a part of schizophrenic illness. Figure 11.1 shows the chronic, progressive course of schizophrenia

FIGURE 11.1. Progressive Deterioration of a Schizophrenic Person

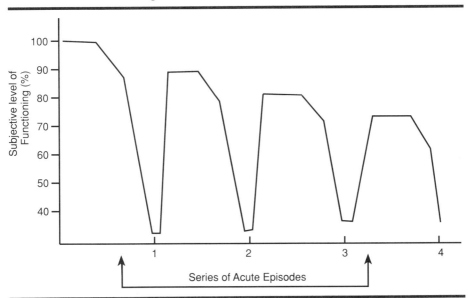

that is more often the norm than the exception. The figure shows an individual who previously functioned at a 100 percent level. The individual reports gradual drop in performance levels before each schizophrenic episode (the prodromal stage) and then a sudden drop in functioning levels during the acute stage. After hospitalization and/or adequate treatment, improvement follows. However, improvement levels off in the residual phase at levels lower than the previous functioning. Each new episode of acute schizophrenia brings a greater loss of functioning that is not regained. The treatment regimen is designed to reduce the number of subsequent relapses as much as possible.

Two features operate that add to the burden of family members. One is the difficulty in alleviating the negative behaviors of the person with schizophrenia. The second is the difficulty in altering the progressive deterioration that follows each acute episode. These considerations make it important for families to understand that the maintenance and rehabilitation of the schizophrenic client requires long-term care and planning. Unfortunately, the attention of health care professionals often focuses on responding to acute episodes rather than constructing a long-range plan. The client may need to be hospitalized during agitated, psychotic episodes, but the current trend is to hospitalize the client briefly. Lengthy hospitalization erodes community and family support and reinforces the belief that the client is incompetent in self-care and daily living.

Abramowitz and Coursey (1989) advise health care professionals not to regard the family itself as a pathological unit. Instead, the family is a resource in need of education, understanding, and support. The emphasis of therapeutic encounters with the family should be on education, direction, and support.

In order to determine what families want, the health care professional should listen to what families say. Hatfield and Lefley (1986) report data obtained from members of the National Alliance for the Mentally Ill, in response to questions concerning what contributions from clinicians would be most helpful. The top responses were: (1) help in reducing their anxiety stemming from the client's irrational behavior, (2) assistance in setting realistic goals and expectations, (3) guidance in learning how to mobilize and motivate the client to do more, and (4) education about the nature of mental illness and support during times of crisis. Abramowitz and Coursey (1989) address similar needs in offering a family support group designed to dispense accurate information about schizophrenia, teach problem-solving and client management skills, and connect families to community systems and resources; group leaders conclude that the group experience reduced family anxiety and led to improved coping skills. Interestingly, the group experience, although positive in some ways, was ineffective in lessening negative feelings felt by family members toward the client. Negative perceptions of the schizophrenic relative seem to be one component of family emotion that may be controllable but tends to persist.

It is unlikely that the families of schizophrenic clients consistently get the help they need. Spaniol and Zipple (1988) cite their study of families of clients and of mental health professionals in which satisfaction with available health services is explored. As might be expected, practitioners report satisfaction with the services they offer, while families make clear their dissatisfaction.

EXPRESSED EMOTION

The emotional climate in the families of schizophrenic persons is of interest to health care professionals trying to help families find a balance between overinvolvement and underinvolvement with the person who is ill. Out of family research a concept has emerged called *expressed emotion.* Expressed emotion includes three aspects of family interaction: (1) criticism of the client, (2) hostility toward the client, and (3) intrusive involvement with the client. The concept of expressed emotion became important when it was learned that chronic schizophrenic males who returned to parents or spouses after hospitalization were more susceptible to relapse than counterparts who lived in community facilities or with more distant relatives (Koenigsberg & Handley, 1986). In differentiating families with high amounts of expressed emotion from families with low amounts, four characteristics prevail (Leff & Vaugn, 1985):

Characteristics of Families with Less Expressed Emotion

- Interested, controlled, concerned but not acutely anxious about the client
- Respectful of the client's need for personal and social distance
- Accepting of the client as a person who is ill rather than a malingerer
- Tolerant rather than critical or impatient with the client's actions

Characteristics of Families with More Expressed Emotion

- Extremely concerned, acutely anxious, and preoccupied with the client
- Disrespectful of the client's need for personal and social distance
- Perception of the client as a malingerer who chooses to be dysfunctional
- Intolerant, critical, and impatient with the client's behavior

The fact that expressed family emotion correlates with repeated relapse offers guidance for family intervention. Some clients who are living with critical and intrusive family members may need to be protected. Merely reducing the hours of contact between the client and the family may be beneficial. The client may be encouraged to find alternative living arrangements or to enroll in a daytime program that gets him out of the house for most of the day. It is better to suggest activities for the client than to recommend that he spend more time in his room. If for some reason the only way to reduce family tension is for the client to retreat to his room, time spent alone should be regulated or activity-oriented to discourage the client's regressive tendencies.

Family intervention is always indicated when caring for a schizophrenic client, and sometimes may be mandatory. Family meetings during which health care professionals can observe interactions are good sources of assessment data. Teaching the family about the illness helps convince family members that the client's strange behaviors are not chosen simply to annoy them. Parents, especially, tend to blame themselves for the illness, but this is actually a form of overinvolvement and intrusiveness. Telling parents and spouses that they did not cause the illness increases emotional distance between them and the client. Support groups and educational programs for relatives are valuable adjuncts to the treatment plan.

The concept of expressed emotion is not limited to the families of persons with schizophrenia. Criticism, hostility, and overinvolvement are impediments to recovery from any illness. It is not yet known at what point low levels of expressed emotion may be detrimental for the schizophrenic client. Additional studies are needed to differentiate family tolerance of the client's actions from family indifference to the client's welfare. Treatment necessitates careful assessment of prevailing family attitudes, and is directed toward modifying emotional extremes that are counterproductive.

Acknowledging the importance of psychoeducation, especially when offered early in the family's encounter with psychiatric illness, the health care professional must then decide what the family should be taught. There are limitations derived from professional confidentiality, but the following information may be freely shared with the family.

- The nature, course, and implications of the illness may be disclosed. It is possible to tell families what to expect without being unreasonably optimistic or pessimistic.
- If neuroleptic drugs are prescribed, the family should know why they are being used, what the effects are, and possible side effects. The same information should be given to the client, so that family and client impressions coincide.
- Families are inclined to dwell on what the client used to be, rather than what he is today. It is advisable to shape family expectations so that they conform to the client's present abilities. This realignment is therapeutic on two fronts. It removes excessive pressure on the client to be what he once was, and it lessens family frustration and disappointment with the client as he is today.
- Emotional confrontation and family conflict should be avoided if at all possible. Many persons with schizophrenia are exquisitely sensitive to the emotional climate of the family and are overly reactive. Clients living in households with high levels of expressed emotion are especially vulnerable and need to be protected (West et al., 1985).

- Families need to deal with concrete, everyday matters and avoid abstraction as much as possible. They need not be encouraged to engage in introspection. Their problem-solving skills should be strengthened through practical advice for dealing with the client, and by gratifying some of their own needs for respite and diversion.
- Family members, especially the primary caretaker, need to be aware of their feelings and responsive to them. It seems hard for devoted parents to turn away even briefly from a child in turmoil. One way of inducing them to attend to themselves is to warn them that destroying their own health will not help the client in any way.
- External sources of support for the family are essential, especially if previous support networks are no longer available. Self-help groups made up of persons with similar experiences are especially helpful for the families of schizophrenic clients, even when the affected individual does not live in the same household.
- In order to cope, families require explanations of what the health care system can and cannot accomplish on behalf of the client. It is useful for them to recognize their importance in helping to stabilize the condition of the client, and also to understand the limits of their responsibility. Because families are usually in closer contact with the client than professionals are, they should be encouraged to observe and report alarming changes in behavior. This should be done with the previous knowledge, if not the full consent, of the client.
- When the family is unsure of how to handle a situation, they should have access to a dependable health care provider. This is especially important when the family feels overwhelmed or emotionally exhausted. Without recourse to professional advice, families at such times may react emotionally in ways that are not in the client's best interests nor their own.
- Even if the health care professional sees that the family may be exacerbating the client's problems, a message should be conveyed that it is possible for them to become allies rather than saboteurs of the treatment plan. This begins by indicating to the family some alternative actions likely to prove more helpful for everyone concerned.
- The outlook for the full recovery of many schizophrenic clients is dubious. Throughout the long course of the disorder, families continue to look for information, guidance, and reassurance from health care professionals. Their search should be rewarded with honesty and generosity.

Clinical Example: Family Involvement in a Schizophrenic Episode

Marlene Woods is 18 years old and a senior in high school. For the past three months she has been increasingly withdrawn. Her mother noticed that at times Marlene seems to be talking to herself and responding to voices that no one else can hear. Recently she became very distressed and revealed to her mother that a voice kept telling her to drive the family car off a cliff. She also expressed fear that her brother wanted to poison her. A few nights ago she woke up screaming, grabbed a carving knife from the kitchen, and ran into her brother's room, yelling that she had to stop him from killing her. Not wanting to involve the police, her father called their family physician, who told them to take Marlene to the emergency department of a general hospital that had an inpatient psychiatric unit.

Marlene soon quieted down and gave up the knife to the father. Her parents argued about whether to take her to the hospital, with father saying no and mother saying yes. Marlene's brother, Mark, said that either they should take Marlene to the hospital immediately or he would pack his belongings and leave home. At this, mother became hysterical; father offered to take Marlene "for a ride" to calm her and instead drove her to the hospital even though she insisted that she neither wanted nor needed treatment. When she realized they had arrived at the hospital, Marlene became very upset and locked herself in the car until hospital security people were called on to unlock the car and bring her into the emergency department.

Assessment

Marlene is the youngest of three children. She has two brothers, Jerry, aged 25 years, and Mark, aged 21 years. It was Mark whom Marlene accused of trying to poison her and whom she attacked. Mark and Marlene have been rivalrous since early childhood; he had often declared that he hated Marlene and wished she had never been born. Their father is a busy contractor, and their mother owns a small art gallery. Both are in their mid-fifties. For as long as the children can remember, their parents' marriage has been stormy and marked by frequent quarrels and separations. When Marlene was 16, her mother left the family home and lived in her own apartment for more than a year.

Although not an alcoholic, the father sometimes drank heavily. At such times he hit his wife and once knocked her down. On this occasion she struck back at him, scratched his face, and broke his glasses. The older son, Jerry, had behavior problems during adolescence but managed to graduate from college and works about thirty miles away from the family home. Mark suffers from severe asthma and presently attends a community college while living at home. In recent years the art gallery managed by Marlene's mother has become quite successful. Although she lives with her husband and family, Marlene's mother has a small apartment in New York City, which she visits often.

The bond between Marlene and her father is very strong and may have incestuous overtones. He has always disapproved of her boyfriends and wanted to know just where she was going at all times. Sometimes he slept in the second twin bed in her room after he and his wife quarreled. There were no signs of sexual abuse, but his emotional involvement and possessiveness toward Marlene seem inappropriate. It is obvious that generational boundaries between father and daughter are blurred.

When Marlene's father was 10 years old, his own father died. His mother, to whom he is close, is 83 years old and lives in a retirement home. Marlene's maternal grandparents are no longer living. Her mother's only sister had spent time in a psychiatric hospital following episodes of a mysterious illness. Marlene's father revealed that his wife's sister had also "heard voices," and he appeared eager to attribute Marlene's distress to her mother's side of the family.

Planning

A psychiatric consultant in the emergency department recommended admission for Marlene. The emergency mental health team then insisted on a preliminary family interview that included Marlene, Mark, and her parents before she was admitted. This was done to enlist family support for the treatment plan and assess the extent of family dysfunction. In this initial family meeting Marlene became agitated and noisy, again accusing Mark of wanting to kill her. This caused the mother to become very distressed. Father ignored his wife's discomfort and was protective only of Marlene, almost refusing to allow her to be admitted to the hospital.

Intervention

After admission to the psychiatric inpatient unit, Marlene was placed on antipsychotic medication. Within a week's time she was calmer and more composed. She was under the care of a young male psychiatric resident, and she flaunted her regard for him to her family. During the first week of her hospitalization, her family canceled three appointments to meet. For father, the crisis was over, and he wanted no further investigation of family interactions. Marlene began pleading to return home, but Mark and her mother opposed this. After resisting briefly, her father could no longer withstand Marlene's entreaties. After fourteen days of hospitalization, he took her home without medical authorization.

Upon Marlene's return home, Mark installed a full lock on his bedroom door, and mother spent a long weekend in her New York apartment. She had a long-distance conversation with her oldest son, who advised her to move out permanently. It was Jerry's contention that both Marlene and her father were "sick in the head." Although Mark's sympathies were with his mother, he did not think he could move out before finishing his college program. Though separated by distance, Marlene's mother and two brothers formed an alliance that excluded father and daughter. The alliance, though understandable in the circumstances, bound father and daughter even closer in their enmeshed relationship.

Evaluation

Although Marlene's stay in the hospital was short, it was long enough for the diagnosis of schizophrenia, paranoid type, to be made. The parents had long avoided dealing with their own troubled relationship, and Marlene had become a buffer between them. Both parents were fearful of what might happen between them when Mark and Marlene left the family home. Marlene herself was unready to face the prospect of her own eventual separation, and had never managed to form a strong or clear sense of self. She saw father as her protector against a harsher mother. Psychological studies administered to Marlene revealed that she saw herself as rescuing father from an unkind creature—her mother. Father could not tolerate her trust in and attachment to a young male therapist, for the relationship symbolized her separation from him. Marlene, also, could not face the loss of her father, and chose him rather than the healthier relationship with her therapist. In begging to be taken home from the hospital, Marlene renounced her wish for improvement and maturation.

When Marlene left the hospital against all professional recommendations, her mother decided to stay in New York. This decision completed the girl's oedipal victory and personal defeat. Mark joined his mother shortly afterwards and finished his schooling in a New York state college. With little need to keep up appearances and no one to object, Marlene's father began to drink more and socialize less. Marlene remained in the family home with father, not blatantly psychotic but phobic and housebound.

MOOD DISORDERS AND THE FAMILY

Transient periods of depression are experienced by everyone, usually as a reaction to the loss of a loved one, to the occurrence of trauma or illness, or to defeats or disappointments over the course of a lifetime. Though hard to endure, negative events are eventually integrated into the pattern of existence after a period of grief and mourning. For some people, however, depression appears as a recurring or long-standing dysfunction, often in the absence of an identifiable less or precipitating event. Depression is the most common kind of mood disruption, but sometimes disruption takes the form of *mania*, a state of hyperactivity, excitement, grandiosity, and euphoria. Clinically, mania seems to be a reversal of depression, but in fact it is a compensatory mechanism that enables the individual to mask or deny the depression that invariably underlies a manic state.

Depression is the most prevalent psychiatric disorder. It is ten times more common than schizophrenia; up to 70 percent of psychiatric diagnoses in general treatment settings are for depression (Cancro, 1985). In some individuals depression is a lasting condition that persists for a lifetime. These persons are a burden to society, to their families, and to themselves. Causes of depression exist at biological, psychological, and social levels (Table 11.1), and the condition is expressed through complex pathways. The process of differentiating depression from normal grief or sadness is often influenced by the orientation of primary care providers and their reaction to the disturbed mood.

TABLE 11.1. Significant Factors in Depression	
Type of Loss or Change	**Typical Examples of Loss or Change**
Loss of meaningful relationships	Alienation or estrangement from a loved one; death, divorce, separation from a loved one
Change in body image or self-image	Physical or functional change in self-concept due to disease, trauma, or aging
Loss of status or prestige	Career demotion or disappointment; social or interpersonal inadequacy
Loss of confidence and self-assurance	Lowered sense of competence, autonomy, and independence
Loss of security and safety	Economic or social reverses; loss of control; unpredictable future outcomes
Loss of dreams, fantasies	Unfulfilled hopes; unrealized and unreachable ambitions

There are two divergent views of depression, with most experts adopting positions between the two extremes. One view is that depression is biologically determined even though situational factors may be present. At the other extreme is the view that depression is psychologically and socially generated, with situational factors being primary causes. Recent studies consistently link chemical imbalances to depression, although these imbalances may not cause depression but may only be associated with its occurrence.

Without a doubt, depressive symptoms affect all spheres of functioning (Keitner, 1985). Somatic manifestations include appetite loss or appetite increase, agitation or apathy, insomnia or hypersomnia, and marked libido loss. Behavioral manifestations include neglect of personal needs, loss of concentration and cognitive abilities, and social unresponsiveness. The depressed individual feels sad and hopeless; often thoughts of suicide intrude and may be acted upon.

Sociocultural factors appear to influence the clinical manifestations of depression. Psychological states of worry, tension, and irritability seem more prominent in higher socioeconomic groups. In less industrialized areas, depressed persons' complaints take somatic forms that are more culturally acceptable. Their complaints center on physical symptoms such as indigestion, constipation, fatigue, and loss of sexual function. Depressed persons in these groups may complain of being mistreated or persecuted but rarely express feelings of guilt or worthlessness. In more advanced industrialized areas, guilt is often present, but even in these societies clinicians have noted a decline in the frequency and severity of guilt feelings expressed by depressed clients. Instead of reporting feelings of guilt, clients are now more likely to voice feelings of personal inadequacy and of unfulfilled hopes (Robert, Hirschfeld, & Shea, 1985). Despite sociocultural differences in the manifestations of depression, race, class, and culture are not correlated with overall rates of mood disorders. Table 11.2 shows some of the demographic risk factors associated with depression.

Primary and Secondary Manifestations of Depression	
Primary	*Secondary*
Hopelessness	Sleep disorders
Helplessness	Digestive disorders
Apathy (low interest and activity)	Weight change (usually loss)
Anhedonia (inability to enjoy)	Loss of libido (low sex drive)
Asthenia (low levels of energy)	Suicide ideation, threats, attempts
Guilt	Somatic delusions
Rumination	Indecisiveness
Feelings of inadequacy	Motor agitation or retardation
Fatigue	Somatic delusions
Inability to concentrate	Delusions of persecution

Statistics regarding rates of depression probably underestimate its prevalence, perhaps because clinical signs vary so much. Some depressed individuals mask their feelings and appear cheerful to the untrained eye. Others manifest their depression mainly in somatic complaints that partly explain their apathy, agitation, or lack of pleasure (anhedonia). Precipitants of depression include accumulated or multiple life events that are perceived negatively by the individual. Rejection by parents in childhood, poor marital adjustment, economic worries, and failed ambitions are only a few of life experiences that contribute to depression. Additionally, some people spend their formative years in homes where there is a constant atmosphere of hopelessness and a sustained expectation of failure. Such family depression can be contagious; members learn to expect the worst and find it hard to be optimistic.

Lowered self-esteem is an overriding feature of depression, which intensifies the discomfort of the client. Whereas depression involves a devaluation of the self in response to an actual or perceived loss, mania represents a denial of loss and temporary restoration of self-esteem. Episodes of mania may be interspersed with periods of normality or of depression. Mania occurs more often before age 35; depression occurs more often after age 35. In any manic-depressive illness, there is little or no deterioration between episodes, which may be separated by weeks, months, or years. Untreated depressive episodes may last months or years without treatment; untreated manic episodes usually last for weeks. The person suffering from mania is

TABLE 11.2. Demographic Risk Factors in Variations and Disruptions of Mood: Depression

Risk Factor	Epidemiological Data
Gender	In almost all industrialized countries more women than men are found to be clinically depressed. Data may be biased because help-seeking behavior is more acceptable for women. Furthermore, alcohol use and aggressive behavior may mask depression in men. Other factors accounting for greater prevalence in women are more precarious thyroid function, use of steroidal contraceptives, and premenstrual and postpartum endocrine changes.
Age	Early studies indicated that incidence of depression in women was greatest between 35 and 45 years of age; in men incidence was greatest between 45 and 55 years of age. More recent studies show that the median age of onset is the mid-twenties for both. High rates of depression are now reported in children and adolescents, due to recognition that depression is not confined to adults.
Race	Black Americans receive less treatment for depression than whites. As health care systems were integrated, diagnosis and treatment of depression in black Americans rose significantly. Community-based studies now indicate that race is not a significant risk factor.
Social class	No association has been reported between social class and clinical evidence of depression. This is a contrast to bipolar disorders (mania) where social class is a significant factor.
Religion	No association between religion and depression has been proved, partly because genetic and cultural factors intrude.
Family influence	Family history of depression doubles or triples the risk. Depression concordance rates for identical twins are less than bipolar concordance rates. Evidence for genetic transmission of depression is less convincing than for bipolar alterations. Family studies are complicated by symmetrical mating (likelihood of depressed persons to have a depressed spouse). It is unclear whether depressed persons choose mates with similar problems or whether depression in one partner is contagious for the other. Children of two depressed parents are twice as likely to be clinically depressed as the children in families where only one parent is depressed.

Source: Adapted from Weissman and Boyd (1985); Kerr, Hoier, and Versi (1985); and Wierzbicki (1987).

more likely to receive treatment either by burning out or by acting so inappropriately that an alarmed family seeks professional help. Table 11.3 shows some of the demographic risk factors associated with mania.

TABLE 11.3. Demographic Risk Factors in Variations and Disruptions of Mood: Mania	
Risk Factor	Epidemiological Data
Gender	Most of the incidence and prevalence studies now show equal rates for men and women. Earlier studies showed higher overall rates for women.
Age	Recent studies show onset occurring most often in late teens or early twenties. Earlier studies showed incidence to rise until age 35, followed by decline. With advancing age, time between manic episodes may shorten and duration lengthen. NIMH (National Institute of Mental Health) studies consistently show earlier onset (late twenties) for mania, and later onset (late thirties) for major depression.
Social class	Bipolar disorder is more common in upper socioeconomic groups. Persons with bipolar disorders usually reach higher educational and occupational status than comparable control groups comprising normal subjects.
Race	No relationship has been found between race and bipolar disorders.
Religion	Because intermarriage within religious groups may introduce genetic and cultural influences, no association between religion and bipolar disorders has been proved.
Family influences	Abundant evidence shows that bipolar disorders are familial and probably genetic. In a study of paired twins, there was three times as much concordance between identical as between fraternal twins. Adopted persons with biological family histories of bipolar disorders were three times more likely to develop the disorder than adoptive parents or siblings with no family history of bipolar disorders.

Source: Adapted from Weissman and Boyd (1985) and Wierzbicki (1987).

While in a manic state, the individual behaves in ways that are not governed by convention or good sense. To maintain the illusion of omnipotence, the individual engages in reckless spending or may embark on grandiose schemes to impress others. The manic person is demanding, exploitive, self-centered, and manipulative, but underneath feels uncertain and anxious. Although the individual seems eager for social interaction, there is extreme fear of intimacy and sensitivity to rejection. Singing, rhyming, dancing, dressing, and undressing proceed in rapid order, until onlookers, but not the manic individual, are exhausted. The limitless energy and excessive responsiveness to all stimuli make it hard for the manic person to maintain adequate nutrition and rest. Unless treatment is given, the individual will suffer dangerous exhaustion and total depletion of energy.

Because mania is apt to be a recurring process, families must be taught to recognize the warning signs and obtain treatment before the client is beyond control. Frequently, an individual in a manic episode will become involved in extravagant purchases and impractical undertakings. When the manic period subsides, client and family must then face the consequences of questionable actions taken by the client. Lithium carbonate is a natural substance that acts as a preventive against recurrences of mania. It is effective for about 80 percent of cases of manic disorder. The person taking lithium must be monitored by means of regular blood testing. The therapeutic range for lithium is narrow; too little is useless, while too much can be toxic or even lethal. This places a heavy responsibility on family members. They must observe the client's behavior for indications of imminent mania, because the client may or may not be reliable about the prophylactic regimen. In addition, they need to know the symptoms of lithium toxicity and the importance of medical examinations that include blood studies and tests for kidney and thyroid function, since lithium may have an adverse effect on these readings.

The DSM-III-R (1987) differentiates Major Depression from Bipolar Disorder. It further classifies bipolar disorder as Mixed, Manic, or Depressed. The essential feature of Depressive Disorders is one or more episodes of depression without a history of manic or hypomanic periods. The essential feature of Bipolar Disorder is the occurrence of one or more manic or hypomanic episodes, usually but not always accompanied by a history of periods of depression. The presence of a depressed person in the family creates many problems for families but is probably less frightening and certainly less dramatic than witnessing a full-blown manic episode. With treatment, the manic client can return home within a comparatively short time. At this point family members are unsure how to behave and fear that their actions may precipitate another manic episode. Persons with bipolar illness can lead relatively normal lives if they are willing to comply with treatment plans. Following a manic period, the patient feels slowed down and is more aware of his limitations. This inevitable reaction worries the client, who tends to blame it on his medication. Both the client and the family need to know that during the manic period the client was like a person experiencing the exhilaration of driving at a hundred miles per hour. The slowdown that the client complains of is only a relative one, and simply means that the client is moving at the same speed as most other people. The family can become a reinforcer of the therapeutic plan by insisting that the client has a physical disorder, much like diabetes, and that discontinuing lithium puts both client and family at risk. After a manic episode the confidence of the client in himself is shaken, and the family is distrustful as well. If the family continues to treat the client in a fearful manner that shows they expect the worst, family relationships will continue to suffer. By offering full, cognitive explanations which convey the same messages to the family as to the client, the clinician can help restore family equilibrium.

Therapeutic Guidelines

It can be valuable for families to learn that the depressed client and the manic client are victims of disorders that are largely physiological. They cannot be blamed for their illness even though the resultant behaviors are stressful for families to endure. It is also advisable to remind families that between episodes of impairment, persons suffering mood disorders return to their previous levels of functioning, especially if the family is supportive and accepting. For some clients, medication may be required for long periods of time. To reinforce compliance and protect the client, families need to know the ramifications, hazards, and precautions accompanying the prescribed medications.

Clear communication between client and family members, and between client, family, and the health care professional is essential. The depressed family member is apt to arouse impatience in the household, and the manic individual is apt to arouse fear or dread. Even when initial treatment is effective, it may take a long time for family members to deal with memories of the acute episode. Emotions continue to run high during the client's convalescence and recovery. Lefley (1987) applied measures and variables in depression similar to those used in research with schizophrenic persons. He found that critical comments made by families to depressed persons correlated with relapse of the depressed persons over a nine-month period. These findings, coupled with what is already known of the negative impact of high expressed emotion in families with a schizophrenic member, suggest that families should respond to persons with a mood disorder in a concerned but objective and dispassionate manner.

The depressed person interprets experiences and events in a self-defeating, self-denigrating way. There is a wide range of depressive emotion, ranging from mildly uncomfortable to severely disabling. All individuals construct their interpretations of reality out of past, present, and future information, using their preferred patterns of thinking. From this accepted construct, Beck (1969, 1972) formulated the cognitive triad present in the thinking of depressed persons: (1) a negative, self-deprecating view of the self; (2) a negative, pessimistic view of the world; and (3) a negative, unpromising view of the future as it relates to the self. These are the distortions that torment the depressed person, and which the clinician and family endeavor to refute.

The depressed mood and disorganization of the depressed client make it difficult for him to mobilize enough energy to share relevant information with the health care professional. Moreover, clinicians committed to theories that mood disorders are biochemical disorders unrelated to life events may be disinclined to make active inquiries into the client's psychosocial history. This is a serious omission, for if there is no exploration of real, symbolic, or fantasied loss experienced by the client, therapeutic outcomes may be jeopardized.

People with moderate to severe depression often have a strong desire to be liked and approved of by others. Because they already tend to blame themselves, they may be unwilling to risk further rejection by revealing too much. Family members may collude with the client to conceal information that casts a poor light on the family. In such situations a series of family meetings will be useful in piecing together a clear picture of events. After obtaining an accurate history, the health care professional is more able to work with the client in correcting the cognitive distortions that perpetuate his hopeless mood.

Somatic therapies, in the form of medication or of electroshock treatment that is sometimes used for intransigent depression, have their place, but so have psychotherapeutic interventions designed to clarify the meaning of the client's losses, to restore the ability to relate to other people and resume productive activities. Depression is often a reaction to life stresses, albeit an extreme one. Extensive assessment must therefore be made of past and present events in the client's life and of relationships with significant others. Frequently the depressed person is a participant in family interactions that contribute to a sense of worthlessness. As the symptoms of depression continue, even the most devoted family members become impatient and angry. In these cases marital or family therapy is an effective component of treatment. In family sessions the family can learn much by observing the clinician's nonjudgmental attitude, and the clinician can learn by observing family interactions. The participation of the family can be crucial to diminishing family confusion and confronting unresolved issues. Even when prolonged family therapy is not indicated, input from family members and occasional communication with them are advisable. Like the client, the family can be told of the favorable prognosis and assured that the future will be different from the painful present. Because of the dark mood of the client, families share the conviction that the depressed state will last a lifetime and never lighten.

If a depressed client is deemed to be suicidal, the family should be informed that an emergency situation exists and that immediate hospitalization is necessary. Here the health care professional becomes a psychological security guard for the client by taking charge and explaining what steps must be taken and why. At this point families are simultaneously worried and relieved. Hospitalization as a precaution against suicide relieves the family of responsibility for protecting the client against self-destructive impulses. More often than not, families and clients feel grateful that their desperate situation has been understood. Resistance to hospitalization usually arises only when the client believes that the measure is punitive rather than protective. Families are sometimes upset if they see hospitalization as a reflection of their inability to meet the client's needs. Everyone involved should be told that the suicide urges are an aspect of the client's illness, and that the client will recover from the illness and no longer be at the mercy of suicidal thoughts.

It is not easy to live with a depressed person, and families need help in managing their feelings and reactions. The implicit message that the family has certain responsibilities is counterproductive unless the family is given explicit advice on how to help. Families that are overly invested in the client's recovery and believe that the family's well-being depends totally on the recovery can create an additional blow to the client's self-esteem. The depressed person can feel under an obligation to stop being depressed in order to help the family. Because the depressed mood is not under voluntary control, the client who cannot stop feeling sad endures yet another failure. Concentrating on the client's condition may be well motivated but may encourage regression in the depressed person and indicate distrust of the client's ability to progress in his own way.

- Families should be encouraged to proceed with their own lives as much as possible. A mater-of-fact attitude is better than forced cheerfulness or false encouragement. Exhortations to "stop brooding" or "get going" are interpreted as judgmental by the client. Specific suggestions (i.e., get dressed or take a walk) are more acceptable.
- Families should make suggestions in ways that give the depressed person freedom to reject the advice. When suggestions are made in a way that allows no options, the client feels helpless and infantilized.
- The apathy and listlessness of depressed persons is extremely distressing to families. Time management is a strategy of which most families are capable. Encourage families to plan pleasant events that include the client. Initially the events should be enjoyable but not too demanding.
- Families can be taught to observe and monitor the client's reactions to certain activities, even to the extent of keeping a record that can be shared with the client. This can be a guide for the family in planning future activities and a reminder to the client of recent experiences that were relatively enjoyable. By considering the client's negative reactions to situations or events, the family can help the client avoid similar experiences in the future.
- In addition to planning positive social encounters for the client, families can arrange for undemanding tasks that are of interest and within the client's current capabilities. Tasks that require great concentration or decision making are inadvisable, but many depressed people can complete selected tasks and experience feelings of accomplishment.
- It is not necessary for families to understand the dynamics of depression in order to be helpful. Most families, however, are capable of taking a behavioral approach in dealing with the depressed person. Deficits in the client's social skills and activities of daily life benefit from specific family strategies that avoid criticizing the client but reward positive moves on the part of the client. Social avoidance may be reduced by offering pleasurable encounters; negativism and feelings of failure may be reduced by arranging graduated tasks at which the client is likely to be successful.

- Decision making on the part of the client should be simplified by offering two rather than a host of options. This gives the client some freedom but focuses his thinking.
- Cognitive errors in thinking can safely be refuted by the family without negating the reality of the client's bleak outlook. The depressed person looks at the world through darkened lenses. It is enough to say that the client's pessimism is not shared by everyone and will pass as the client's illness improves.

Clinical Example: Intergenerational Depression Issues

Mr. Cody is a 42-year-old insurance salesman, married and the father of two sons, ages 14 and 12 years. He was hospitalized following a self-inflicted wrist-slashing episode. At age 38 Mr. Cody was evaluated psychiatrically for depression and treated with antidepressant medication. Medication was recommended by a psychiatrist and continued by his family physician. At the time of the initial depression, Mr. Cody refused further psychotherapy, saying he thought medication was sufficient.

Assessment

Mr. Cody is a shy, retiring man who seems to be unemotional and reserved. His suicide attempt followed a number of painful incidents that occurred about the same time. He became involved in a rare argument with his wife, who frequently complained that there "never was enough money around here." Usually Mr. Cody overlooked her complaints, but in this instance he reacted angrily. A week before, he had been passed over for promotion at work in favor of a younger man. His 14-year-old son had been caught exposing himself at school, and counseling was urged by the school principal. In addition, it was the month of the fifteenth anniversary of his daughter Lucy's death. Lucy, their first child, had died at three years of age from a chronic kidney ailment. Lucy had been named for Mr. Cody's mother, and he had loved her dearly. When Mr. Cody was 14 years old, his father had died by his own hand. He and his younger sister were raised by their mother, who worked hard inside and outside the household to support her children.

Mr. Cody's wife had only a high school education; he had a bachelor's degree in economics and had completed some graduate-level courses. Mrs. Cody was employed as a department store clerk; she was a driving, dissatisfied woman, perhaps somewhat depressed herself. She was more verbal than her husband and tended to criticize him in front of their sons. Mike, the older boy, was born only a year after Lucy's death, and both parents were disappointed that he was not a girl to replace the lost child. Mike suffered from a lack of confidence and was effeminate in his mannerisms. This annoyed and disgusted both parents. Pete, the 12-year-old boy, was an aggressive child with temper outbursts who was very tied to his mother.

Planning

The psychiatric inpatient unit to which Mr. Cody was admitted, after spending two days in an intensive care facility, used a family orientation to care. The interdisciplinary mental health team arranged meetings with Mr. Cody, his wife, and their children. His antidepressant medication was changed, and he was told that medication was not a magic answer to his problems. Instead of relying solely on medication, he was told that he needed to talk about his feelings, which he had heretofore kept hidden. Family meetings were recommenced to clarify the family's strengths and to learn to what degree Mr. Cody's depression represented family pathology.

Intervention

At first, the family meetings focused on members expressing their solicitude and concern for Mr. Cody. A little later, family members began to express their anger at his suicide attempt. Second, the focus was on allowing Mr. Cody to talk individually with the unit therapist to whom he had been assigned. Unit staff members began to move him gently away from his emotional avoidance patterns and to encourage him to verbalize his feelings. Soon it became apparent that his long-time sadness had obscured his underlying anger — mainly toward his wife for her complaints and attacks on him. For his wife, also, anger was a mask for her own sad feelings, and in the sessions she wept as she talked about the death of their first child. Clearly, neither parent had mourned adequately for the dead child, and this had prevented them from truly accepting their second child. On an intuitive level, Mike, the older son, sensed the parents' distance from him. Thus, in early adolescence he was desperately struggling for validity; he exposed his genitals to others for confirmation of his maleness. The younger son, Pete, was rebelling against mother's control, and both boys demonstrated in their behavior a need for a father who could be a strong male role model. Out of Mr. Cody's brief psychiatric hospitalization came a recommendation for individual outpatient care for him, for marital sessions, and for family meetings that included the children. In family meetings emphasis was on helping the parents communicate in a more open fashion with their boys. In marital sessions emphasis was placed on helping the parents bond as partners so they would be able to develop confidence in their parental roles, and present a united front to the sons. The mixed therapeutic approach was useful and for the most part productive.

Evaluation

Mr. Cody in all likelihood will not be able to give up his reticent, self-controlled stance completely, but he is less frightened of his strong inner feelings. His sons welcomed his efforts to share activities with them; in time they came to enjoy fishing or camping together. It was an opportunity for all three to be buddies, and the boys saw a new side of their father. Mrs. Cody joined a women's athletic club where she learned to become an expert swimmer. Since swimming was a hobby at which Mr. Cody and the boys were proficient, the whole family shared this interest. Little had been said in the family about Lucy, yet both boys felt that they were poor replacements for the beloved daughter. With the new emphasis on sharing emotions, the parents were able to acknowledge their grief at Lucy's death and also reassure the boys that they too were loved and valued.

EATING DISORDERS AND THE FAMILY

Anorexia nervosa and bulimia are eating disorders that are very prevalent today among women and girls. Ninety-five percent of the cases of anorexia nervosa occur among young women; an estimated 5 to 15 percent of adolescent girls are thought to be affected. On some college campuses 20 percent of the female students fit the psychiatric definition of anorexia nervosa (Brumberg, 1988). In anorexia nervosa the afflicted individual is obsessed with losing weight; in bulimia the afflicted individual is obsessed with eating and its consequences. In both disorders the lives of the individual and the family are disrupted. For the person with anorexia nervosa, the disorder can be life-threatening. Social and family influences are thought to be significant in anorexia nervosa and in bulimia.

Anorexia Nervosa

The person with anorexia nervosa is convinced that she is fat even though she has starved herself to the point of emaciation. The disorder was once thought to be an upper- and middle-class aberration found mostly in adolescent females. Recently it has been discovered to be quite common among lower-class females as well, and among women over 25 years of age (Shisslak et al., 1987). The term *anorexia* is misleading, for the individual does not lose her appetite until the disorder is far advanced and the body no longer sends hunger signals. Even then, the individual remains preoccupied with food and food preparation for others, while she continues to deny herself nourishment. Intensive exercise programs become food substitutes; the individual is usually active and energetic in spite of starvation, until finally the body succumbs. The extreme weight loss and the amenorrhea accompanying it are of no concern to the anorectic person.

Cultural preferences for slimness in women undoubtedly play a role in the prevalence of anorexia nervosa and of bulimia also. Society persuades women that to be attractive they must not exceed stated weight standards. They are instructed to diet and exercise in order to be healthy and beautiful. Brumberg (1988) believes that anorexia nervosa is prevalent today because women increasingly use their bodies as instruments of competition and participate in a dangerous game to become as thin as possible. She adds that for women who lack a strong sense of self-identity, the cult of diet and exercise assumes a religious importance, and brings "coherence" that otherwise might be absent from the women's lives.

A late-nineteenth-century French neurologist, Charles Lasègue, developed an approach to the treatment of anorexia nervosa that is curiously modern. Lasègue described a sequence of events familiar to the families of anorectic persons. The sequence consists of presenting food to the individual who refuses to eat. This is followed by entreaties to eat as proof of love for the parents. The pleading is met with stubborn rejection by the individual, whereupon both sides engage in manipulative actions that become a domestic battle. Warfare continues until the individual is so undernourished that medical help is summoned (Brumberg, 1988). Lasègue attributed the Victorian girl's refusal of food as a weapon against family pressure on her to make a socially approved, conventional marriage. What better methods were available to the girl than to develop a malady that would remove her from social competition?

In treating a person with anorexia nervosa, the immediate aim is restoration of the client's nutritional state. Extreme emaciation causes irritability and depression, so that psychotherapy and behavioral programs may be useless until the client's physical status improves. Outpatient treatment may be effective with clients who have had the disorder less than six months and whose family is cooperative. Otherwise the client should be hospitalized for a time. This has the advantage of removing the client from the battleground existing in the household. Sir William Withey Gull, the personal physician of Queen Victoria, was often consulted by parents dealing with anorexia nervosa in their daughters. Sir William recommended that "the patients should be fed at regular intervals, surrounded by persons who would have more influence over them, relatives and friends being generally the worst attendants" (Halmi, 1985, p. 1147).

During hospitalization, full bed rest is prescribed and gradually relaxed through a program of rewards as the client progresses. The use of behavioral reinforcement is facilitated by hospitalization. It is widely used and is usually supplemented with family therapy. Family collaboration is a necessary component of treatment for anorexia nervosa but is usually supplemented by individual psychotherapy and by behavioral modification. Anorexia nervosa can range from mild to severe; prognosis may range from complete recovery to death.

The person who is anorectic believes that there are few areas of life under her control. Eventually she learns that one area she can control is what she eats. Many anorectic persons are obsessive-compulsive in various aspects of their lives, are of above average intelligence, and are high academic achievers. Bruch (1973) depicts the mother of the client as often controlling and a perfectionist in her own right. Anorectic persons display three consistent characteristics: (1) distorted body image, (2) distorted sensations of hunger and fatigue, and (3) underlying feelings of inadequacy. Bruch (1983) attributes the disorder in part to parental neglect during the child's formative years or inappropriate responses to the child's needs. As a result of the control exerted by parents, the child experiences herself in a distorted, unrealistic fashion.

Minuchin, Rosman, and Baker (1978) identify patterns in the families of persons with anorexia nervosa that contribute to the occurrence of the disorder:

- *Family enmeshment*: All family members are excessively involved with one another.
- *Family rigidity*: Family members have a strong need to maintain outward appearances at all costs.
- *Family authority*: Family members, especially parents, discourage autonomy in the child, to the detriment of the child's social skills and relationships.
- *Family conflict resolution*: Family members deal with conflict by avoiding rather than resolving disagreements.

Beyond these patterns, Minuchin and his associates note that the family of an anorectic child tend to emphasize food and body functions such as digestion and elimination. Therefore, it is not surprising that in this climate a child yearning for autonomy might use anorexia nervosa as a weapon that enables her to control others in the family who want to control her. Clients with anorexia nervosa need long-term help. The prognosis is better for younger persons than for older ones, and family intervention is always indicated. The long-range goal is to stop the individual and the family from judging success or failure in terms of pounds lost and food not eaten.

Family resistance to participating in treatment may be a problem. Forisha, Grothaus, and Luscombe (1990) find that families refuse involvement unless they think the individual is dying. Researchers report family dropout rates of 50 to 60 percent (Szmukler et al., 1985). Several clinicians (Minuchin et al., 1978; Bauer & Anderson, 1989) observe families eating together or share meals with families in order to shift attention from the identified patient to the family, and to assess family interaction at mealtime. Minuchin, however, curtails mealtime sessions as soon as the client attains minimally acceptable weight, in order to deal with other family issues.

Mealtime sessions are considered advantageous from the perspective of family assessment, intervention, and evaluation. Bauer and Anderson (1989) state that in some families mealtime has become so horrendous that members no longer eat together. This is a strategic tactic that helps the client avoid eating and the family avoid dissension. The mealtime session is presented as a therapeutic tool. During the meal family conflict becomes evident. Role performance is visible, and the power struggle in the family is clearly shown. Whenever possible, two health care professionals are present at the mealtime sessions; this allows them to validate their impressions concerning family interaction.

When using a mealtime session, the family is asked to start the meal as if they were at home. The seating arrangement of the family is easily seen and is assessed in terms of boundaries and subsystems. In subsequent sessions various family members might be asked to select seating arrangements more to their liking. During the meal, the health care dyad can see who is eating or not eating, who stops eating when disagreement surfaces, and what the tempo of eating is for different members. The person with anorexia nervosa usually demonstrates childlike eating habits, pushing the food around the plate, rearranging it, and cutting it into smaller and smaller particles. The client is usually silent at mealtime, especially at the beginning of therapy. Parents inadvertently collude in this by cajoling the client, commenting on the eating behavior, and treating the client like a recalcitrant child. The health care dyad is committed to separating the issue of food from the issue of family transactions, and will deemphasize eating behaviors as soon as possible. As the mealtime sessions are repeated, client and family become more comfortable. Forisha, Grothaus, and Luscombe (1990) report that sharing meals with the client and family gradually "desensitizes" the client to food and reduces her obsessiveness about controlling her weight. As family members gain an understanding of the impact their mealtime actions have on one another, they are more receptive to therapeutic interventions that alter destructive facets of their behavior. Frequently the client will describe herself as "unable" to eat while the health care professional quietly describes the client as "choosing" not to eat. This opens family discussion of choices available to all members in the realm of eating and other unrelated activities. Specific interventions are selected to improve communication processes, comment on scapegoating or other power maneuvers, and encourage behavioral changes to reduce conflict around eating. Often the family of a person with anorexia nervosa is uncomfortable with open disagreement, except that which surrounds the client's refusal to eat. Whether mealtime therapy is available or not, these families need to learn that disagreements are not life-threatening if faced openly and discussed honestly. This is preferable to anorexia nervosa, in which individual and family conflicts can assume life-threatening proportions.

Bulimia

This eating disorder is manifested by binge eating followed by purging and/or vomiting. Unlike the person with anorexia nervosa, the bulimic individual has no body image distortion. She realizes that her eating behavior is abnormal, and she is less resistant to treatment than her anorectic counterpart. Food eaten during a binge is often sweet and of a texture that is easily regurgitated or vomited. The eating, vomiting, and purging are done in secret. Because the bulimic person is generally of normal weight, her aberrant behavior is unknown to those around her. In searching for the cause of bulimia, the etiology is best summarized by Strober and Humphrey (1987, p. 654) who state that ". . . it seems likely that certain personality factors, which may be genetically determined, predispose the individual to greater sensitivity and vulnerability to powerful familial and social experiences that impinge adversely on self-esteem and self-efficacy." In the explanation cited here, both a cultural factor and a genetic factor are thought to be present in bulimia. A number of investigators locate the chief etiological factor in the family. The family of an anorectic person is reputed to be enmeshed, critical, intrusive, and unresponsive to the emotional needs of children. In most cases families of anorectic individuals are judged to be more dysfunctional than families of bulimic persons, although parents of the latter are described as lacking in affection, hostile, disengaged, and impulsive. Alcoholism and obesity are prevalent in the families of bulimic persons. Strober and Humphrey (1987) caution that the contribution of families to anorexia nervosa and bulimia is speculative at best, and suggest that families may be unfairly blamed for contributing to the onset of eating disorders.

Therapeutic Guidelines

Orbach (1986) points out the inherent conflict that is expressed in eating disorders, and calls it a metaphor for our society. The conflict is about starving oneself in the midst of plenty, about suppression of appetite, and about striving to be invisible while wishing to be acknowledged. The pressure on women in Western life is to live up to a stereotype of the perfect female form, regardless of its cost.

In the absence of clear evidence of the family's role, it is imperative to refrain from premature assumptions. The dynamic explanation that is most acceptable is that the core conflict in eating disorders is powerlessness. It is therefore advisable to allow the anorectic and the bulimic person control over other aspects of her life, so that she eventually becomes willing to give up her obsession about the one thing she can control, namely her weight.

- If disruptive patterns are identified in the family, these should be addressed, while avoiding any semblance of blame.
- As soon as possible in treatment, the defensiveness of the family should be modified. This can be done by enlisting the family as an ally and by expressing hope that they will become part of the solution. In language appropriate to the family's level of comprehension, the health care professional might begin by saying, "We are not here to judge anyone but to help deal with a family problem. My impression is that you care deeply about one another and are upset by what is happening in your family. Some things that families do work out well, but other things don't work

so well. So today we will look for the things that work well, so you can do them more often. As we go along, we may recognize some things that are not helpful to see if we can improve them."

- Cognitive restructuring is a preferred approach for clients with eating disorders. Nutritional information should be given to correct misconceptions that the client and the family may have about food. And a challenge must be made to the overvaluation of slimness placed upon women. The key to successful treatment is patience and flexibility on the part of the health care professional in determining the family's unique needs.
- As always, what is known about eating disorders must be divulged to the worried family. Anorexia nervosa and bulimia are complex, multidetermined disorders. There are no hard and fast rules for proceeding. Assessment and intervention must be individualized for each clinical situation.
- The client with anorexia nervosa is more likely to be living with her family of origin; the bulimic is more likely to be living on her own or with a spouse. This means that family intervention is more feasible for the anorectic person; individual or marital therapy may be more suitable for the bulimic client. Persons with bulimia are seldom emaciated and are more often treated on an outpatient basis. For any eating disorder, lengthy treatment is usually needed.

SUMMARY

Severe psychiatric illness represents ongoing trauma for the client and for the family. Factors contributing to the trauma of psychiatric illness include unpredictability, recurrence, chronicity, stigmatization, and fears of family members that somehow they caused the illness. Disorders of thought known as schizophrenic illnesses are very hard for families to manage, largely because of the progressive deterioration that occurs. The concept of expressed emotion and its association with relapse and rehospitalization can be used to alter the way some families react to the behavior of the schizophrenic client.

Mood disorders, especially depression, can be as difficult for the family as for the client. Families need specific instruction about medication regimens and about coping with the client's negativism. Family members should go on with their own lives as much as possible. They need not understand the dynamics of the client's depression. More important is teaching the family a behavioral-cognitive approach aimed at reducing regression and improving the client's hopeless viewpoint.

Eating disorders such as anorexia nervosa and bulimia may be adversely affected by family patterns, but data on this is still speculative. Cultural and social influences play a significant part in the prevalence of these two eating disorders. In the absence of proven information about family contribution to the etiology of eating disorders, it is wise not to make premature assumptions. The prevailing dynamic explanation for eating disorders, especially anorexia nervosa, is that the core conflict is struggle for control. It is therefore advisable to give these clients all possible control over other aspects of their lives, so that they can become less obsessive about eating and weight.

It is quite possible that family dysfunction is the effect rather than the cause of eating disorders. The presence in the home of a member who is slowly starving is not conducive to family harmony. Regardless of whether the family is part of the problem, the clinician should try to make family members part of the solution. Distracting the client and the family from preoccupation with eating can be done in several ways. In cases of advanced anorexia nervosa, hospitalization may be necessary to restore the client's nutritional status. During hospitalization, the primary care provider may wish to arrange mealtime sessions attended by client, family, and one or two health care professionals. This increases opportunities for assessment and intervention, and may desensitize the individual to the experience of social eating so that she is more willing to relinquish her obsession with controlling her weight by starving herself.

REFERENCES

Abramowitz, I. A., & Coursey, R. D. (1989). "Impact of an Educational Support Group on Family Participants Who Take Care of Their Schizophrenic Relatives." *Journal of Consulting and Clinical Psychology*, 57(2):232–236.

American Psychiatric Association. (1987). *Diagnostic and Statistical Manual of Mental Disorders*, third edition, revised (DSM-III-R). Washington, DC: American Psychiatric Association.

Bateson, G., Jackson, D., Haley, J., & Weakland, J. (1956). "Toward a Theory of Schizophrenia." *Behavioral Science*, 1:254–264.

Bauer, B. G., & Anderson, W. P. (1989). "Bulimic Beliefs: Food for Thought." *Journal of Counseling and Development*, 67:416–419.

Beck, A. T. (1969). *Cognition and Psychopathology in Depression: Clinical, Experimental and Theoretical Aspects*. New York: Harper & Row.

Beck, A. T. (1972). *Depression: Causes and Treatment*. Philadelphia: University of Pennsylvania.

Brumberg, J. J. (1988). *Fasting Girls: The Emergence of Anorexia Nervosa as a Modern Deviance*. Cambridge, MA: Harvard University Press.

Bruch, H. (1973). *Eating Disorders: Obesity, Anorexia Nervosa and the Patient Within*. New York: Basic Books.

Bruch, H. (1983). "Psychotherapy in Anorexia Nervosa and Developmental Obesity." In R. K. Goodstein (Ed.), *Eating and Weight Disorders*. New York: Springer.

Cancro, R. (1985). "History and Overview of Schizophrenia." In H. I. Kaplan & B. J. Sadock (Eds.), *Comprehensive Textbook of Psychiatry*, 4th ed. Baltimore, MD: Williams and Wilkins.

Faloon, I., Jeffrey, R. H., Boyd, J. L., & McGill, C. W. (1984). *Family Care of Schizophrenia*. New York: Guilford Press.

Forisha, B., Grothaus, K., Luscombe, R. (1990). "Dinner Conversation: Meal Therapy to Differentiate Eating Behavior from Family Process." *Journal of Psychosocial Nursing*, 28(11):416–419.

Fromm-Reichmann, F. (1948). "Notes on the Development of Treatment of Schizophrenia by Psychoanalytic Psychotherapy." *Psychiatry*, 11: 263–273.

Halmi, K. A. (1985). "Eating Disorders." In H. I Kaplan & B. J. Sadock (Eds.), *Comprehensive Textbook of Psychiatry*, 4th ed. Baltimore, MD: Williams and Wilkins.

Hatfield, A. D., & Lefley, H. P. (1986). *Family of the Mentally Ill: Coping and Adaptation*. New York: Guilford Press.

James, B. (1988). *Treating Traumatized Children: New Insights and Creative Interventions*. Lexington, MA: Lexington Books.

Kietner, G. I. (1985). *Bipolar Illness: A Guide for Families*. Butler, RI: Butler Veterans Administration Center. (Videotape)

Kerr, M. M., Hoier, T. S., & Versi, M. (1985). "Methodological Issues in Childhood Depression: Review of the Literature." *American Journal of Orthopsychiatry*, 57(2):193–198.

Koenigsberg, H. W., & Handley, R. (1986). "Expressed Emotion: From Predictive Index to Clinical Construct." *American Journal of Orthopsychiatry*, 143(1):1361–1373.

Leff, J. P., & Vaugn, C. E. (1985). *Expressed Emotion in Families*. New York: Guilford Press.

Lefley, H. P. (1987). "Culture and Mental Illness: The Family Role." In A. B. Hatfield & H. P. Lefley (Eds.), *Families of the Mentally Ill*. New York: Guilford Press.

Lidz, T., Fleck, S., & Cornelison, A. R. (1965). *Schizophrenia and the Family*. New York: International Universities.

Minuchin, S., Rosman, B. L., & Baker, L. (1978). *Psychosomatic Families*. Cambridge, MA: Harvard University Press.

Orbach, S. (1986). *Hunger Strike: The Anorexic's Struggle as a Metaphor for Our Age*. New York: Norton.

Robert, M., Hirschfeld, A., & Shea, T. (1985). "Affective Disorders." In H. I Kaplan & B. J. Sadock (Eds.), *Comprehensive Textbook of Psychiatry*, 4th ed. Baltimore, MD: Williams and Wilkins.

Romano, J. (1979). "The Chronically Ill Schizophrenic Patient." Paper presented at the annual meeting of American Psychiatric Association, Chicago, May 17.

Seeman, M. (1986). "Heterogeneous Needs of Families of Schizophrenic Patients: Gender Differences." In *Family Involvement in the Treatment of Schizophrenia*. Washington, DC: American Psychiatric Association.

Shisslak, C. M., Crago, M., Neal, M., & Swain, B. (1987). "Primary Prevention of Eating Disorders." *Journal of Counseling and Clinical Psychology*, 55(5):660–669.

Spaniol, L., & Zipple, A. M. (1988). "Family and Professional Perceptions of Family Needs and Coping Strengths." *Rehabilitation Psychology*, 31(1):37–45.

Strober, M., & Humphrey, L. (1987). "Family Contributions to the Etiology and Course of Anorexia Nervosa and Bulimia." *Journal of Counseling and Clinical Psychology*, 55(5):654–659.

Szmukler, G., Eisler, I., Russell, F., & Dare, C. (1985). "Anorexia Nervosa: Parental Expressed Emotion and Dropping Out of Treatment." *British Journal of Psychiatry*, 147:265–271.

Terkelson, K. G. (1987). "The Meaning of Mental Illness in the Family." In A. B. Hatfield & H. P. Lefley (Eds.), *Families of the Mentally Ill*. New York: Guilford Press.

Weissman, M. M., & Boyd, J. H. (1985). "Affective Disorders: Epidemiology." In H. I. Kaplan & B. J. Sadock (Eds.), *Comprehensive Textbook of Psychiatry*, 4th ed. Baltimore, MD: Williams and Wilkins.

West, K., Cozolino, L., Malin, B., McVey, G., Lansky, M., & Bley, C. (1985). "Involving Families in Treatment of Schizophrenia: The Role of Family Education." In *Family Approaches to Major Psychiatric Disorders*. Washington, DC: American Psychiatric Association.

Wierzbecki, M. (1987). "Similarity of Monozygotic and Dyzygotic Child Twins in Level and Lability of Subclinically Depressed Mood." *American Journal of Orthopsychiatry*, 57(1):33–40.

PART
SIX

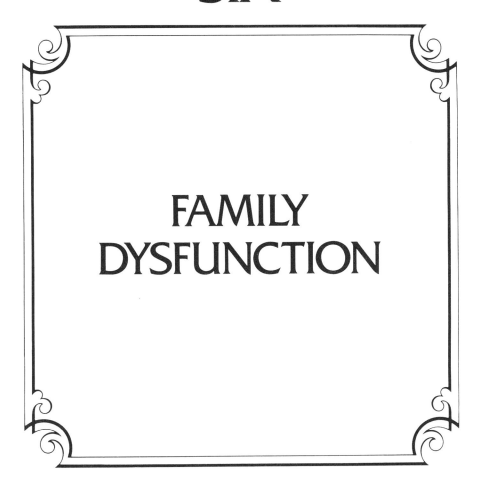

FAMILY
DYSFUNCTION

CHAPTER TWELVE

Abuse, Violence, and Neglect in the Family: Perpetrators and Victims

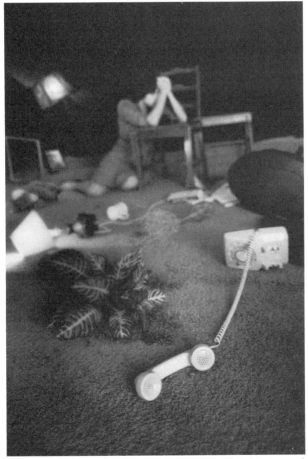

Anger is inevitable when our lives consist of giving in and going along; when we assume responsibility for other people's feelings and reactions; when we relinquish our primary responsibility to proceed with our own growth and ensure the quality of our own lives; when we behave as if having a relationship is more important than having a self.

Harriet Goldhor Lerner

The problem of family violence is not a new one. What is new is that it is now being recognized as a major social problem. Violence in the family is a multidimensional phenomenon affecting wives, husbands, children, extended family, and even pets. Its causes are rarely simple or linear; they are complex. More recently, abuse of elderly persons by adult children and by nursing home personnel has come to public attention. Violent acts receive prominent coverage in newspapers and the other mass media. Few aspects of violence are overlooked in portraying assaultive behavior between individuals and between groups of people. Within families, violence is widespread and is not limited to any social milieu, although family violence is often associated with alcohol and drug addiction. Of all countries in the Western world, the United States is considered the most prone to violence and its people the most likely to kill one another (Pittman, 1987).

This chapter reviews some relevant theories of violent behavior within the family offered by Lyman Wynne, Blair and Rita Justice, and Frank S. Pittman III. Three sections are concerned with child abuse and neglect, spouse abuse, and the abuse of the elderly. The section on child neglect and abuse discusses sexual abuse; the section on spouse abuse discusses retaliatory spouse murder. In the three sections, characteristics of the abusers and the victims are presented. The special features of father–daughter sexual abuse and sibling incest are described. The chapter includes content on child abuse as it relates to the single-parent family. There is also discussion of legal aspects related to these issues.

The section on spouse abuse concerns the social problems of battered women and chronologically traces representative theories regarding the abuse of women. Characteristics of men who batter and of women who ultimately kill their abusing husbands are included in this section.

In the section on abuse of the elderly, the loss of status of aged persons in American family life is noted, as well as the impact on elderly people of the divorce and remarriage of their adult children. The predicament of middle-aged children, often called the "sandwich" generation, is described here. These adults are caught between caring for aged parents and raising adolescent children, and sometimes find the dual burden too onerous to bear. The rising incidence of violent acts against older persons is noted and its origins traced. The chapter concludes by exploring pertinent issues for health care professionals in working with the abused population and the abusers. Therapeutic guidelines are formulated for each of the three major sections.

THE ABUSING FAMILY SYSTEM: THEORIES OF FAMILY VIOLENCE

Family theorist Lyman C. Wynne discusses developmental and familial origins of vengeance and violence (Saunders et al., 1984). He states that there are three connecting links between feelings of vengeance and acts of violence in the family: (1) a constant feeling of strong, vindictive anger; (2) integration of this feeling into a belief system; and (3) a setting of disillusionment and deprivation of a relationship or an unsuccessful relationship leading to vengeful, violent behavior. Wynne emphasizes the presence of intense resentment and the enduring wish to right what is wrong. Like any other social group, large and small, families can structure belief systems that are based on the need for revenge. In most social groups there is a close relationship between the cognitive and emotional aspects of what is defined as fair and just.

It is in the family setting that members have well-fixed expectations that their emotional needs will be met or fail to be met, Wynne continues. Abusive and violent behavior occur more often than not within a group whose members have primary relationships with each other—that is, the family. Because of our experience in the family, we develop a sense of whether we are likely to be loved and cared for or to be hurt, neglected, and abused. Failure to have our basic needs met produces feelings of inferiority, disillusionment, sorrow, anxiety, and humiliation. Family therapist Rodney Shapiro reminds us that there are numerous acts of nonphysical violence that produce their own trauma. The expression of hostility through taunting and belittling, especially when heaped upon young children, can be as devastating as physical abuse (Shapiro, 1984).

Blair and Rita Justice (1976) identify several characteristics of the abusing family. Its violent behaviors are carried from one generation to another; its individual members are for the most part undifferentiated, lacking a feeling of belonging or a sense of separateness. Dysfunction of one marital partner erupts into abusive behavior toward offspring. In these fragile families the anxiety level is quite high, while the ability to contain and control intense emotions, such as rage, is extremely poor. Ties to families of origin are often unbroken and infantile. There is great competition between the abusing parents for gratification of their unmet emotional needs. Often abusing parents were themselves emotionally deprived or physically abused as children. Thus, these authors concluded that the victims in one generation become perpetrators in the next.

Although some experts such as Blair and Rita Justice subscribe to theories of intergenerational transmission of family violence, this is not always the case. Some adults who become parents learn from their painful experience to be better parents and to give their children a safe and wholesome home environment. Kaufman and Zigler (1987) find that although family abuse sometimes continues over time, it is unfair and unwarranted to assume that this always happens. They further claim that the unquestioned hypothesis that abused persons become abusers has a negative impact and impedes the process of learning more about the origins of family abuse. Furthermore, the hypothesis may lead to inappropriate legal sanctions and social policies. It is crucial for investigators to learn more about the specific circumstances that are likely to perpetuate family abuse from one generation to another.

Family crises are frequently a factor in violent and abusive behaviors. Pittman (1987) outlines four categories of family crises:

- *Unexpected crises:* These are brought about by uncontrollable external forces.
- *Developmental crises:* These are brought about by predictable maturation and transitions.
- *Structural crises:* These are precipitated by marital turmoil.
- *Caretaker crises:* These follow changes or disruption of role enactment.

In discussing structural crises, Pittman asserts that the behavior of family bullies serves a family function and that seemingly frail spouses may complain but, in reality, protect the person who terrorizes them. They may even take responsibility for having caused the violent behavior of the partner. In Pittman's view, such spouses are not impotent victims but, rather, are strong, influential fellow conspirators.

CHILD ABUSE

Definitions Seen in Historical Perspective

What constitutes child abuse changes from one decade to another and even from year to year. What is considered acceptable practice in one generation becomes abuse in the next. For many centuries harsh treatment of children was justified by the belief that severe physical punishment was needed to maintain discipline and teach children their place in the social and working world. Because children were considered property, parents had the right to inflict any measure deemed necessary to enforce their control (Helfer & Kempe, 1968). At various times and in many cultures, such practices as clitorectomy, castration, and the ultimate abuse, infanticide, were routine.

Children have been mistreated in the workplace to the extent of slavery and forced labor; they have been abandoned in times of war, sold into bondage, and starved in times of meager harvests. The Society for the Prevention of Cruelty to Children was founded in 1971, long after the Society for the Prevention of Cruelty to Animals. In the early 1960s, Henry Kempe introduced the term "battered children syndrome" and led a well-attended symposium at the American Academy of Pediatrics in 1961. This became the stimulus for increased public interest in child abuse as a national problem.

Incidence of Child Abuse

Surveys that have been conducted are probably unreliable, but it is estimated that about three million children are abused every year. Statistics on the sexual abuse of children indicate that one-third to two-fifths of reported incidents involve other family members, and one of every twelve involve a father or stepfather. There were 123,400 cases of child sexual abuse reported in 1984, and this is probably only a fraction of actual cases (Kissel, 1986).

A number of factors contribute to child abuse, including characteristics of the abusing parent, the nonabusing parent, and the child. These are discussed in the sections that follow.

Characteristics of the Abusing Parent

Most abusing parents do not have overt psychopathology that distinguishes them from nonabusing parents, but they do have some common characteristics. Often they seem to be depressed at times and to demand a great deal from their children. Their expectations are usually beyond the comprehension and abilities of the child. Abusive parents deal with children as if they were older than their actual age and are both ignorant of and intolerant of age-appropriate behavior. Many of them feel insecure and unloved themselves, and they look to their children for comfort and assurance that they are respected. For the abusing parent, infants, children, and adolescents exist primarily to satisfy parental needs, and the needs of their offspring are not important. Kaufman (1966) states that abusing parents project their own problems onto their children and are convinced that the child is the cause of their difficulties. Instead of confronting their problems, they relieve feelings of anxiety by attacking the child.

In many instances abusing parents are recreating the pattern of their own upbringing, although this is not always true. They frequently experienced intense demands from their own parents which they could not fulfill. Accompanying these demands was constant parental criticism, so that they grew up feeling inadequate and inept. Within their family of origin, interaction was oriented toward satisfying the demanding, critical parent.

Helfer and Kempe (1968), in their classic work on child abuse, suggest that abusing parents cannot enact the parental role adequately because they never experienced a satisfying, confidence-building relationship with their own parents. This deficient relationship creates disbelief in the possibility of good parent–child relationships, which persists after they have children of their own. For the abusing parent, most relationships tend to be distant, barren, and unrewarding. Their basic lack of confidence, originating in poor parenting in early life, is reiterated in subsequent life experiences and impairs marriages and parent–child interaction. Convinced that their needs were not met by parents, spouse, or friends, the individual then turns to sons or daughters for the reassurance and acceptance that are desired so desperately.

Contribution of the Nonabusing Parent

Usually only one parent attacks the child, but the other parent may contribute either by openly accepting the abusive behavior or by tolerating it. If the nonabusing parent shows undue interest or attention toward the child, feelings of envy and resentment may generate more abusive behavior from the other parent. Any perceived rejection from the nonabusing partner may also be a stimulus to attack. In some families abuse is directed either toward the wife or toward the children; in other families all are targets of abuse. There are families where the pattern of abuse is so entrenched that when one parent tries to change, the other parent then becomes abusive. Sometimes the child is a scapegoat for conflict between parents who are dissatisfied with one another but displace their feelings on the child. Invariably, the abusing parent has unrealistic expectations that the child cannot meet. These expectations may lie in the realm of performance or may consist of parental needs for affection and comfort that the child cannot and should not be asked to meet.

Contribution of the Child

Innocently and unwittingly, the child may contribute to his own mistreatment. Unwanted infants are often targets for abuse, as are infants who do not live up to parents' idealized images. Parents who expected an active child may be disappointed with a placid one and vice versa. Children who cry a great deal threaten the parents' self-esteem and self-control. They may fear that the baby is irritable because they are not good parents or because the baby is sick. Any child who is different or special may be a target for abuse. This is especially true of children born with congenital defects whose needs require much attention and constitute a drain on family resources of time and money.

Sometimes, but not always, children have strong feelings of loyalty for the abusing parent. Such feelings should not be underestimated or denied by health professionals. This writer worked with a single-parent family consisting of a mother and six children. Previously the mother and all the children were severely abused by the father. On one occasion he had beaten a 10-year-old son, thrown him across the room, and broken the boy's shoulder. After the father deserted the family, this same boy hitchhiked from a northeastern state to Florida, searching for his lost father. Some abusing parents can be strong and caring at times, and this boy seemed to be in search of that aspect of his father.

Child Sexual Abuse

The sexual abuse of children is another term whose connotations change over time and from culture to culture. What never changes is the fact that children are relatively helpless and, like most helpless people, may be mistreated and exploited by adults charged with their care. In general, child sexual abuse may be defined as the involvement of developmentally dependent, immature children and adolescents in sexual activities they do not fully comprehend, or for which they are unable to give informed consent (Kempe, 1978). A child who is the object of sexual abuse is doubly powerless: The perpetrator is usually a person on whom the child must depend in other ways, and the child suffers from a lack of choice (see Table 12.1). Lack of choice is evident whether coercion, seduction, or bribery is used to involve a child in sexual activities. Often the offender is known to both child and parents. Relatives who abuse children sexually or in other ways may be found in every socioeconomic stratum. They may live in urban or in rural areas, and their educational level may range from grade school dropout to advanced graduate degree. They represent a wide variety of religious affiliations and ethnic groups.

Finkelhor (1985) reports several critical differences that have been found in patterns of physical and of sexual abuse. First, the physical abuse of children takes place at the hands of men and women in almost equal proportions, whereas those persons who commit sexual abuse are 85 to 90 percent male. In cases of physical abuse the primary offenders are most often the parents. This is less true of sexual abuse, which occurs both inside and outside the nuclear family system. Sexual offenders may be members of the extended family, neighbors, coaches, and teachers. Although sexual abuse occurs between stepparents and children, allegiance on the part of the child toward the perpetrator is infrequent, and the nonabusing parent is rarely inclined to countenance the behavior. Therefore, sexual abuse is likely to be confronted earlier and more openly in stepparent families. This point is expanded in Chapter Six.

Incest Patterns

Incest practices and prohibitions date back to premodern times and vary according to culture, locality, and historical moment. Sometimes incest was permitted between family members in order not to dissipate the wealth of a family through numerous heirs. More often, early taboos against incest

---

TABLE 12.1. Consequences of the Sexual Abuse of Children

Physical consequences:
  Rectal fissures
  Rectal sphincter damage
  Anal and vaginal lacerations
  Gonorrheal infections of the genitals, tonsils, larynx, and pharynx
  Pain and discomfort

Emotional consequences:
  Sense of betrayal
  Guilt and shame
  Need for secrecy and concealment
  Loss of trust in others
  Anger toward both parents; generalized hostility
  Feelings of helplessness and powerlessness
  Confusion and mystification

Behavioral consequences:
  Withdrawal into a fantasy world; reclusiveness
  Aggressive actions outside the home
  Promiscuous sexual behavior
  Phobic reactions to sexuality
  Poor school performance
  Inability to set limits for self or others
  Running away from home

Source: Adapted from Janosik and Davies (1989).

---

were invoked to prevent internecine feuds and jealousies in primitive family systems. The ancient royal families of Egypt practiced incest as a religious and patriotic duty. The pharaohs were considered gods. Only gods could marry gods; therefore, divine pharaohs could marry only their divine sisters. Incest was practiced in Rome by certain emperors, among them Caligula. In Greek mythology incest was rampant both among the gods and between gods and mortals. However, usually at least one of the participants was unaware of the true identity of the other. The ambivalence of the early Greeks toward incest is revealed in the legend of Oedipus, who slew his father and committed incest with his mother. Even though this was done unknowingly, Oedipus was blinded for his deeds. Parricide seemed to be more abhorrent than incest with his mother, but perhaps to the Greeks the crimes were one and the same. In some cultures men were forbidden to marry the widow of a dead brother, whereas in other cultures men were expected to marry and provide for the widow of a dead brother. In general, taboos against incest between blood relatives were stronger than those between in-laws, perhaps because observant primitive people saw the effects of inbreeding. This may explain why advances in genetic knowledge and awareness of dominant and recessive traits have reinforced incest taboos.

The dynamics of incest are reviewed by Forward and Buck (1978), who state that the father who sexually abuses a daughter frequently has no need to use brutal force because of the parent–child bond and the emotional strength of the relationship. A daughter looks up to her father and usually sees him as a provider and authority figure. Therefore, she is inclined to try to please him or to do his bidding without resistance. Added to his influence is the threat of reprisal unless she submits voluntarily. The punishment the daughter fears may not be specific or harsh, for the greatest fear of children is that a parent will withhold love and approval if the child disobeys. It is the threatened loss of love that coerces children into cooperating in their own sexual victimization.

When victims equate incestuous behavior with attention, caring, or pleasure, they derive some gratification from the relationship. In contrast, many young girls experience physical pain, anxiety, and feelings of helplessness and repugnance. Fear of being punished, of being unloved, or of not being believed deters many young girls from reporting the sexually abusive behavior. Shame and guilt for their reluctant participation prevails into adulthood; the victims' search for relief from their anguished feelings often leads to self-punitive behaviors such as substance abuse, promiscuity, prostitution, or avoidance of sexual relationships. Periods of depression, intermittent or chronic, are common, as is a pervasive sense of worthlessness. Many victims of incest exhibit a pattern of poor interpersonal relationships, often fraught with repetitive self-destructive actions. Having experienced victimization at the hands of a significant person who did not respect limits, these children tend to become adults who are unable to set limits for themselves or others.

Incest between father and son is particularly abhorrent in our society, perhaps because it violates heterosexual values. Forward and Buck (1978) attribute this form of incest to paternal decompensation rather than to family dysfunction. On the other hand, there are sources that declare all forms of incest to be an indication of family dysfunction, especially father-daughter incest (Machotka et al., 1967). In their view incestuous behavior does not occur unrelated to poor marital adjustment, including a mother's indifference and abdication of her parental role. Mothers have been known to aid and abet the father's sexual liaison with the victimized daughter by isolating themselves and withdrawing from parental responsibilities and from sexual relations with their husbands. One middle-aged father was hospitalized because of depression. In interviews with the wife, she disclosed a seven-year history of his sexual abuse of their 12-year-old daughter. She also revealed that she had told the father he could break the lock on the girl's bedroom door if he chose as "it was a weak lock." The mother was fully aware of her daughter's sexual relationship with father and did not support the daughter in her resistance to father. The daughter, who had reached puberty, was attempting to oppose her father's sexual overtures.

Sibling incest is thought to be fairly common but is largely unreported. The game of body exhibition and exploration between young siblings of opposite sexes occurs frequently. It is usually harmless and is most often the result of their natural curiosity. Many variations of sibling incest are possible: older brother–younger sister, older sister–younger brother, and homosexual sibling incest. The greater the age difference between the siblings, the stronger the likelihood that the sexual behavior is imposed on the younger sibling by the older one. This is true of both heterosexual and homosexual encounters. A harsh parental attitude toward very young siblings about their innocent curiosity and exploration can be traumatic for children and detrimental to normal development. Older siblings, however, are usually aware of prohibitions against this form of sexual expression. If it continues, professional help may be needed. Sibling incest, like other forms of incest, constitutes a problem for the entire family, and the victimized child is in real danger when there is no one to turn to for help.

The Single-Parent Mother and Abuse

Single parents are thought to be at risk for committing violent acts against their children, for a number of reasons. The mother may transfer her anger at her husband to a son, who then becomes a target for the mother's displaced rage. The stresses of raising children as the sole parent are compounded in the setting of a painful separation and divorce. Research corroborates the belief that abusive behavior is more frequent in single-parent households because of economic deprivation and the absence of a second parent (Gelles, 1989).

Legal Issues

Although there are criminal penalties for incestuous behavior in every state, the legal definitions of incest vary. Many states have laws that require incestuous behavior (termed child abuse) to be reported by any school, medical, legal, or social agent who suspects abuse. Persons who report suspected incest or other forms of abuse are protected from being sued for slander or libel. The legal procedures that follow reporting can provoke emotional distress in the child victim. Testifying in court can be very intimidating; children and adolescents often have very mixed feelings about accusing a parent for whom a child holds ambivalent feelings of loyalty and distrust. In some states a child's testimony alone is not enough to bring about a guilty verdict. When a sexually or physically abusive father is removed from the home, the mother may press for his return, either for economic reasons or from her pathological need to perpetuate the dysfunctional but familiar family system.

Therapeutic Guidelines

It is not easy to work with abusing families, for most health professionals must first deal with their own feelings of outrage. Although it is rewarding to rescue abused children, to comfort and protect them, it is less gratifying to deal with parents who taunt, hurt, and even kill their children. For these reasons it is sometimes recommended that the same health professional not work with the abused child and the abusing parent. Identification with the child victim and negative feelings toward the abuser can be obstacles to establishing a therapeutic alliance with the abuser (Justice & Justice, 1976).

Learning about the abuser's life stresses and hearing about the abuse experienced early in life, can enable health professionals to develop empathic responses for the perpetrator. Single-parent mothers are often young women who need parenting themselves and are likely to respond positively when their pain and emotional neediness are recognized. A nonjudgmental attitude on the part of the health professional is essential in working with abusing families. This does not mean dismissing or excusing the abuser's behavior by saying that "he is mentally ill" or that "she has had a hard life." It is possible to reject the behavior without rejecting the abuser. Abusers, if they are to be helped, must learn to take responsibility for their actions and have a desire to change. Although the health professional does not punish or reject the abuser, neither should he or she condone or rationalize it in any way. No health professional can make up for the emotional deprivation abusing parents may have suffered as children, but it is possible to help them work for more self-control and a higher level of self-esteem. Because many abusing parents have little knowledge of developmental stages or acceptable child-rearing tactics, cognitive teaching on these issues is helpful. Parents who know how a 2-year-old or a 10-year-old is likely to act may react by reducing their excessive expectations. Techniques for handling a child's temper tantrums or unruliness can be taught by health professionals who have established rapport with the parent. For potential and actual abusers who are highly motivated to change, group treatment is often successful. Long-term, supportive community groups such as Parents Anonymous and Parents Without Partners can also be effective. Removal of a child from the home may be necessary to provide protection for the child. At times it is not the child but the abusing parent who is ordered to leave the home and not return until authorities are convinced that the abuser's attitude and behavior have changed for the better.

SPOUSE ABUSE

In the last decade or so, the predicament of the battered wife has received increasing attention from health care professionals, as well as from the media and the criminal justice system. The phenomenon known as the "battered wife syndrome" was used successfully in Rochester, New York, in the mid-1980s as the defense for a battered wife who eventually killed her chronically abusive husband. It has also been used unsuccessfully by other women who have killed their mates. These women are found guilty by courts, and are imprisoned. According to the Federation of Organizations for Professional Women (1977), two million Americans have used a lethal weapon against their spouse, and an additional two million couples report beatings between husband and wife. Data from the early 1980s indicate that between 20 and 25 percent of adult women, or between 12 and 15 million, have been physically abused at least once by a male intimate (Kissel, 1986).

Although family violence is often assumed to be more prevalent in lower socioeconomic groups, studies show that wife battering transcends ethnic groups and social classes. DeLorto and LaViolette (1980), operating a shelter for battered wives in California, found that their clients were 62 percent white, 13 percent Chicano, 3 percent Asian, and 2 percent other. The abusing husbands represented almost every profession and occupation. Battering appears to be more frequent in families at lower socioeconomic levels because these families are more apt to come to the attention of protective and law enforcement agencies. When upper- or middle-class husbands abuse their wives, the behavior is hidden from public view, partly because wives are too embarrassed to tell others (DeLorto & LaViolette, 1980).

Wife abuse exacts a great toll from its victims, physically, emotionally, and socially. Marital violence is frequently cited as grounds for divorce (O'Brien, 1971) and is often associated with child abuse and problem child behavior (Hilberman & Munson, 1978; Rounsaville, 1978). Why do husbands beat their wives? A number of theoretical explanations have been advanced by members of the health care disciplines. Each emphasizes different concepts as crucial in understanding spouse abuse. Practitioners may draw appropriate concepts from various theories so as to enhance their understanding and develop a framework for providing care to battered women.

Intrapsychic Theories

Traditional explanations of wife battering rely on Freud's theory of feminine masochism. According to Freud, the masochist wants to be treated like a small, dependent, helpless, naughty child. The true masochist holds out a cheek whenever there is a chance of receiving a blow. The continuation of suffering is all important; punishment is used to eradicate feelings of guilt. In the Freudian paradigm, this self-destructive behavior results from failure to resolve the female version of the oedipal romance. The girl competes with mother for father's attention, but fears losing mother's love. To show she is not interested in her father, she unconsciously provokes aggression from him, thus reducing the guilt she feels for desiring father. Learned in childhood, this pattern persists in adult relationships with men.

Sociocultural concepts have been incorporated in explanations for wife battering (Shainness, 1979). Some men use violence as ego-enhancing behaviors, and resort to violence because their repertoire of nonviolent responses is limited. These are the kind of men to whom masochistic women often relate. In this formulation, masochism in women and sadism in men are influenced by intrapsychic forces and sociocultural influences.

In psychoanalytic theory, such factors as helplessness, plasticity, and prolonged dependency make infants susceptible to the masochistic process. The masochistic person is afraid to resist, offend, or set limits. In addition, sociocultural circumstances like superior male strength and poor control of reproduction have contributed to submissiveness in women. Tacit acceptance of male dominance has induced many women to enact the gender-determined role in ways that avoid conflict.

The psychoanalytic stance has been criticized on several fronts. Symonds (1979) refutes the idea of the victim's masochism and challenges society's tendency to blame the victim. She suggests that violent marriages fall into one of two groups: those in which violence precedes the marriage and those in which violence follows the marriage. In the first group, the man has a history of violence; his tendencies toward violence erupt early in the courtship and grow progressively worse. For these men, aggression and violence are ego syntonic. There is an underlying sense of powerlessness, often originating in a childhood marked by violence and lack of control. According to Symonds (1978), the wives of such men react in three phases: the impact phase, the infantilization phase, and the depression phase. It is the second stage that is crucial to understanding the battered wife. In this stage the wife resorts to the coping mechanisms of childhood; she becomes obedient and cooperative, trying desperately to please and placate her husband. Later she feels that no outside support network can rescue her; isolation, hopelessness, and depression follow. Unluckily for the wife, there is little she can do to avoid provoking her husband. She is the convenient, available recipient of the husband's entrenched violence.

In the second group of marriages where violence occurs later, the behavior may be a last resort when other communication attempts have failed. These are dysfunctional marriages in which the behavior of one partner threatens the defenses of the other. Projection of their own shortcomings onto the partner is used by both to justify their behavior. The eruption of violence makes both partners feel worse, not better, and these marital relationships can be improved through counseling or therapy. A literary example of this kind of interaction is found in D. H. Lawrence's autobiographical novel, *Sons and Lovers*. Here, the upwardly oriented wife is married to a coal miner who is limited but well meaning. Her aspirations threaten him, and he takes refuge in alcohol, which releases his aggressive impulses, causing him to behave in ways that acutely distress his genteel wife.

In a study of 60 battered women attending a medical clinic, Hilberman (1980) developed a stress–response theory compatible with the psychoanalytic approach. In this formulation, battered women are likened to women who have been raped, except that the threat of assault is ever present and their stress is unending. These women are exhausted, depleted, and emotionally numbed. They see themselves as inferior, unworthy, unlovable, and powerless to alter their situation.

On the basis of case study examinations, Steinmetz (1978) reformulates some psychoanalytic explanations. Contrary to the notion that some women are at risk for battering because of their personality traits, Steinmetz argues that it is the dynamics of beating that produced the traits, and compares chronic battering to brainwashing techniques. In brainwashing the subjects are isolated and deprived of their usual rewards and comforts. This results in hypersuggestibility and in receptivity to new values and behavioral standards. The only validation of the subject's worth comes from persons enforcing the isolation and reward system. Inconsistent, confusing, punitive measures, interspersed with kindness, produce the effects of brainwashing.

Seligman (1975) explains that people who are exposed to negative reinforcement unrelated to their actions learn that what they do does not determine what happens to them. The result is that they learn to be helpless; their survival instincts are extinguished, and depression follows. Learned helplessness is reinforced by the patriarchal nature of society. Women are conditioned to believe that their personal worth and well-being depend to a great extent on their physical beauty and appeal to men. This places women at a disadvantage in marriage and perpetuates historical ideas of male supremacy.

Sociological Theories

In proposing sociological explanations for family violence, Straus and Hotaling (1977) state that the popular image of the family as a place of love and gentleness is a myth. The aspects of family life that contribute to intimacy and attachment also facilitate expression of violence. Added to this is the belief in the United States that violence is an acceptable solution to many problems. Approval of violence in other spheres of life influences what happens in the family. Indeed, it is a circular process that is self-perpetuating. The violence that takes place in the family is a factor contributing to a society in which violence is common and often meets with approval. Gelles (1974) states that people in certain structural positions experience great frustration and deprivation, which stimulate violent reactions. Gelles lists several factors that are prominent in family violence (Table 12.2).

Gelles emphasizes that acts of family violence are not sporadic or unilateral. The role of the victim is an active one, with the victim often serving as verbal instigator. Pagelow (1976) uses social learning theory to explain wife battering, and suggests that persons raised in abusive households learn to respond to frustration or stress in violent ways. A man who

TABLE 12.2. Contributing Factors in Family Violence

- Experiences in the family of origin: Abusive family patterns
- Socialization in childhood and adolescence: Violent social group patterns
- Negative family structure: Unwanted children, religious differences
- Superimposed stresses: Unemployment, illness
- Social and geographic isolation: Inaccessible support systems
- Situational events: Drinking, gambling
- Permissive norms and values: Legitimization and acceptance of violence

Source: Adapted from Gelles (1974).

has been socialized to believe that physical aggression is acceptable, that patriarchy is undisputed and male dominance is admirable, will be likely to abuse the female(s) in his life. If the female conforms to the same gender concepts, she will make a great investment in her relationship with men and will accede in her own victimization.

Maria Roy, social worker and founder of Abused Women's Aid in Crisis in New York City, believes that wife beating is passed from one generation to the next and that the cycle could be interrupted by a gestalt approach involving social, educational, and legislative changes. She claims that in a violence-prone society like that of the United States, everyone is capable of violent acts. When violence is condoned and victims blamed, everyone comes to believe that physical aggression is permissible and often useful. Roy (1977) calls for city, state, and federal governments to become more accountable. Not only government but also religious institutions, schools, and media outlets must respond to the problem with new programs, new laws, and new interpretations of marriage contracts and relationships.

Shelters for battered women and their children have proliferated across the United States, but additional support and research are needed. More data are needed to identify causal factors and tailor programs to the needs of the client population. Theoretical explanations tend to be fragmented in the absence of definitive studies regarding causation and the needs of battered women. Most rewarding is the fact that spouse abuse is now a visible issue and that greater efforts are now being made to reduce the isolation and hopelessness that battered women experience.

Feminist Viewpoints

The feminist movement has done a great deal to publicize and sensitize us to the plight of the battered woman. Chapman (1978) mentions the economic victimization of women and claims that limited resources are a significant factor in the inability of women to extricate themselves from violent relationships. Many battered wives are unprepared to be breadwinners, especially if children are involved. Even when women try to be economically independent, they cannot escape being victims because of the way they are treated by men in authority positions in the working world. Chapman considers sexual assault, sexual harassment, pornography, prostitution, and medical and media exploitation to be methods used by society to continue the victimization of women.

Another strong feminist is Del Martin (1977) who asserts that all social institutions are designed to keep marriages intact, regardless of the dangers to women. Martin believes that men beat their wives because they are allowed to do so, and that women are beaten because they are conditioned to be submissive. They are taught from childhood that marriage and motherhood are women's primary goals. To catch a husband, a woman must be subordinate, passive, and submissive. She must submerge her own personality in order to appear "normal" and "well adjusted." Her passivity then makes her an underling who is subject to her husband's whims. If she "steps out of line," she is abused to put her "back in her place." Excuses are often made for the abusing husband. The wife is described as too passive, too assertive, too educated, too ignorant, or "too" anything, to justify the husband's behavior toward her. True, the husband is criticized, but the tone is different. He is overworked, unemployed, exhausted, or drunk, and thus the behavior is condoned.

Men Who Batter

While shelters and programs for battered women and their children are being maintained, much less is being done for abusing men. Edelson (1984) describes one group program of which he is the founder. Located in Albany, New York, the program offers cognitive restructuring, interpersonal skills training, and relaxation techniques using a small-group format with two male leaders. Early in the program of twelve two-hour sessions, the group members analyze events that precipitate their violent behavior. They are asked to record their angry feelings on a chart and are taught ways to counter their feelings during times of stress. As the program advances, the men begin to describe specific situations that are labeled "critical moments." These situations are discussed and alternative behaviors explored to replace their customary violent reactions. The program utilizes an approach that combines cognitive, behavioral, and emotional repatterning.

Wives Who Kill

In the 1970s and 1980s a case was reported in Lansing, Michigan, and another in Rockford, Illinois, in which a wife murdered an abusive husband. One of the women was given a light sentence; the other went free because her behavior was judged a "justifiable action." Family quarrels are the cause of one-quarter of all U.S. homicides, according to the FBI Uniform Crime Reports. Meyers (1980) reviewed California records and found that 52 percent of women killed in the state in the course of a year were killed by a husband or lover. Meyers also noted that police often ignore the beating of women by husbands, and that lawyers or judges may blame the woman because she may have "deserved what she got." Angela Browne's study of 250 abused women, 42 of whom murdered their lover or husband, appears in her book *When Battered Women Kill*. Browne (1987) writes, "Abuse of women by male partners is imbedded in and grows out of society's laws and practices denying women equal self-determination and protection in their relationships with men" (p. 179). Browne compares two groups of abused women: those who endured abuse without resorting to violence, and those who ultimately killed their abusing mate. No significant differences were found between the two groups of women; instead, the difference lay in the men and in their actions. From these data it seems possible to identify situations in which there is a high risk that the woman will murder her abuser. The findings point to a series of determining factors: the frequency of violent acts by the man, the man's abuse of alcohol or other drugs, the severity of injuries to the woman, threatened or actual sexual assaults to the woman, threats by the man to kill the woman and/or the children, and the woman's suicidal tendencies. From the study we can conclude that it is essential to learn more about the pattern of abuse and the characteristics of the abuser. Until a clearer picture can be drawn, effective programs cannot be provided for these men.

Therapeutic Guidelines

Battered women need help in overcoming the guilt and shame they feel for having been abused. They also need to be convinced that the fault is not theirs. Overwhelmed and frightened, they need encouragement to seek legal counsel and other forms of assistance. In addition to psychological help, these women need guidance in locating housing and in obtaining child support or public assistance. The central focus is on helping the battered woman achieve autonomy and self-confidence as she begins to build a new life. If the woman's partner is available for rehabilitative or preventive measures, he should be referred for help for himself. Some abused women repeatedly attempt unsuccessful reconciliations and return again and again to the shelter. Many shelters have a policy of limiting the number of times a woman may return to the shelter within a certain time frame. The personnel confront the repeater about her self-destructive behavior. She is strongly encouraged to extricate herself and her children from the abusive environment before someone is seriously hurt or killed. When the man's abuse is associated with alcohol or other drugs, the woman needs to be told that abuse will continue as long as alcohol and drugs are used (Walters et al., 1988).

Unlike the child or elderly person who is abused, the battered wife who does not leave her husband, or who leaves and returns, does not receive much sympathy from the public or even from some care providers. Police and professional persons in the legal system are usually informed about various aspects of family violence and can carry out their responsibilities without displaying hostility or indifference toward battered women. It must be remembered that much spouse abuse is unreported, because women feel they are in a no-win position. Many suffer in silence and loneliness, afraid for themselves and for their children. Those who are abused beyond their ability to endure sometimes retaliate by killing their husband or lover. Dreadful as this is, it may seem the only recourse available, and it serves to remind health professionals of the value of early intervention.

Group work with battered wives has the advantage of providing a support group in which the woman can, perhaps for the first time, realize that she is not alone. This realization has several meanings, not the least of which is that there are many other women who have experienced and are experiencing similar traumas. Her isolation is also reduced because she now has the opportunity to share with sympathetic listeners her traumatic experiences. This supportive group network is in a position to help with basic services such as financial advice, job counseling, and legal advice.

Because a major offering of the group is peer support and crisis intervention, the access to the group is open-ended, with new members accepted as they are referred or as they seek entry on their own initiative. In this way, older members in the group can function in supportive, cotherapy roles. Women who are referred to the group may join it, but they will need special attention and concern if they are to continue in the group long enough to derive benefit. First and foremost, neither the group leaders nor other members should encourage or urge the woman to leave her partner. Other people have probably attempted this strategy in the past, but to no avail. The abused wife will not leave her partner until she has developed enough self-confidence and trust in the community at large to be able to do so. Initially, she needs help in recognizing that she has alternatives. Elbow (1977) listed these alternatives: The woman can leave, she can continue in the relationship while hoping that her husband will change, or she can continue in the relationship while giving up hope that he will change. When women opt for the second or third alternative, they are encouraged to recognize that this is a conscious, deliberate choice. After becoming involved in counseling, during which self-esteem is fostered, the woman is better able to carry out plans to leave.

The major goal of group work with battered wives is *not* basic personality change. It is likely that a reasonable number of these women would benefit from treatment aimed at ameliorating neurotic patterns and improving ego functioning. These women should be informed of the professional's assessment of this need and be made aware of the community resources available to them.

Because the battered wives' group is open-ended, the members will at any given time be in different phases of progress. Because of vacillation caused by ambivalence that most of these women experience, the group itself goes through recurring phases of progression and regression, typified by the pendular life cycle model of groups. Experiencing these recurring phases gives the group members the opportunity to see others face temporary setbacks and to function as role models for newer members in the group. In addition to these benefits, the group approach for helping the battered wife uses a pool of problem-solving resources to meet the basic survival needs that many of the women face.

ELDER ABUSE

In 1960 the U.S. Census Bureau reported that 9.3 percent of the population was 75 years old or more; in 1990 the estimated percentage of persons in this age group was 12.7 percent. In the year 2030 projections indicate that one-third of the United States population will be over 65 years of age, or an estimated 77 million people. It is believed that by the year 2000, four-generation families will be the norm. These trends will have significant psychological, emotional, and financial impact on American family life.

The average American couple does not marry with the idea of taking an aged parent into their home then or later. When a decision is made to care for an elderly parent in the household, it is usually after other options have been exhausted. In contemporary American society, older people do not have much status once their productive years are over. This is in contrast to Asian societies, where old people are respected, even revered. Another trend influencing the situation of older Americans is the later marriages of adult children, especially daughters. Not only do marriages occur later in life, but they also produce fewer children. This means that the care of elderly parents is shared among fewer people, most of whom are themselves middle-aged or older. The situation is even more complex for adult children who divorce. If they remarry, they create an extended family network that may include several older persons. If they do not remarry, they may be burdened with alimony or child support, or they may have to function as single parents. Among this group there may be no financial or emotional surplus to expend in caring for a frail, elderly parent.

Definition

Mistreatment of elderly persons may take many forms, such as physical and psychological abuse, neglect, violation of rights, and financial exploitation. Giordano and Giordano (1984) report the following distinctions, taken from the 1981 Select Committee on Aging.

Physical abuse:
  Physical assault

Sexual abuse

Murder

Restrictions on freedom of movement

Denial of rights

Psychological abuse:

Provoking fear of violence or isolation

Verbal assaults

Threats of institutionalization or nursing home placement

Negligence:

Breach of duty or carelessness resulting in injury

Breach of duty or carelessness resulting in violation of rights

Violation of rights:

Breach of rights guaranteed to all citizens by the Constitution, federal statutes, federal courts, and state laws

Financial exploitation:

Theft or conversion of monies or objects of value belonging to an elderly person by a relative or caretaker, accomplished through either force or misrepresentation

Self-neglect:

Self-inflicted physical harm, failure to take care of one's bodily needs, stemming from the elderly person's diminished ability to cope, or from negative attitudes and actions of relatives or caretakers

Psychological abuse could include infantilizing the elderly person through isolation or exclusion from family meals and activities. Financial abuse could include coercion or persuasion of the elderly person to rewrite wills or sign over property. Neglect could take the form of provision of inadequate food and clothing, or of failure to provide appropriate medical treatment and/or medications.

Incidence of Elder Abuse

The American Medical Association indicates that between 500,000 and 2.5 million instances of elder abuse take place every year (Kissel, 1986). A survey conducted by Pillemer and Finkelhor (1989) revealed that 32 out of every 1,000 elderly persons in the Boston metropolitan area suffered abuse. Their study covered three forms of elder abuse: physical abuse, neglect, and chronic verbal aggression. The researchers found that 58 percent of the abuse was inflicted by a spouse; males were abused in 52 percent of the cases, females in 48 percent. A significant finding was that the characteristics of the abusers were more important predictors of abuse than the characteristics of the victims. Abusers of the elderly were troubled persons with a history of instability and socially maladaptive behavior. Steinmetz (1981) reports that violence is exhibited not only by the adult son or daughter providing care but also by the elderly parent. Their frustration takes the form of violence because both the caretaker and the aged parent fear that nothing else will be effective. *Both* resort to violence to gain control in the situation or control in the family. The demands of the older person are perceived as selfish and excessive; the efforts of the caregiver are perceived as restrictive and insensitive.

Adult Children as Caregivers

If the older person and the caregiver bring to the situation many unresolved conflicts from the past, or if they had a poor relationship, the attenuation or reversal of customary roles is intolerable for both. Perhaps the parent behaved in ways that did not promote the self-esteem of the child who is now the adult caregiver, or perhaps the caregiver was not able to separate or individuate from the parent. Parent–child relationships are always complex and are made more difficult when dissatisfaction and rage have smoldered for years. Caring for a beloved parent can be very demanding, and feelings of resentment are compounded when ties between the aged parent and the caregiver are ambivalent at best. The dependence of the elderly person is even more onerous when financial resources are meager and respite care unavailable. In many families the burden of caring for an elderly parent is not shared among siblings but is left to one or two persons to handle. This inequity increases the anger of the caregiver toward siblings and toward the parent as well. The elderly parent, for physical or emotional reasons, may have poor impulse control or react to increased dependence by lashing out at the caregiver. Yelling, profanity, hitting, pinching, and throwing things may characterize the behavior of the parent, with the caregiver the nearest available target. All this tries the patience of the caregiver, so that frustration levels and the potential for physical retaliation escalate.

In some circumstances physical violence does not erupt, but abuse of the elderly person is manifested in negligence. Good nutrition and personal care, as well as medical evaluation and treatment, are essential for the elderly, but some of these caretaking responsibilities are not met. The writer can recall a situation in an urban teaching hospital when a very confused old man was simply dropped off at the emergency department by those responsible for his care. He had severe bronchitis and was so weak he could hardly walk. There were no identifying papers on his person, and he could not recall his name or his address. Pinned inside his coat pocket, unsigned, was a note bearing the name of a funeral home to which his body could be taken, should he die. His abandonment is an extreme example of neglect and indifference, but variations of this sort of treatment are encountered by many health professionals in the course of their work.

Unfortunately, most abused or neglected older people do not solicit help from police or other community resources. They may be embarrassed, ashamed, or simply unsure of how and where to look for help. Their plight is discovered only when they are hospitalized or if a neighbor notifies the police. Even then, they seldom are willing to complain or bring charges against the person on whom they must depend for survival. Some caregivers are astute enough to realize that the needs of the elderly person have become overwhelming and therefore seek help before conditions worsen, but many do not. And the elderly person often has neither the energy nor the fortitude to obtain help on his or her own behalf.

Many times the family caregiver for an elderly person is well past middle age or has other responsibilities. Regardless of their age or capabilities, caregivers need care too. When an elderly parent comes to live with a son or daughter, the situation is new for everyone, and additional sources of help must be found. Day care programs for the ambulatory elderly are becoming more widely available, especially in urban areas. Nursing home care is expensive and is not usually sought by families until the elderly person is physically or mentally disabled. The primary caregiver and others residing in the household should be encouraged to live as normally as possible and to accept whatever help is available. Sometimes the primary caregiver is unwilling to delegate or accept respite care. These virtuous people can be told that taking care of their own needs is another way of taking care of the elderly person. If caregivers replenish their own supply of energy, they ultimately can give better care to their charge. They also need permission to express some of their feelings of fatigue and even desperation. Referrals to appropriate support groups are often helpful and can reduce the sense of aloneness that primary caregivers may experience.

Therapeutic Guidelines

Some health professionals become involved with the home care of an elderly person early on, but often their services are not sought until there is a crisis. Regardless of the circumstances, there is need to establish rapport with family members who have been involved, however inadequately, with the older person's care. It may be difficult to achieve a nonjudgmental attitude if evidence points to abuse or neglect of the older person. These feelings of anger or revulsion may be inevitable, but the health professional must put them aside in order to learn more about the condition of the elderly person and about the stresses that may exist for the caregiver. A comprehensive family history that includes the family's strengths as well as its deficiencies may give the health professional a more objective perspective and dilute countertransference reactions. Looking for some family strengths sheds light on what persons or attributes can be mobilized on behalf of the elderly person. Knowledge of community resources can be shared with family in order to introduce a more hopeful atmosphere. It may be appropriate for the health professional to give permission to the caregiver to say that "it's just too much." Medical and psychiatric evaluation may be needed and should be facilitated. Caretakers should not be required to do more than they feel they can do. They should be assured that both they and the elderly person are *entitled* to whatever outside services are available. Such assurances have the effect of easing some of the caretakers' guilt for accepting help. If serious abuse or neglect are present, it may be necessary to remove the elderly person from the household. This may be met with resistance from the family and from the elderly person who dreads change more than the current situation. The criterion is whether removal is needed to prevent further injury to the elderly person and further deterioration of conditions within the household. The health professional may ask for consultation or verification from colleagues to support a decision to remove the elderly person from the household. Until appropriate arrangements can be made, home visits by nurses, social workers, or protective personnel may be used to maintain close supervision while a new placement is pending.

Working with the Abused and the Abuser

Like child abuse, abuse of the elderly represents mistreatment of weaker persons by those who are stronger. In their struggle to overcome their distaste for abusive behavior, health professionals may search for intellectual explanations so as to "understand" the abuser. Shapiro (1984) urges caregivers, family, and professionals to come to terms with their own fears and dark impulses. The health professional with no personal experience of family violence may see this as alien territory, which arouses revulsion. The health professional who has experienced family violence first hand may find that old memories are reactivated, and the strong feelings that are evoked may impair professional judgment. Self-awareness is crucial in dealing with these families. The health professional's first response may be outrage, but this must be joined by objectivity and assessment of all aspects of the situation. Only then can work begin on improving the situation of everyone involved. Self-awareness means being open about personal emotional reactions so that judgmental interventions are avoided. Working in teams made up of health professionals from several disciplines validates assessment, provides mutual support, and coordinates planning for what is, after all, a family problem involving more than one person.

CLINICAL EXAMPLE: COMPLEMENTARY ROLES OF TWO BATTERED WOMEN

A shelter for battered women offers a sixty-day residential program for abused women and their children. Agnes and Joyce came to the shelter in the same week and soon became friends. Joyce was 18 years old, the mother of a 10-month-old boy, and six months pregnant. She is an attractive young woman, somewhat shy, and her dark eyes reflect her sadness. Agnes is in her mid-twenties, a fast-talking, outgoing young woman who is an attentive mother to her 8-year-old son and 6-year-old daughter. The two women appear to have little in common except motherhood and a history of being beaten. Despite outward differences, they enjoy each other's company. Agnes looks out for Joyce much as an older sister might look after a younger one.

Assessment

Joyce is a dependent young woman whose religious beliefs oppose divorce. She married a few months before her first child was born and became pregnant again when this child was a small infant. Until her second pregnancy her husband had been inattentive but not abusive. He continued to socialize with his buddies and lavished more attention on his motorcycle than on Joyce. He blamed Joyce for the second pregnancy and accused her of "trapping" him. The battering began almost as soon as he learned of the second pregnancy. Violence escalated, and nothing Joyce did seemed to appease him. She arrived at the shelter after her husband pushed her down the stairs. Fearful for herself, her son, and her unborn child, Joyce gathered a few belongings while her husband was out with his friends and came to the shelter. She telephoned her parents to tell them where she was, but they advised her to return to her husband "where she belonged."

Agnes works as a waitress while her children are in school. Her relationship with her husband was stormy even before they were married. He drank to excess and always resented Agnes's willingness to laugh and joke with other men. Her explanation that she flirts with male customers only to win larger tips does not satisfy him. Many of the quarrels between the couple are brawls rather than beatings. Agnes uses any available weapon to defend herself and attack her husband. Once she hit him with a broken bottle, causing a laceration that required sutures. Agnes is proud of not being the one to strike the first blow, and until recently she was not overly distressed by the frequent battles and reconciliations. But recently her son, in trying to protect Agnes, received the blow intended for her and was knocked unconscious. The boy was hospitalized for a week and expressed fear of returning home. The incident was investigated by a children's protective agency; for the first time Agnes realized that she and her children might be seriously hurt. She states that she has come to the shelter to think things over and deal with her son's fear of his father.

Both Agnes and Joyce are in the early stages of defining the problems in their respective marriages, and neither is quite ready to divorce the abusive partner. Joyce's situation is more difficult. With one small baby and another on the way, she is not able to hold a job. She has no financial resources, and her parents and husband are unwilling to extend financial or emotional support.

Planning

The workers at the shelter watched with interest the growing friendship between the two women, and noted that Agnes seemed able to help Joyce relax and even laugh occasionally. With help from the staff, Agnes sought a restraining order against her husband. She was referred to legal aid and filed for child support. At this point Agnes's husband is asking to be reconciled, but she insists that he stay sober for at least a year before she will even consider reunion. Agnes's husband has agreed to move out and give her sole access to the apartment they had shared. Joyce's husband has not communicated with her and shows no interest in reconciliation. Despite pressure from her parents to return to him, Joyce is afraid to do so.

The two women talked at great length, both alone together and in the presence of staff members. It was a great relief for Joyce when Agnes suggested sharing her apartment. In return for free housing, Joyce plans to take care of Agnes's children when their mother is at work and the children are not in school. This will enable Agnes to work more hours, since she knows that her children will be looked after.

Implementation

When the staff learned of the plan, they assisted with the logistics of the move. Joyce applied for a support order and supplementary welfare. Some furniture for her little boy and the baby-to-be was provided from donations made to the shelter. Agnes and Joyce met frequently with a worker who encouraged them to work out specifics of their living arrangement. Anticipatory guidance was used to clarify their expectations of each other and avoid future problems.

Evaluation

Sudden friendships are common among residents of shelters for battered women. Some of these friendships continue, but many are short-lived. Because of the complementary temperaments of Agnes and Joyce, shelter workers predicted that this friendship might endure. Each woman is able to offer something that the other needs. Agnes is the executive of the household, and Joyce is content with this. Although she is less assertive than Agnes, Joyce feels that she will be a valuable contributor to the operation of this newly organized household. Her worries about her labor and delivery have lessened because of Agnes, whose hard-boiled veneer conceals kindness and a strong maternal drive. There is a chance that Agnes will return to her husband if he solves his drinking problem. Joyce's marriage is less likely to be resumed, but living with Agnes solves her most urgent problems and gives her more time to plan for the future. With independent Agnes as a role model, Joyce may learn to be more self-sufficient. As ex-residents, both women are planning to participate in support groups offered at the shelter.

SUMMARY

Abuse in families is perpetrated upon weaker members such as women, children, and elderly persons. Despite wide attention in the media, violence and its counterpart, deliberate neglect, do not seem to be abating in American family life. The violence-prone family is one in which anxiety and tension are joined by poor impulse control. These conditions are aggravated by the physical and emotional intimacy of family life.

There is some debate as to whether the majority of abusive persons were themselves abused when they were children. What is not debatable is that much of our behavior in adult life has been learned in the family of origin and persists. In some families, abuse is aimed only at the wife or at a selected child. In other families no one escapes, and all members are vulnerable to the onslaught of the abuser. Incest is a behavior whose definition changes over time and varies from one culture to another. In most Western countries incest is thought to be a moral and legal transgression that inflicts lasting damage on the individual who is victimized. Because the instigator of the sexual relationship violated standards of acceptable behavior, the victim in adulthood may continue to have difficulty in adhering to certain behavioral standards or in setting limits for others.

Potential for abuse is intensified by several factors present in contemporary life. The overworked single parent may feel trapped by responsibilities and discharge frustration by treating children harshly, either physically or psychologically. The remarried family in which one parent and some of the children are not related by blood may produce a climate for the sexual abuse of stepchildren or stepsiblings.

Explanations for wife battering range from psychodynamic to sociological to learning theories. The feminist view is that wife abuse reflects the patriarchal structure of the family and the secondary status of women. Each viewpoint contains some but probably not all of the truth. Abused women who ultimately kill their husbands or lovers seem quite similar to abused women who do not retaliate by killing. The chief difference between the two groups seems to be in the extent and chronicity of the abuse they suffer, rather than in their own characteristics.

Elder abuse is becoming more common as the aged population increases. Although abuse of the elderly outrages the sensibilities of most health professionals, it is important to include the caretaker and other aspects of family life in the assessment. Many caretakers have reached the limit of their endurance, are themselves in poor health, and are desperate to find a way out of their dilemma. In most instances the caretaking family has

insufficient knowledge of sources of assistance or of eligibility requirements. An objective, nonjudgmental stance by the health professional en-
hances problem solving and does not overlook the legitimate needs of the
elderly person. When a decision is made to remove an elderly person from
the home, it may take time to find a suitable placement. In the interim,
close supervision of the home situation should be maintained through
frequent home visits by various health professionals working as a team.

REFERENCES

Browne, A. (1987). *When Battered Women Kill.* New York: Free Press.
Chapman, J. R. (1978). "The Economics of Women's Victimization." In J. R. Chap-
    man & M. Gates (Eds.), *The Victimization of Women.* Beverly Hills, CA: Sage
    Publications.
DeLorto, D., & LaViolette, A. (1980). "Spouse Abuse." *Occupational Health Nurs-
    ing,* pp. 17–19.
Edelson, J. J. (1984). "Working with Men Who Batter." *Social Work,* 29(3): 237–242.
Elbow, M. (1977). "Theoretical Considerations of Violent Marriages." *Social Case-
    work,* 59(9): 515–526.
Federation of Organizations for Professional Women. (1977). *Women and Health
    Roundtable Report,* 10: 1–4.
Finkelhor, D. (1985). "Sexual Abuse and Physical Abuse: Some Critical Differences."
    In E. H. Newberger & R. Bourne (Eds.), *Unhappy Families: Clinical and Re-
    search Perspectives on Family Violence.* Littleton, MA: PSG.
Forward, S., & Buck, C. (1978). *Betrayal of Innocence: Incest and Its Devastation.*
    Middlesex, England: Penguin Books.
Gelles, R. J. (1974). *The Violent Home.* Beverly Hills, CA: Sage Publications.
Gelles, R. J. (1989). "Child Abuse and Violence in Single Parent Families: Parent
    Absence and Economic Deprivation." *American Journal of Orthopsychiatry,*
    59(4).
Giordano, N. H., & Giordano, J. A. (1984). "Elder Abuse: A Review of the Litera-
    ture." *Social Work,* 29(3): 232–236.
Helfer, R. E., & Kempe, C. H. (1968). *The Battered Child.* Chicago: University of
    Chicago Press.
Hilberman, E. (1980). "Overview: The Wifebeater's Wife Reconsidered." *American
    Journal of Psychiatry,* 137: 1336–1347.
Hilberman, E., & Munson, R. (1978). "Sixty Battered Women." *Victimology: An
    International Journal,* 2: 460–470.
Janosik, E. H., & Davies, J. L. (1989). "Situational Alterations: The Crises of Suicide
    and Violence, the Crisis of the Violent Family." In *Psychiatric Mental Health
    Nursing,* 2nd ed. (Chapter 15, pp. 556–576). Boston: Jones and Bartlett.
Justice, B., & Justice, R. (1976). *The Abusing Family.* New York: Human Sciences
    Press.
Kaufman, I. (1966). "Psychiatric Implications of Physical Abuse of Children." In
    Protecting the Battered Child. Denver: American Humane Association.
Kaufman, J., & Zigler, E. (1987). "Do Abused Children Become Abusive Parents?"
    American Journal of Orthopsychiatry, 57(2): 186–192.
Kempe, C. H. (1978). "Sexual Abuse, Another Pediatric Problem." *Pediatrics,* 62:
    382.

Kissel, S. J. (1986). "Violence in America: An Emerging Public Health Problem." *Health and Social Work*, 11: 153–155.

Machotka, P., Pittman, F. S. III, & Flomenhalf, K. (1967). "Incest Is a Family Affair." *Family Process*, 6(1).

Martin, D. (1977). "Society's Vindication of the Wife Beater." *Bulletin of the American Academy of Psychiatry and the Law*, 5: 391–410.

Meyers, L. (1980). "Battered Wives, Dead Husbands." In A. Skolnick & J. H. Skolnick (Eds.), *Family in Transition*, 3rd ed. Boston: Little, Brown.

Newberger, E. H., & Bourne, R. (Eds.). (1985). *Unhappy Families: Clinical and Research Perspectives on Family Violence*. Littleton, MA: PSG.

O'Brien, J. E. (1971). "Violence in Divorce Prone Families." *Journal of Marriage and the Family*, 33: 692–698.

Pagelow, M. (1976). "Preliminary Report on Battered Women." Paper presented at the Second International Symposium on Victimology, Boston, September.

Pillemer, K., & Finkelhor, D. "Causes of Elder Abuse: Caregiver States versus Problem Relatives." *American Journal of Orthopsychiatry*, 59(2): 179–187.

Pittman, F. S. III. (1987). *Turning Points: Treating Families in Transition and Crisis*. New York: Norton.

Rounsaville, B. J. (1978). "Battered Wives: Barriers to Identification and Treatment." *American Journal of Orthopsychiatry*, 48: 487–494.

Roy, M. (Ed.). (1977). *Battered Women*. New York: Van Nostrand Reinhold.

Saunders, S., Anderson, A., Hart, C. A., & Rubenstein, G. (Eds.). (1984). *Violent Individuals and Families: A Handbook for Practitioners*. Springfield, IL: Charles C Thomas.

Seligman, M. E. (1975). *Helplessness: On Depression, Development and Death*. San Francisco: W. H. Freeman.

Shainness, N. (1979). "Vulnerability of Violence: Masochism as a Process." *American Journal of Psychotherapy*, 33: 174–188.

Shapiro, R. J. (1984). "Therapy with Violent Families." In S. Saunders, A. Anderson, C. A. Hart, & G. Rubenstein (Eds.), *Violent Individuals and Families: A Handbook for Practitioners*. Springfield, IL: Charles C Thomas.

Steinmetz, S. K. (1978). "The Politics of Aging: Battered Parents." *Society*, July-August, pp. 54–55.

Steinmetz, S. (1978). "Wife Beating: A Critique and Reformulation of Existing Theory." *Bulletin of the American Academy of Psychiatry and the Law*, 6: 322–334.

Steinmetz, S. K. (1981). "Elder Abuse." *Aging*, 315–316: 6–10.

Steinmetz, S. K. (1984). "Family Violence toward Elders." In S. Saunders et al. (Eds.), *Violent Individuals and Families: A Handbook for Practitioners* (pp. 137–163). Springfield, IL: Charles C Thomas.

Straus, M. A., & Hotaling, G. (1977). *The Social Causes of Husband-Wife Violence*. Minneapolis: University of Minnesota Press.

Symonds, A. (1978). "The Psychodynamics of Violence Prone Marriages." *American Journal of Psychoanalysis*, 38: 213–222.

Symonds, A. (1979). "The Myth of Masochism." *American Journal of Psychotherapy*, 33: 161–173.

Walker, L. (1979). *The Battered Woman*. New York: Harper & Row.

Walters, M., Carter, B., Papp, P., & Silverstein, O. (1988). *The Invisible Web: Gender Patterns in Family Relationships*. New York: Guilford Press.

CHAPTER THIRTEEN

Substance Abuse in the Family: Dependents and Codependents

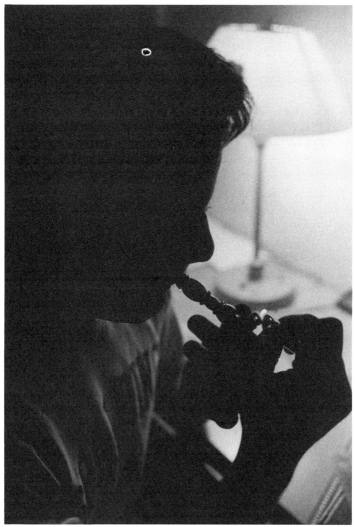

© David C. Conklin, Monkmeyer Press Photo Service

It is good to put behind one the desire to live the life of the surroundings, get to know oneself better, understand the reason for one's needs. Perceive more clearly the motivations of others, and recognize my own fear and insecurity in them.

Liv Ullmann

The term *drug abuse* is applied to several different kinds of behavior that may or may not deserve the label. Davies (1989) defines drug abuse as the use of any drug in ways that differ from the medically or socially approved purpose. This is a broad definition that is open to subjective interpretation. It implies that using a barbiturate to fall asleep may be acceptable but using it to escape everyday stress is not. Using a narcotic to relieve pain may be acceptable, but employing the same drug to produce euphoria is not. Obviously, drug abuse is definable mostly in the context of societal disapproval and includes such behaviors as (1) occasional use of drugs for recreational, experimental purposes; (2) use of drugs to alter one's state of consciousness; and (3) use of drugs to prevent the discomfort of withdrawal symptoms.

Drug dependence may be physical, psychological, social, or a combination of the three. Physical dependence occurs after the user develops tolerance so that progressively larger doses are needed to achieve effects once produced by smaller amounts of the same drug. Physical dependence is accompanied by manifestations of a withdrawal syndrome when the user is abstinent. Physical dependence and tolerance are not characteristic of all forms of drug dependence. Social dependence indicates that the drug is used because of ongoing peer pressure, or because the user has become part of a drug counterculture.

Psychological dependence consists of feelings of pleasure and satisfaction so great that there is a powerful desire to reproduce the sensation over and over. This psychological response is involved in the repeated use of psychotropic (mind-altering) drugs. Compulsive drug use occurs when users develop dependence (physical and/or psychological) on a drug and feel that they must have the drug. If the drug of choice is an illegal or controlled substance, it may be hard to obtain. Users then become preoccupied, even obsessed, with getting it. Frequently, though not always, compulsive drug use is associated with tolerance and physical dependence.

Addiction is a word once applied only to drug abuse but now associated in a superficial way with any activity or object of which individuals grow

[406]

fond. People who exercise every day are said to be addicted to jogging or aerobics. Bibliophiles are glibly accused of being addicted to books and philatelists to stamps. This popularization of the term is unfortunate, for genuine addiction has other connotations. For our purposes, addiction refers to an ongoing pattern of drug abuse marked by compulsiveness, frantic efforts to maintain a supply source, and tendencies to resume drug use after going through withdrawal.

Addiction is not the same as physical dependence, although it has similar features. It is possible to be physically dependent without being addicted. For example, a person in pain might be given morphine several times a day for less than a week. When pain lessens and the drug is abruptly discontinued, this person may suffer withdrawal symptoms but is not addicted psychologically and will experience no craving once the pain that necessitated the drug disappears. Similarly, about half the U.S. soldiers who used heroin regularly while in Vietnam were able to discontinue its use without treatment after they returned home (Davies, 1989).

DEPENDENCY

Drugs causing dependency are those that act on the central nervous system (CNS) to produce one or more of the following effects.

- Lowered levels of tension and anxiety
- Pleasurable mood states of elation or euphoria
- Enhanced physical and mental abilities
- Altered sensory perception

Some drugs cause only psychological dependency; some drugs cause physical and psychological dependency. Table 13.1 lists some frequently abused drugs, their potential for physical and psychological dependency, and likelihood of tolerance.

Many persons abuse more than one drug for a variety of motives. If tolerance to one drug develops, the user will combine it with another substance to achieve greater effect. The preferred drug may be unavailable, and the user will resort to whatever substance is at hand to avoid withdrawal symptoms. Cross-addiction refers to the ability of one drug to suppress symptoms of physical dependency produced by another drug. Discomfort may be avoided by this practice, but the user remains physically dependent. Sometimes cross-addiction is used therapeutically. Barbiturates, for example, can suppress symptoms of alcohol withdrawal, and alcohol can suppress symptoms of barbiturate withdrawal. Some persons addicted to alcohol try to maintain sobriety by using Librium or Valium, and cross-addiction is a factor in methadone maintenance programs, where heroin addicts are offered a substitute drug.

TABLE 13.1. Frequently Abused Drugs: Their Potential for Dependence and Tolerance

	Physical Dependence	Psychological Dependence	Tolerance
CNS depressants:			
Opioids	+ + + +	+ + + +	+ + + +
Synthetic narcotics	+ + + +	+ + + +	+ + + +
Barbiturates	+ + +	+ + +	+ +
Alcohol	+ + +	+ + +	+ +
Minor tranquilizers:			
Meprobamate	+ + +	+ + +	+
Benzodiazepines	+	+ + +	+
Stimulants:			
Amphetamine	?	+ + +	+ + + +
Methamphetamine	?	+ + +	+ + + +
Cocaine	0	+ + +	0
Hallucinogens:			
LSD	0	+ +	+ +
Mescaline, peyote	0	+ +	+
Marijuana	0	+ +	?

Key:
LSD: Lysergic acid diethylamide
0: No effect
+: Slight effect
+ +: Some effect
+ + +: Considerable effect
+ + + +: Extreme effect

ALCOHOL AND SOCIETY

Alcohol has been used for centuries by great numbers of people, but attitudes toward alcohol and alcoholism are ambivalent and contradictory. In some religious circles any drinker is considered a sinner or morally corrupt. In some social settings a person who drinks to excess is a bore, a nuisance, or perhaps a menace. And in certain circumstances a drinker is a pal, a real man, and a member in good standing.

It was Benjamin Rush, physician and signer of the Declaration of Independence, who first called the immoderate use of alcohol a disease. Concern about alcohol abuse gained support for the temperance movement in the latter half of the nineteenth century and eventually resulted in the Eighteenth Amendment to the Constitution, passed in 1919, which imposed Prohibition on the nation. Paradoxically, the enactment of Prohibition made alcohol consumption fashionable and popular. Speakeasies opened, which for the first time allowed women to drink in public places along side of men. After thirteen years the great experiment failed, and Prohibition was repealed. In the time since then, the proportion of drinkers has increased steadily.

Two developments of the 1940s are worth mentioning. In that decade articles describing alcoholism as a disease began to appear with some regularity in respectable journals. Local committees of professional people and private citizens met to discuss alcoholism as a public health problem. By the 1960s the concept of alcoholism as an illness rather than a crime or a moral weakness had gained wide acceptance. During the 1940s a small group of self-confessed alcoholics joined together in an attempt to stay sober and to help others to do the same. Their program, which is based on the idea that alcoholism is an illness, became known as Alcoholics Anonymous (AA). Since its inception AA has grown from one small chapter with a handful of members to over 12,000 groups meeting in ninety countries.

Alcoholism is a severe, progressive disorder that has adverse effects on an alcoholic's physical health, psychological outlook, job performance, and family life. There are abundant physiological, psychological, and cultural theories about the etiology of alcoholism; research continues on many fronts, but as yet no one knows definitively why some people can drink socially while others cannot. What is known is that alcoholism is the nation's third largest public health problem and contributes to gastrointestinal disorders, heart disease, organic brain deficits, automobile accidents, suicides, homicides, and other forms of violence. Recent figures show that alcoholism adversely affects the lives of 70 million Americans. An estimated 14 million are themselves alcoholics, and 56 million others are affected by the drinking of a family member or loved one. Alcohol-related illnesses account for 30 to 50 percent of all hospital admissions (Franks, 1985).

The Male Alcoholic

The percentage of male alcoholics is about three times greater than that of women, although alcoholism rates for women are increasing. About three and one-third million teenagers from 14 to 17 years of age are thought to be problem drinkers (Lewis et al., 1989). In trying to explain the nature of alcoholism, Kaplan, Freedman, and Sadock (1980) classified problem drinkers as either reactive or addictive. The reactive alcoholic craves alcohol whenever he feels overwhelmed by external stressors. Sometimes temporary relief from outside forces is all that is needed. When stressors diminish, the drinking diminishes. However, some reactive drinkers consume alcohol for extended periods of time in order to deal with stress that may be physical or psychological. As a result, physiological dependence follows, and the individual continues to drink in order to avoid suffering from withdrawal. Still, for reactive drinkers previous adjustment was relatively satisfactory, and sobriety may be within reach.

In contrast, the addictive alcoholic probably had poor interpersonal relationships and personality disturbances before becoming a problem drinker. The addictive alcoholic is a problem drinker almost from his first encounter with alcohol, and drinks without apparent reason. He drinks when things are going well and when things are going badly, and he will continue to drink as long as alcohol can be had.

Despite the foregoing typology of addictive and reactive drinkers, there is little solid evidence to support alcoholic personality profiles. Because most clinicians encounter alcoholics who are in trouble, it is difficult to say whether characteristic personality traits preceded or followed alcohol abuse. A dominant "alcoholic personality" has not been identified in spite of earnest research. What have been identified are a number of conflicts that seem to be associated with alcoholism.

Dependent/Independent Conflict

Many alcoholics seem to be in conflict between the need to be dependent and the need to be independent. To avoid facing this conflict, the alcoholic chooses to express one need but not the other. It is the dependency need that is most often apparent in the behavior of an alcoholic. Dependency is expressed not only in drinking behavior but also in interpersonal relationships. The unexpressed wish to be independent instead of dependent gives rise to inner tensions that are relieved by drinking. Alcohol lends a temporary sense of autonomy, which makes the conflict disappear for a while.

Aggressive/Submissive Conflict

Persons with strong dependency needs are often reluctant to express negative feelings openly lest they lose the relationships that support them. Alcohol frees them to express negative feelings of anger or resentment.

Powerful/Powerless Conflict

The alcoholic tries to eradicate feelings of personal inadequacy by drinking. For the moment, the alcoholic feels competent and in charge of himself and his surroundings. Once sober, he is again aware of reality and his shortcomings. Embarrassment and guilt are added to his sense of inadequacy, until he resumes drinking.

Depressed/Euphoric Conflict

Many alcoholics are depressed, and depression can be the initial impetus to drink. Excessive drinking impairs interpersonal relationships and job performance, causing depression to deepen. Using alcohol to escape or disguise depression is self-defeating. Alcohol is a depressant, which may give momentary feelings of relief, but soon intensifies the depression.

Defense Mechanisms

Denial, along with the rationalizations and projections that support it, is the primary defense mechanism of alcoholics. Most alcoholics deny they have any problem controlling their drinking and often claim that they are not drinking at all. Even when confronted with evidence of their drinking, they will minimize the amount they actually consume. When they suspect that they can no longer control their drinking, they refuse to acknowledge this. They project blame to others who, they allege, drove them to drink. Another ploy they use is to devise reasons for drinking, no matter how trivial or unbelievable these reasons may be.

One of the first effects of alcohol is to release inhibitions and reduce psychological controls. Alcohol acts like an anaesthetic; uncomfortable feelings of loneliness, insecurity, and fearfulness disappear. Although there is some debate about the role of alcohol in releasing aggression, there is no doubt that it plays a part. Some theorists subscribe to the idea that alcohol generates fantasies of power and dominance over others as reality testing weakens. Another factor linking alcohol and aggression is the tendency of the alcoholic and others to attribute aggressive acts solely to being intoxicated. Proponents of this explanation believe that drinking provides a socially acceptable reason for acting violently toward others. An alcoholic may beat his wife and children but be excused even by the victims because the behavior took place when "he was drinking and not himself." When family violence erupts and the alcoholic is inebriated, the first goal is the removal of the alcoholic from the home or the removal of the wife and children. It is essential not to try to counsel or initiate therapeutic measures until the alcoholic is sober and, if willing, enrolled in a detoxification and rehabilitation program.

Therapeutic Guidelines

When an alcoholic enters treatment, it is advisable to include the family, especially the wife, in making an assessment. The alcoholic may continue to deny the extent of his drinking, but the family may be more forthcoming. A family is likely to talk more frankly if they are interviewed privately, but the alcoholic should be informed of this and understand the purpose. Following the private interview, the family and the alcoholic should be seen together (Lewis et al., 1989). A history should include the following information:

- Age at time of first drink and length of time drinking has been a problem
- Patterns of drinking: Is drinking a daily, weekend, or monthly occurrence?

- Effects of drinking in the following areas:
  Family life
  Employment
  Social relationships
  Health problems
  Sexual problems
- History of blackouts, delirium tremens, or alcohol hallucinosis
- Record of violence toward others or driving while intoxicated
- History of suicide attempts, threats, or ideation
- Availability of support systems:
  Family
  Employer
  Church affiliations
  AA membership
- Willingness to acknowledge a drinking problem and accept help

Because alcoholism is a condition affecting every family member, all should be involved in the rehabilitation process. The wife must stop protecting and rescuing the alcoholic husband, and allow him to experience the consequences of his drinking. She should neither condone nor criticize his drinking since there is nothing she can do to stop it. In short, the wife must disown the husband's alcoholism and establish emotional distance from the problem. This will have a beneficial effect on her self-esteem, reduce her guilt, and improve her self-image of being an autonomous, inner-directed adult.

Many alcoholics become willing to enter a treatment program only after pressure from family members, employers, or the courts. After detoxification, which may be offered on an inpatient or outpatient basis, long-term treatment should begin immediately. A multidisciplinary team of medical, psychological, nursing, and social work professionals is usually given responsibility for restoring physical health, dealing with the psychological aspects of alcoholism, and untangling the web of family relationships. Problem-solving techniques are taught to the alcoholic and the family, to discourage the alcoholic from turning to alcohol as a solution to life's difficulties.

The long-term treatment goal is sobriety, but the alcoholic is instructed to take one day at a time. Referral to AA and other programs that emphasize social events without alcohol helps the alcoholic discover sources of pleasure that do not include drinking. AA members will make themselves available to alcoholics and families and provide transportation to meetings. Phone numbers for local AA chapters are listed in every telephone directory. Family members should be encouraged to participate in Al-Anon and Alateen programs to increase their understanding of alcoholism and to differentiate themselves from the alcoholic relative. Gradually the alcoholic should take more responsibility for himself. This begins with establishing short-term goals such as keeping appointments, getting to work on time, and continuing in a rehabilitation program. For virtually all alcoholics, total abstinence must be strongly advocated because alcoholism can be arrested but seldom cured. Relapses are almost inevitable and should be used to remind the alcoholic that complete abstinence is the route he must take. Regardless of how often an alcoholic resumes drinking, he should be accepted by caretakers without blame or censure. Rejection by caretakers further jeopardizes an alcoholic's efforts to remain sober. When relapses occur, a cognitive approach can be helpful. This consists of looking at how and why renewed drinking took place, in order to avoid similar circumstances and thought patterns in the future.

Lewis et al. (1989) describe a process referred to as "Bud-ing" or building up to drink. This is a period of increased temptation to return to drinking, and it occurs frequently in the first two years of sobriety. There seems to be a cyclical aspect to "Bud-ing." Clinicians have observed that after a month of sobriety, after two to three months of sobriety, and after one year of sobriety the alcoholic enters a period of extreme vulnerability. One explanation may be that these periods are due to physical agitation caused by prolonged withdrawal. The pattern develops slowly; moodiness, restlessness, and irritability become evident. Frequently the alcoholic complains of physical discomfort. The family becomes aware of the alcoholic's rising tension and anxiety but does not know how to respond except with impatience. If the family has been warned that such behavior may arise, they are better able to handle it. At these times it is better for family members to be supportive than to ignore the behavior or respond harshly.

The Female Alcoholic

Alcoholism is not confined to one particular gender, age, or segment of society, but research in the past tended to concentrate on the adult male drinker. Throughout the twentieth century the incidence of alcoholism among women has risen steadily. The highest rates of alcoholism among women are found in those over 55 years of age, in young women with small children, in women working in stressful occupations, and in wives with an alcoholic husband (Nathan, 1983). The literature suggests that the causes of alcoholism in women lie in specific events such as divorce, widowhood, and role changes. Three types of events are thought to be important contributing factors:

- Biological events unique to women, such as premenstrual tension, abortion, unwanted pregnancy, and menopause
- Psychosocial changes, such as the empty nest syndrome and midlife identity crisis
- Stresses not unique to women, such as marital problems, job problems, family problems, physical problems, and aging

Allan and Cooke (1985) evaluate the hypothesis that stressful life events increase alcohol consumption in women and report that studies supporting this idea are inadequate from a methodological standpoint. They conclude that problem drinking does increase the frequency of stressful life events but is perhaps the cause more than the result of life problems. Busch et al. (1985), in a sample of women with obstetrical/gynecological difficulties, state that 31 percent were potential or active drug and alcohol abusers. This incidence is significantly higher than the 5 percent estimated for the general population.

One of the chief concerns regarding the drinking habits of women is the danger of fetal alcohol syndrome (FAS). According to the National Clearinghouse of Alcohol Information, between 2,000 and 4,000 infants are born each year with FAS, and another 36,000 may be afflicted with less severe alcohol related defects (Anderson et al., 1986). Fetal alcohol syndrome has three basic characteristics:

- Central nervous system damage resulting in lowered intelligence, hyperactivity, and peripheral motor disturbances
- Growth deficiencies resulting in low birth weight, slowed growth, and below average size for their age
- Unusual facial features, including low nasal bridge, drooping eyelids, small chin, thinned upper lip, and strabismus

In addition to FAS, drinking during pregnancy is associated with stillbirths, reduced activity levels, and congenital malformation. A safe amount of alcohol consumption during pregnancy has not been established. For the fetus the first trimester is the most crucial period. In the second trimester alcohol consumption is associated with spontaneous abortions, and in the third trimester with low birth weight. Even social drinking is questionable during pregnancy. Because FAS and other alcohol related fetal problems are preventable, health care professionals should actively counsel women about the hazards of drinking while pregnant. Public education and family cooperation are strongly indicated.

Therapeutic Guidelines

Alcoholics who are housewives are often secret drinkers who manage to function after a fashion and conceal the extent of their drinking from family members. Usually their drinking grows progressively worse until concealment is no longer possible. When family life is seriously disrupted, father and children may join forces to preserve a semblance of family life. They may feel this is the only course open to them, but their realignment tends to exclude the woman from meaningful family interaction and increases her lonely dependence on alcohol. A better course is to encourage openness within the family so that the problem can be confronted and help obtained.

If the woman is willing to admit being an alcoholic and to accept treatment, her progress is likely to resemble that of male alcoholics. Abstinence is the prime objective, but there will be periods of sobriety broken by occasional relapse. Like the male alcoholic, she needs to learn that she is a valuable, worthwhile person whose recovery lies in her own hands. The interest and support of family members is crucial, since for most women these relationships are very important. Education about the nature and dangers of alcohol abuse is essential because morbidity and mortality related to alcoholism are higher for women than for men. Death rates from accidents, suicide, and liver disease are higher for female alcoholics, as are rates for cardiovascular disease, brain damage, and alcohol related malignancies (Davies, 1989). This suggests that education and early intervention may be even more crucial for the female alcoholic.

The Teenage Alcoholic

Alcohol is the substance most widely abused by young people between 12 and 17 years of age. Problem drinking that may develop in some children markedly increases with the onset of adolescence, and is frequently accompanied by antisocial acts such as stealing and vandalism. In addition, teenage problem drinkers are much more likely to use illicit drugs than their nondrinking counterparts. Many reasons are given for widespread drinking among today's teenagers, and the reasons reflect different social viewpoints. Secular society, broken homes, and working mothers are held responsible by some social critics, as well as peer pressures and media influences.

Many young people drink from motives of curiosity and a desire to belong, and do not become problem drinkers. In families where a mother or father drinks to excess, the danger to the child is heightened. It is estimated that 28 million American children have at least one alcoholic parent. The children of alcoholics have a high risk of becoming addicted to alcohol themselves. Moreover, alcohol abuse is believed to be a factor in 90 percent of child abuse cases. Latency-aged children just entering the teen years have special problems in dealing with an alcoholic parent, for to identify with the sober parent means rejecting the drinker (Davies, 1989). As they reach their teens, some of these children solve their dilemma by becoming problem drinkers themselves.

Therapeutic Guidelines

For young people showing signs of alcoholism, group programs are especially helpful. They relieve the isolation of a youngster who may be living with an alcoholic parent and who sees in the parent intimations of his or her future. Groups can be a means of educating the teenager about alcohol and alcoholism by providing factual information and removing the attractive mystique that surrounds alcohol in many settings. Expressing opinions, sharing experiences and feelings, gives the teenager a sense that others understand. For the children of alcoholics, who may or may not have an alcoholism problem of their own, AA offers a range of group programs. Alateen helps children differentiate themselves from a drinking parent. Similar groups are available in rehabilitation programs that provide services to problem drinkers of different ages. Community mental health centers across the country offer group therapy and support groups to problem drinkers still in their teens.

The Elderly Alcoholic

The older person who turns to alcohol as a refuge from the distress of aging has been recognized only recently. Alcoholics who have been drinking all their lives should be distinguished from the elderly person who begins drinking in later years. The elderly person who starts to drink is usually influenced by external factors, such as living alone or being unable to manage everyday tasks. In some ways it is easier to modify drinking habits in these individuals than in persons whose alcoholism is entrenched.

Many of the complaints expressed by elderly persons are assumed to be part of the aging process and are not attributed to drinking. Depression, paranoia, and organic brain syndrome may be indications of excessive alcohol consumption but are unrecognized as such. All too often the care given to an elderly person is fragmented and superficial. There are even times when the elderly alcoholic is excluded from alcoholism programs because of advanced age and from gerontology programs because of alcoholism (Gulino & Kadin, 1986).

Therapeutic Guidelines

The elderly alcoholic can be helped if appropriate measures are taken, but any assistance must be coordinated to make sure the person is not lost in the system. Many elderly persons use alcohol as self-medication for the infirmities of old age. A complete medical assessment is needed so that symptoms can be identified and relieved by proper medication. Caution must be used in prescribing drugs for an elderly alcoholic because of metabolic and other changes associated with aging. Disulfiram (Antabuse) is contraindicated for most elderly persons. This is a drug that interferes with the metabolism of alcohol, so drinking while taking Antabuse creates a physical reaction similar to shock, with deep flushing, a rise in blood pressure, labored breathing, and violent vomiting. Although Antabuse has no ill effects unless a person drinks alcohol, it can be lethal for persons with medical problems who drink while on an Antabuse regimen. Elderly persons who abuse alcohol usually respond to social and environmental improvements. They need help in meeting people and in establishing and maintaining interpersonal relationships. For many of them alcohol is a way to fill a void, but this need can be met in other ways. Home visitors, day care programs, phone calls, and occasional outings can replace excessive drinking. The eventless lives of many elderly persons can be changed in small ways that produce large dividends. Family members and old friends need to become reinvested; church affiliations can be reactivated to bring new interests to the elderly person. Measures that seem unimportant can be very therapeutic for an elderly person trying to live without relying on alcohol. Referral to an alcoholism support group may be necessary if the individual does not respond to environmental and social interventions.

The Alcoholic Family

The alcoholic organizes his or her life around alcohol, and the family organizes itself around responses to a member's alcoholism. With few exceptions, people living with an alcoholic become reactors who adjust their own behaviors in response to the offensive and defensive behaviors of the drinker. Their attitudes, decisions, beliefs, and habits are shaped by the presence of alcoholism. Any family member, adult or child, who is dominated or controlled by the drinking patterns of the alcoholic is a *codependent*. In families where the husband is an alcoholic, it is most often the wife who becomes a codependent. Kaufman (1986) describes stages in the formation of this reaction, which was originally labeled coalcoholism. The onset of alcoholism in a family member upsets family equilibrium and produces dysfunctional responses in the codependent member. The alcoholic is dependent on a chemical substance but is also dependent on another person, namely the codependent. Persons who become codependents experience a loss of selfhood as they find themselves accommodating more and more to the behaviors of the dependent family member. Because they spend their lives responding to another rather than obeying the dictates of their own mind or conscience, they have no authentic, separate identity. The codependent person is neither independent nor interdependent, for service is devoted to a dependent person tied to alcohol who can give nothing in return. The actions of the codependent are determined by a heavy sense of responsibility and by willingness to discharge massive role obligations.

There is an all-or-nothing quality to life in an alcoholic family. The codependent is always afraid of losing control of whatever normality still exists in family life. The actions of the alcoholic become something to which the codependent constantly adjusts. The codependent, whether husband, wife, or child, adapts his or her view of the world to conform to that of the alcoholic. More often than not the codependent is a wife who hears over and over that her nagging and distrust make her husband drink. She tries for a while to interact differently with him, but in vain. Because she cannot control her husband's drinking, she feels guilty, helpless, and somehow at fault.

To oppose her feelings of being devalued, the wife may adopt a superior, moralistic manner. Like the alcoholic, she may use denial and pretend to herself and others that there is nothing really wrong in the family. As family life spins out of control, denial fails her. She becomes preoccupied with the desire to protect her family and her husband from the consequences of his drinking. Because her best efforts are futile, the wife lives in a constant state of anxiety, depression, and resentment. As her codependency and her psychological turmoil grow, she has less time and energy to expend on behalf of herself or her children.

At first the spouse of an alcoholic uses the mechanism of denial to avoid admitting there is a problem; as the dimensions of the problem grow, the spouse may deny to avoid direct confrontation. Then the spouse may begin to plead, lecture, accuse, and try to extract a promise from the alcoholic not to drink any more. When all this fails, the spouse begins to hide liquor, withhold money, and engage in various power struggles. At this point the whole family is in turmoil and living from crisis to crisis. The struggle for control permeates every corner of family life so that rational communication becomes impossible.

No matter how affluent a family is or how well physical needs are met, the children in an alcoholic family suffer neglect if not abuse. They become junior codependents or parent surrogates for their younger siblings. Like the spouses of alcoholics, children may be blamed or blame themselves for the drinking problems. A father may tell the children that if they helped more around the house, mother would not drink. A mother may tell the children that father drinks because they fight too much and this bothers him. Children cannot see the illogic in this and are inclined to accept blame. They may believe that since they caused the drinking, they can stop it by being very good. When their best efforts fail, this increases their feelings of not amounting to much.

Because of the global denial existing in the home, children are confused by the discrepancy between what they see and what they are told is happening. Neither the drinking parent nor the sober one is much of a role model. Brown (1988) writes of the problems children in an alcoholic family have in emulating either parent: "The nonalcoholic may be seen as strong and dependable, but a martyr without joy. The alcoholic is commonly seen as weak, full of needs, yet perhaps carefree and loving as well" (p. 65).

Children of Alcoholics

Families with an alcoholic member want to appear normal to outsiders. This perpetuates the pattern of denial and creates for children the feeling of living simultaneously in two worlds. Brown (1988) explains that in order to seem normal, the family must detach itself to a considerable extent from the external world. For children, there is an outside world of friends, church, school, and neighborhood. There is also a family world of secrets, deviance, and conflict. The child learns early not to let the outside world intrude much into family life; to allow this endangers the pretense that the family is like all other families. In order to sustain denial, many children of alcoholics strive to be models of adjustment and apparent happiness. This semblance of normality is often a mask worn to conceal the family problem from outsiders. Other children living with an alcoholic parent learn not to expect much and to fend for themselves as much as possible. This path may lead to delinquency and rebellion, and in some cases to indifference, distrust, and flattened affect. Tesson (1990) writes that adults whose parents were alcoholics have a history of more marital disruption than is found in the general population, and notes the frequency of incest between an alcoholic father and a daughter. Parker and Harford (1988) attribute high rates of depression among women raised in alcoholic households to the presence of an alcoholic parent and estimate that two-thirds of children raised in an alcoholic home suffer some form of physical abuse. Living with alcoholism and the abuse that often accompanies it creates emotional problems in children that persist into adulthood. Even in the absence of violence and incest, sexual indiscretion, nudity, and false accusations of promiscuity are frequently present in the family, and cause lasting trauma for the adult children of alcoholics (ACOAS).

Violence is endemic in alcoholic households. The alcoholic is often the perpetrator, but sometimes it is the nondrinking parent, frustrated and angry, who abuses the children. In families like this there is no one to protect the children. Older children may try to protect younger siblings and take the brunt of abuse on themselves. When an older child eventually leaves the alcoholic household, he may carry feelings of guilt for abandoning younger siblings. The legacy of every child of an alcoholic parent is suspicion of others, especially authority figures, and problems with assertiveness.

In spite of the pathology in alcoholic families, the children remain emotionally connected to the family even in adulthood. After leaving home as adults, they continue to have troubles separating. For many of them, breaking emotional bonds means renouncing the pretense that the family was normal. Staying connected preserves denial and prevents the individual from seeing the family realistically. For some children, remaining attached to the family means becoming alcoholics themselves as they grow up. For others it means assuming the role of rescuer, continuing the reliable behaviors of childhood. The alcoholic needs rescuers who erase the full consequences of drinking. Although rescuers may temporarily cope with emergencies, they are also "enablers" whose efforts permit the alcoholic to go on drinking.

Unfortunately, failure to separate emotionally from an alcoholic family of origin prevents adult children of alcoholics from forming healthy attachments in the new families they establish. They tend to replicate their relationship with the drinking parent by choosing a mate who is dependent and/or alcoholic. Even after they marry and become parents, they may feel that their primary commitment is to the family of origin, which remains crisis-prone and is the repository of unresolved emotional problems (Brown & Beletsis, 1986). Table 13.2 shows some residual behaviors of adult children of alcoholics.

Therapeutic Guidelines

Problem drinking is a behavior that is reinforced by a social climate that condones drinking. Except for public outrage over drunken driving, there is no arbitrary division between problem drinking and drinking that is considered acceptable. The notion that alcoholics end their lives on Skid Row is giving way to realization that there are many alcoholics who live outwardly normal lives until extreme behaviors or alcohol-related illness reveal the secret. They are assisted in concealment by the fact that alcohol is a legitimate substance which is easily obtained.

The care of an alcoholic person is divided into two phases: the acute phase and the rehabilitation phase. It is during the rehabilitation phase, after the alcoholic has detoxified, that family participation should be invited. Any therapeutic relationship between an alcoholic person and a health care professional is apt to be lengthy and intense. Therefore, the caregiver must discourage excessive dependency by the alcoholic on any single caregiver. One way to avoid fostering extreme dependency is through family involvement. For the same reason, group programs are often the treatment of choice for alcoholics. Group experiences dilute the dependency

---

TABLE 13.2. Residual Behaviors of Adult Children of Alcoholics (ACOAS)

- ACOAS are more comfortable reacting to others than interacting with others.
- ACOAS feel responsible for their family of origin and have trouble separating.
- ACOAS are approval seekers who often feel guilty if they put their own needs first.
- ACOAS tend to confuse love with pity, choosing to love those they can rescue.
- ACOAS have trouble recognizing and expressing feelings because they have denied and repressed their own feelings for years.
- ACOAS distrust spontaneity, tend to be aloof from others, and have problems with authority figures.
- ACOAS may become alcoholic, marry an alcoholic, or both.
- ACOAS judge themselves harshly, have low self-esteem, and fear being abandoned by significant others.
- ACOAS become accustomed to excitement and turmoil; they tend to become compulsive about work, eating, gambling, or other activities.

Source: Adapted from Wortitz (1983) and Tesson (1990).

of the alcoholic client and also provide opportunities for confrontation of the alcoholic by his peers. This is important because the alcoholic person is more likely to accept confrontation by another alcoholic than by a non-alcoholic caregiver.

Interpersonal counseling with alcoholic clients centers on marital and family patterns as they currently exist. In some marriages the nonalcoholic spouse has accepted primary responsibility for the family and is reluctant to give up these responsibilities as the alcoholic starts to recover. Because family life is organized around the drinking habits of the alcoholic member, a return to sobriety requires massive family reorganization. Close attention should be paid to the interactional patterns between the alcoholic and the spouse. As previously mentioned, many partners reinforce problem drinking by repeatedly rescuing the alcoholic, thus becoming enablers. The rescuing partner may be motivated by a wish to protect the alcoholic and the family from further deterioration. However, some partners act from mixed motives and are actually more comfortable when the alcoholic is incapacitated because then they are powerful and in charge. In one group meeting for alcoholics, a member remarked: "When I am drinking my wife is an angel. She takes care of everything—the house, the kids, the business. When I have been on the wagon a while, my wife starts to worry about things and gets depressed." Family adjustment to a sober alcoholic may introduce new problems into the system, especially if the nondrinking partner feels like a dethroned monarch or an out-of-work executive. Role shifts that take place because the alcoholic has stopped drinking need attention, partly because resistance to sobriety on the part of other family members is unconscious. Appealing to the self-interest of all family members, especially the nonalcoholic spouse, is an effective way to encourage the realignment made necessary by the rehabilitation of the alcoholic.

Eels (1986) presents an approach to dealing with the alcoholic family based on systems theory. In this approach the dysfunctional behaviors of children are interpreted as a consequence of alcoholism in the family. Children in alcoholic families see faulty adaptation in both parents. The child has no parent with whom to identify, and because the family is a closed system the child lacks a supportive external network. Whether the child sees himself as a victim or a rescuer, he is unable to negotiate age-appropriate tasks in such a household. Instead of developing adequate coping mechanisms, the child acts out by withdrawing, rebelling, underachieving, or overachieving. Although it is the child who is labeled the identified patient, it is probably the alcoholic and the spouse of the alcoholic whose problems should be addressed. In effect, the child is acting in ways that detour conflict between the parents. By behaving in ways that draw attention to himself, the child lowers tension between parents and fortifies the family system.

In alcoholic families a child frequently is "triangled" into the marital relationship by becoming dysfunctional. A useful intervention is to teach the alcoholic and the spouse about triangles, to help them understand their own interactions and the importance of dealing with the essential family problem which is alcoholism. Detouring or deflecting marital conflict to a child allows the partners to ignore or minimize problem drinking, which is the basic family problem.

Family work is most beneficial when a codependent, usually a spouse, is willing to participate in treatment. As a rule the spouse accepts treatment only after trying unsuccessfully to control the partner's drinking and reaching a point of desperation. To encourage change, the health care professional must deal with codependency and undifferentiation existing between the spouse and the drinking partner. Separateness can be fostered by teaching the spouse to use the pronoun "I" when stating personal beliefs and attitudes. The spouse is urged to express only what he or she thinks or feels, and not to describe what the drinker thinks and feels. If the spouse is taking total responsibility for the family, the health care professional suggests that these responsibilities be gradually narrowed to exclude those that the recovering alcoholic should be assuming.

Emphasis is placed on relinquishing any feelings of guilt and embarrassment on the part of the spouse, since control of drinking lies only within the power of the alcoholic. Differentiation of self by the spouse is further encouraged by a referral to Al-Anon, where separateness and disowning the alcoholism (but not the alcoholic) are encouraged. When the spouse begins to put distance between himself or herself and the alcoholic, family dynamics are altered. The drinking of the alcoholic may grow worse; the alcoholic may deteriorate greatly and still refuse treatment. More often, however, the alcoholic becomes alarmed by rapid deterioration and by feeling abandoned. The only recourse that holds any promise for the alcoholic at this point is to join the spouse in treatment. Whether the spouse continues in treatment alone or with the alcoholic, a major objective for both of them is differentiation of self. For the children of alcoholics, Alateen is available. Here again the thrust is not on helping the alcoholic but on living with an alcoholic parent without losing one's selfhood and identity in the process.

Alcoholism is a lifelong illness that can be treated successfully if the therapeutic regimen is tailored to the alcoholic's needs. In most instances treatment is facilitated by family participation. AA is a worldwide and very successful group program for alcoholics, but its inspirational approach is not acceptable to everyone. For persons who do not accept the AA approach, other group programs, such as those given by Veterans Administration agencies and by community mental health centers, are available. Although total abstinence is the goal in AA and other treatment programs, periodic relapses are almost inevitable. Relapses should be explored to discover the alcoholic's perception of events and emotions preceding the drinking; this cognitive exploration can be used for anticipatory planning to avoid future relapses. Family members need counseling when the alcoholic is sober and encouragement when the alcoholic resumes drinking. Like the alcoholic, family members can be told that change takes time, that something can be learned from each relapse, that the alcoholic has demonstrated some ability to stay sober and must begin again. For the health care professional and for the family, condescension, anger, or refusal to acknowledge the alcoholic's painful struggle are counterproductive and increase the likelihood of additional relapses.

CLINICAL EXAMPLE: ALCOHOL ABUSE AS A FAMILY ISSUE

The Burton family consists of a 56-year-old wife who is a college graduate and full-time homemaker, her 58-year-old husband, and three grown children. Tony, the only son, is married and lives with his wife and child in the same town as his parents. Sally is the middle child. She is 27 years old, a psychologist who lives and works in another city. Jane, who is 18 years old, is the last child to leave home and will soon attend college in another city. Mr. Burton is a professional man who works long hours and frequently travels to other regions for conferences and meetings. Some colleagues jokingly say he is "married" to his work.

Assessment

For years Mrs. Burton has been a secret drinker. She presents a good front, is socially personable, and is a warm neighbor. She grew up in a farm family and has deep feelings of inadequacy, which are hidden behind her friendly but rather self-effacing manner. She drinks mostly vodka, in the belief that it is harder to detect. She usually has several martinis between breakfast and lunch, two or three before dinner, and two jiggers of brandy before bedtime. As a rule she manages to function despite her garbled speech and occasional bumping into furniture. She denies the extent of her drinking, even to her physician, who has noted her enlarged liver.

Her family fosters her denial, ignoring her drinking habits or condoning them by saying, "Mama loves to party and is just relaxing." When she is not drinking as much as usual, Mrs. Burton vacillates between fault-finding and making sarcastic remarks to family members, or withdrawing into sullen silence. Over the past six months her drinking has increased, and she is functioning less well. Her increased intake coincides with Jane's decision to live away from home while attending college. In the last three months Mrs. Burton had several blackout spells and two episodes of driving while intoxicated for which she was apprehended by police. As a result, neither she nor the family can continue to overlook the impact of her heavy drinking. When arrested, Mrs. Burton was ashamed and embarrassed. Her family now feels publicly disgraced and for the first time is expressing anger toward her. A major family crisis seems to loom on the horizon.

All three children, especially Jane, are embittered and now can openly express their hidden feelings about their mother's alcoholism. Jane is especially angry about a recent scene her mother created by falling headlong from her chair and spilling her drink while friends were visiting. In the family confrontation that followed, Tony told his mother to "cut out the histrionics and stop drinking immediately." He emptied the house of all alcohol, searching his mother's closet and dresser drawers for bottles. The middle child, Sally, was present but was more detached from the family turmoil. She adopted a very intellectual approach, and made clinical-sounding statements about the family's "blindness to the fact that mother has been an alcoholic for years." Sally's superior tones conveyed blame and reproach, and indicated that she was less involved in the family problem. Mr. Burton was present but said little, yielding leadership to Tony. The only decision reached by the family was to consult their family physician for help.

Planning

The family physician had considerable sophistication regarding the diagnosis and treatment of alcoholism, and was not surprised that a family crisis had developed. He and his nurse clinician, with whom Mrs. Burton had a good relationship, insisted on a referral to an alcohol treatment program. This, of course, was a condition of Mrs. Burton's second driving while intoxicated charge. With encouragement and guidance from the physician and the nurse clinician, all the family members gathered at a meeting and confronted mother with her behavior. Although the session was painful for everyone, it was a beginning on the long road to recovery for Mrs. Burton.

Intervention

Mrs. Burton and her family participated in virtually all the activities the alcohol treatment program offered in group, marital, and individual counseling. At first Mr. Burton resisted involvement, saying that his work prevented him from attending meetings. Only when his wife asked him directly to attend did he agree. For many years she had made no demands on him, nor had she indicated that his companionship was meaningful to her. Jane, the child who was closest to her mother, felt guilty and remorseful for planning to leave home at this point but was reassured by counselors and her family that it was appropriate for her to get on with her life. The imminent departure of Jane was used to remind Mr. Burton of his continued importance in family matters. Sally remained somewhat intellectual in her reactions, and this was permitted to some extent by treatment staff, who interpreted her attitude as defensive in nature. As Mrs. Burton continued in the program and Sally saw her father, brother, and sister become involved, she became less distant and self-protective. Tony seemed to recognize that his mother's alcoholism and her recovery depended on the participation of the whole family. His behavior mobilized other family members and increased their commitment. Throughout the crisis and afterwards, Tony exhibited genuine concern for his mother as well as anger at her actions. The combination of his caring and his tough approach was therapeutic for mother and for other family members.

Evaluation

Mrs. Burton completed the alcoholism treatment program and joined AA, where she met a circle of nondrinking friends. After Jane left for college, Mr. Burton made an effort to attend AA occasionally with his wife, and Tony frequently accompanied her. His openness about his mother's drinking problem and his pride in her sobriety did much to reduce any embarrassment felt by his father or sisters. As a couple, the Burtons began taking short trips together to visit Jane and Sally. Although her manner with others remained self-effacing, through counseling Mrs. Burton learned to be less tentative and more direct in dealing with her husband.

CLINICAL EXAMPLE: ADJUSTMENT AND READJUSTMENT IN THE FAMILY OF AN ALCOHOLIC

Fred is a 45-year-old salesman whose commissions have dropped recently because of his drinking. He is a friendly, energetic man who has been a top salesman for many years. Lately, however, he has begun to miss appointments and antagonize buyers who are offended by his excessive drinking. Fred has always prided himself on his ability to handle alcohol, and his conviviality is partly responsible for his effective salesmanship. Buyers have begun to complain to Fred's boss that he has become a nuisance, drinking too much at business luncheons, telling the same old stories, and poorly informed about the products he is selling. Fred's boss recognizes deterioration in his ace salesman and has told Fred to get into treatment or lose his job.

The medical workup Fred's boss insisted on showed hypertension and some liver damage. Because his boss was adamant, Fred entered an alcoholism treatment program paid for by the company and stayed with it long enough to make a commitment. For the last eight months Fred has been sober and says he feels like a new man. Lately, however, Fred feels nervous and depressed. His wife Janet and his two teenage daughters attribute these feelings to the fact that Fred is not drinking. Janet usually has a cocktail at dinner and at bedtime; she comments laughingly that she never thought she would have to drink alone.

Assessment

At work Fred feels happy and fulfilled. His boss is supportive and is very pleased with Fred's progress. It is only at home that Fred feels uncomfortable. In his alcoholism group meetings he has complained of feeling "like a fish out of water" when he is at home. Concerned over Fred's growing restlessness and nervousness, his counselor arranged a family meeting. In the meeting Fred's wife and daughters talked about Fred's heavy drinking in the past. They spoke of embarrassing incidents and of family celebrations Fred was too drunk to attend. June and the two girls repeatedly said how much better family life was now.

Planning

As the counselor interacted with the family, two facts became apparent. One was that there was considerable anger toward Fred, which until now had not been verbalized. The second fact was that although Fred's drinking had been a problem for the family, they had adjusted to it over the years. June and her daughters had successfully kept up a façade of being a happy, normal family. They had organized their lives so that Fred's participation was unnecessary except as a wage earner. Fred's job required some traveling, and he was frequently absent from the home. The pivotal family member was Janet. Since Fred had stopped drinking, he was spending more time in the house and wanted to have a more active role in family activities. His newfound interest in family matters was hard for Janet, who had become accustomed to taking the managerial role in the family. Although she said she was pleased by Fred's sobriety, she resented this intrusive husband who had stopped seeing his drinking friends and wanted to become reacquainted with his family.

Fred's daughters had formed a comfortable alliance with their mother. They rejected and resented Fred's well-meant inquiries about their activities. New problems arose that were not present when Fred was drinking. Janet felt that her freedom was threatened. She had grown used to living without much social or sexual exchange between herself and Fred. Her early pleasure in his sobriety turned to resentment at what she interpreted as interference. Realizing this was unfair, she reacted by being irritable and passive-aggressive in her behavior toward Fred.

Intervention

Tensions at home tempted Fred to resume drinking, but his alert counselor chose to intervene before Fred succumbed. After congratulating the whole family for helping Fred stay sober, the counselor explained to them the phenomenon of "Bud-ing," which makes alcoholics very vulnerable at times. The goal of the meeting was explained as helping the family adjust to Fred's sobriety as effectively as it had adjusted to his problem drinking. The long-term consequences to Fred and the family if he resumed drinking were briefly described. Most important, explained the counselor, was the need by the family to accept Fred as a husband and father. Janet's cooperation in this was emphasized, along with acknowledgment of her accomplishments in maintaining the family when Fred was drinking. The counselor suggested that the strengths that sustained Janet and her daughters when Fred was drinking were still available and should be mobilized on his behalf.

The counselor used the concept of triangulation, explaining that alcohol had been like another woman in the marriage of Fred and Janet. His problem drinking had come between them, creating a dysfunctional triangle. Just as Fred had become too involved with alcohol, Janet had become too involved with the girls. As a result, the marital subsystem was weakened. An effective marital and sibling subsystem could be reestablished only if Janet and the girls permitted this. The counselor recommended some future family meetings to be attended only by Fred and Janet, because she was the key to his reentry into the family. This was a nonverbal way of reinforcing natural subsystems (marital and sibling) in the family.

Evaluation

At first Janet and the daughters were hesitant to give Fred a more active role in the family. It did not take long for the girls, who were engaged in forming their own identity, to realize that the family will be stronger if the parents become reconciled in the true sense of the word. The daughters know that in a few years they will leave home. If Fred is an integral part of the family, their separation from home and mother will be eased. They agree that future meetings should include only their parents, although they are willing to be involved at times. A number of long-range goals have been formulated and agreed to by all four family members:

- To increase communication and closeness between Fred and Janet through shared activities and interests.
- To negotiate changes in family life so that Janet does not feel threatened and Fred does not feel excluded.
- To establish new ways of solving problems and making decisions so that every family member is involved.
- To recognize and reinforce natural family subsystems so that the marital subsystem is the primary coalition, the sibling subsystem is the secondary coalition, and the subsystem comprising parents and children is the tertiary coalition.

Some progress toward these goals is already apparent.

DRUGS AND SOCIETY

Throughout recorded history people have used drugs to alter their state of consciousness. Contemporary society is highly drug-oriented; drugs are taken to relieve anxiety, to alleviate pain, to relax or stimulate, and just to escape the monotony of daily life. As with alcohol, the dividing line between the use and abuse of drugs is determined by social attitudes. In addition, the legal system decides what constitutes drug use and drug abuse. The Harrison Narcotics Act of 1914 was the first national legislation designed to control traffic in narcotics, especially opiates. This attempt to regulate importation of drugs led to the beginning of illegal drug traffic. Physicians could no longer prescribe narcotics to addicts in ways that monitored their dependency, thus forcing them to find illegal sources of supply. In 1925 the Harrison Act was challenged when a guilty verdict for a physician who had prescribed a narcotic for a known addict was overturned by the Supreme Court. For the first time drug addiction was described as an illness that could be legally treated.

In 1937 the Uniform Narcotics Law created a consistent method of record keeping at federal and state levels, but left penalties for use, possession, and sale of narcotics up to the states. In 1956 the Federal Narcotics Control Act increased penalties for narcotic and marijuana violations, imposing sentences ranging from ten to forty years. In 1962 a court case in California established the precedent that a person could not be punished as a criminal solely on grounds of being a drug abuser. This decision reinforced the idea of drug dependence as an illness, not a crime. In 1966 Congress formulated policies for the treatment of narcotic abusers. Abusers guilty of violating federal drug laws could be sentenced to prison or to a drug treatment center. Before disposition the offender must be deemed capable of rehabilitation and of responding to treatment. More recent legislation is the Compulsive Drug Abuse Control and Prevention Act, which provides that violations be considered in light of the dangers and intended uses of the drug. Under this law a judge is free to arrive at alternative penalties such as volunteer work or community service rather than imprisonment.

Over time various mind-altering drugs have gained and lost popularity. For a while heroin addiction was considered the greatest drug problem in the nation, but the number of heroin addicts is said to have decreased in recent years (Lewis & Feldman, 1989). Cocaine is one of the most widely abused and dangerous drugs in vogue at present. Conservative estimates indicate that 10 million Americans use cocaine regularly and another 5 million have used it experimentally. For the addict, cocaine has the advantage of being cheaper than heroin and less likely to produce tolerance. It does, however, lead to psychological dependence, characterized by a compulsion to use the drug, loss of control over the amount used, and continued use despite frightening consequences (Smith & Wesson, 1985).

Davies (1989) reports that about 51 percent of drug addicts in the United States are white, with the average age being 23 years. The illicit use of drugs is greatest in the 18- to 25-year-old age group and is the leading cause of death among this group.

Psychotropic prescription drugs are the most frequently abused medications, and women are the most frequent abusers of this category of substances. The most common form of abuse is the medication borrowed from another person for whom the drug was prescribed. Women who use amphetamines for weight control often go on to become abusers. Sedatives and tranquilizers are frequently prescribed for women who ultimately become addicted and use subterfuge to obtain supplies from various physicians. Persons over 65 years of age use more legal drugs than any other age group. A task force studying prescription drug abuse found that the average individual over 65 years of age uses three times as many prescription drugs as do younger people (Bennett et al., 1983). Reliance on prescription drugs contributes to drug abuse in this age group.

No single explanation covers all forms of drug abuse, but there seem to be factors that produce addiction or protect against it. If an addictive substance is given to relieve pain, persons receiving it rarely become addicted unless a personality predisposition already existed. Most drug abusers never enter the health care system. Drug abuse occurs in all classes of society, and the practice is growing among middle- and upper-class groups. Many noted athletes and entertainers have been found to abuse drugs, both legal and illegal substances. Some drug abusers manage to contain their habit within the bounds of a functional life-style, but many more do not. For a large group of addicts, the appeal of the chosen drug is enhanced by a deviant life-style that contributes to dysfunction and alienation from the mainstream culture. These are the addicts who come most often to the attention of health care professionals. Often they suffer from severe medical problems and from legal difficulties arising from drug abuse.

Some emotionally vulnerable persons have a low tolerance for discomfort of any kind. The use of mind-altering substances gives them a temporary sense of well-being that ignores reality. The chosen drug may deaden the senses, or it may produce high, orgastic feelings of satisfaction. Before long the life of the addict is taken over by a single purpose, the need to obtain the substance that alters his level of consciousness and gives such pleasurable sensations. Because alcohol is a legal substance and is socially accepted if used in moderation, it is likely that abusers of drugs other than alcohol are more deviant than the alcohol abuser, and they are obviously more daring.

Young people who use illegal drugs are impelled by curiosity, excitement, danger, and the lure of the unknown and the forbidden. It has been said that many young people who take drugs are rebelling against their parents, but that young people who use alcohol are emulating their parents.

In general, abusers of prescription drugs are less deviant than the younger users of illegal substances, and try to stay within socially imposed limits.

Easy access to drugs influences the pattern of abuse and the choice of a drug. Physicians, nurses, and pharmacists who have access to controlled substances are likely to abuse opiates. The pharmacological properties of a drug influence the rapidity with which addiction develops. Most persons using opiates become dependent in a week or two. Addiction to barbiturates and tranquilizers takes longer to acquire, usually from two to three months. Injectable drugs tend to produce dependency sooner than drugs taken by mouth. Interestingly, alcohol does not produce physical dependence until months or years of excessive consumption have elapsed.

An essential factor in drug abuse is the ability of a drug to be its own reinforcer. Mind-altering drugs produce pleasurable effects through either tension release or euphoria. With each pleasurable experience the drug becomes more precious. Many times drug abuse begins for social reasons, but the effects of the drug itself soon become paramount. After addiction, the fear of withdrawal symptoms adds negative reinforcement that supports continued use.

The strength of social and psychological reinforcers should not be overlooked. Drug-dependent persons often revert to drug abuse long after physical dependency has disappeared through treatment. Relapse is likely to occur when a former addict reconnects with friends in the drug culture. Sometimes an addict returns to old haunts because he has nowhere else to go or because he is more comfortable in the drug environment. Former heroin addicts have reported feeling withdrawal symptoms upon seeing drug paraphernalia such as syringes and needles, even after undergoing detoxification. It seems safe to assume that for many addicts social and psychological dependency outweighs physiological dependency.

An individual's choice of a drug is largely determined by the kind of person he is and the kind of image he wishes to project to others. It has been suggested that responsibility for drug abuse rests with society rather than with individual users. Old values have eroded without new standards to replace them. As a result, the search for pleasure and for escape leads all too often to chemical substances that offer instant gratification. Fear of symptoms caused by abstinence is, for drug abusers, a persuasive reason to continue to use the drug. Many addicted persons resist treatment because they are afraid of undergoing "cold turkey" detoxification, which is withdrawal without the provision of alternative medications. The media have done a disservice to the public and the addict by portraying withdrawal as a fearsome experience. Most detoxification centers help addicts withdraw gradually by offering substitute drugs, carefully prescribed and administered in decreasing amounts.

Long-term drug abuse is associated with many medical complications. If drugs are injected, sclerosing of veins, thrombophlebitis, and even gangrene can develop. Many addicts live in squalid surroundings and eat poorly. Many develop pneumonia, tuberculosis, and pulmonary abscesses. Liver damage such as hepatitis often results from the use of contaminated or shared needles. Some addicts develop AIDS, transmitted through sexual intercourse or unclean needles and syringes.

Opiate Withdrawal Syndrome

- Within 12 hours of last dose: Physical discomfort, tearing of the eyes, runny nose, sweating, yawning
- Within 12 to 14 hours: Agitation and restless sleep
- Within 2 to 3 days: Dilated pupils, anorexia, goose flesh (cold turkey effect), back pain, tremor
- Within 3 to 4 days: Insomnia, incessant yawning, gastrointestinal symptoms, chills, muscle spasms, abdominal pain, and other flulike symptoms
- After 5 days: Symptoms decrease, usually disappearing completely in a week to 10 days

---

Commonly Abused Drugs and Their Street Names

Trade Name	Street Name
Heroin	horse, smack, "H," junk
Morphine	morph, monkey, white stuff
Codeine	schoolboy
Dilaudid	lords, little D
Percodan	perkies
Dolophine	dollies
Demerol	demies
Talwin	Ts
Combined heroin and cocaine taken intravenously	hot shot
Free-based cocaine	crack

The Adult Drug Addict

Many drug-dependent persons who enter treatment are in some form of crisis, medical, social, or legal. They tend to abuse more than one substance, frequently combining heroin with cocaine, or augmenting cocaine with marijuana or alcohol use. A good way to begin treating a drug addict is to realize at the outset that these are passive-aggressive individuals. They are passive in their reluctance to confront problems in living directly, and aggressive in their efforts to continue taking the substance which to them represents freedom from care. In his classic treatise on alcoholism and gamesmanship, Steiner (1974) comments on differences and similarities between alcoholism and other forms of drug abuse. Although he admits there are differences, he states that a health care professional who works successfully with alcoholics can transfer considerable knowledge to the treatment of an opiate or amphetamine abuser.

Like alcoholics, drug addicts are often untruthful and manipulative. Their behavior can veer from apathy to chaotic activity, usually in an attempt to implement their own hidden agenda. The addict attempts to modify the treatment regimen to achieve his own goals. For example, an addict who combines cocaine, heroin, and alcohol may acknowledge that cocaine addiction is a problem but not mention heroin or alcohol abuse. Sometimes an addict will undergo detoxification merely in order to lower the amount of the drug he needs to obtain the desired effect. This reduces the cost of his habit for a time, although his need for larger amounts will return shortly. It is quite common for addicts to conceal information or give false details. Therefore, it is advisable to validate facts by interviewing family members and other significant persons.

Continuity of care is essential in treating anyone who is drug-dependent. The following information should be obtained as soon as possible when an addict enters treatment:

History and Assessment Data on Drug-Dependent Clients

Reason for entering treatment at this time: Health problems, legal charges, unavailable supply, etc.

Drugs currently being used: Types, frequency of use, and amounts

Drugs previously used (information obtained from client may be unreliable; usage may be underestimated or overestimated)

Educational and employment history

Family history: Family of origin and family of procreation, including family drug use

Living arrangements: Household members currently living with client; household members formerly living with client

Significant relationships: Past and present

Source of drug supply: How does the client support the habit?

Health status: Nutrition, infection, etc.

Sexual history: Current and past sexual habits; presence of or exposure to sexually transmitted diseases, including AIDS

Current and past legal charges: Disposition of previous charges and explanation of pending charges

Psychiatric evaluation: Deferred until client has detoxified and been abstinent for a period of time, because psychiatric symptoms may be due to the drug itself or the life-style of the client before detoxification

It may not be possible to elicit all the data initially, but assessment can be ongoing throughout treatment. Here again, corroboration by family members and significant others continues to be crucial.

Therapeutic Guidelines

Drug-dependent clients present many challenges to the health care professional. The addict, especially the user of illegal substances, often tries to dictate the terms of his own treatment. He already has moved beyond the limits of society and brings to therapy a contempt for establishment values. Any drug is chosen by the addict because its effects and properties fill a need. By choosing substances that are outside the law, the drug addict demonstrates behavior that is more reckless, more deviant, and more provocative than that of the alcoholic.

Rehabilitation of a drug addict is greatly affected by his personal commitment to be free of addiction. Many addicts enter treatment unwillingly, feeling that they are being asked to make a great sacrifice, and unwilling to tolerate much frustration or discomfort. Although all clients have the right to participate in formulating a care plan, this should be done very cautiously when the client is an addict. Addicts want their own way and will use devious means to achieve their objectives. When guile and charm fail, they often resort to demands and threats. They attribute most of their problems to the actions of others, and accuse caretakers and family members of misunderstanding or failing them. They have an uncanny ability to play on the sympathy of caretakers, especially those who are inexperienced. Family members are more familiar with the tactics of the addict, even though they too are often exploited.

At the beginning of treatment the addict should be told that withdrawal and recovery are not the same thing. Permanent recovery means renouncing addiction and adopting a different life-style. Lewis and Feldman (1989) present a program of drug treatment and rehabilitation that is divided into stages, which they describe as parts of a continuum:

Stage One: Withdrawal and detoxification
Stage Two: Long-term residential treatment
Stage Three: Long-term outpatient aftercare through recovery groups

Stage Four: Education and treatment of codependents provided in sessions with the addict and his family, through multifamily groups such as those offered by Narcotics Anonymous

In offering care to drug addicts, a multidisciplinary team approach is recommended. Because this group of clients is so difficult to deal with, health care professionals involved with them need the support of colleagues. If nothing else, other caregivers help one to become aware of one's own feelings and reactions toward the client. A designated approach to care must be implemented consistently by all team members. Rules must be enforced, and therapeutic distance should be maintained. Legitimate complaints of discomfort need attention, of course, but emphasis should be placed on means other than drugs to alleviate discomfort. Drug-dependent clients need to be confronted when they exhibit unproductive or regressive behavior, but confrontation should be cognitive and instructive rather than accusatory. Rates of recidivism are very high among drug-dependent persons. It is important that caregivers not equate therapeutic failure with their own personal failure. Recovery from drug addiction is a lifelong process, and the allure of mind-altering substances is always present.

Education is a basic component in the prevention of drug dependency, and should start with parents who show children that it is possible to live well without resorting to drugs. Schools are excellent places to offer drug education programs, and students can be encouraged to develop habits and skills that make drug abuse unnecessary. Assertiveness training and relaxation techniques are admirable coping methods that can be taught before and after drug dependency occurs, as either a primary or a secondary prevention mechanism.

Employers are in a good position to offer prevention programs and to induce addicted employees to enter treatment. The wish to hold on to one's job can be a powerful motivator to accept treatment. Many drug treatment programs include vocational counseling and job training in the services provided. The unemployed addict is less likely to resume drug use if he has the hope of developing a marketable skill and becoming employable. Trying to live without drugs leaves an emptiness in the lives of former addicts. Successful treatment programs are those that substitute something that compensates the addict for what was lost. Family participation, job prospects, and educational initiatives may be used to show the addict that there can be life after addiction.

The Female Drug Addict

Therapeutic measures suitable for male drug addicts are also appropriate for female drug addicts, but the plight of the female addict, like that of the female alcoholic, is bound to the plight of her children, born and unborn. A 1990 survey by the National Association of State Alcohol and Drug Abuse

Directors found that only 10 percent of pregnant women who need treatment for alcohol and drug dependency receive it. The survey indicates that about 30,000 pregnant women with drug and alcohol problems were currently receiving treatment, while over 250,000 pregnant women remained in need of treatment. Numbers of pregnant women in need of treatment for drug or alcohol problems were highest in Puerto Rico, Michigan, New York, Illinois, Virginia, Florida, and Georgia (Wentzel, 1989).

Cocaine is the illegal drug that is currently preferred by a majority of addicts, either alone or in combination with other substances. For most addicts cocaine is interchangeable with "crack," which is free-based cocaine. Crack is, in effect, a smokable and concentrated form of cocaine freed of its hydrochloride base.

For some years drug addiction has been blamed for much of the crime and devastation found in inner-city neighborhoods. Women, the source of stability for many inner-city families, make up the fastest growing group of drug abusers, especially of cocaine. A national drug hotline that used to receive only one-third of its calls from women now reports that over half of its calls are from women, many of whom are pregnant (Hansen, 1989). The number of addicted babies born in urban areas is awesome, and the rising incidence of pediatric AIDS cases is related to increased drug addiction among women.

Although some drug-exposed newborn infants have no visible symptoms, others are very jittery and are prone to tics and spasms. Some studies link cocaine use in early pregnancy to genital and urinary defects in infants, and to serious gastrointestinal problems that keep the babies from thriving (Frishman, 1989). Possible effects of prenatal exposure to cocaine are shown in Table 13.3.

Residential treatment for pregnant addicts is advisable, but such programs are limited in number. Hansen (1989) deplores the lack of residential drug centers for this group of addicts but says that outpatient treatment is better than no care at all. Many health care professionals working with

---

TABLE 13.3. Prenatal Effects of Cocaine on the Fetus

- Cocaine crosses the placental barrier and appears in fetal circulation two to three minutes after inhalation or injection by the mother. Within five minutes, cocaine blood level in the fetus is about 15 percent of the mother's cocaine blood level.
- Cocaine affects uterine blood flow and reduces transfer of oxygen to the fetus; this increases the risk of fetal brain damage.
- Cocaine causes maternal hypertension, sometimes leading to cardiac arrhythmia and erratic heartbeat. These factors increase the risk of premature separation of the placenta, a condition that may lead to hemorrage in the mother and stillbirth of the infant.

cocaine addicts believe that outpatient care is unrealistic. They have learned from experience that cocaine addiction is so compelling that the addict cannot say no unless she is enrolled in a twenty-four-hour-a-day protective program.

Therapeutic Guidelines

Although some pregnant addicts want to withdraw from drugs to safeguard their babies, many are unable to do so. Outpatient programs complicate the addicts' lives because they have no transportation to clinics, no one to care for older children, and no support group beyond the treatment staff. When they do manage to keep appointments, they must return to the drug-infested neighborhoods where they live. Some drug-positive babies are so sick that they are hospitalized for long periods, but the majority are not. Contrary to popular belief, most babies are sent home with their mothers unless there is a history of severe negligence or abuse. Addiction alone is not currently considered sufficient cause to place a child in foster care. Genuine efforts are made by hospital social workers and child protective services to formulate a safe discharge plan for the baby. If foster care is recommended, the status of the child and the mother is reviewed periodically, with the goal of reuniting mother and child if possible, and of persuading the mother to accept treatment for her addiction.

Some states, like Florida and Connecticut, file criminal charges against pregnant women who take drugs on the grounds that they are guilty of child abuse, but the outcome of these cases remains doubtful. Many health care professionals working with pregnant addicts fear that criminalizing pregnant drug users will scare them away and make them less likely to seek treatment. Most clinicians agree that the best strategy is to provide prenatal care along with drug treatment programs, and to uphold the policy of removing the child from the mother whenever abuse or neglect are obvious. Punitive measures are likely to defeat the goal of protecting the child. As long as the addict remains in the health care system, supervision of mother and child is facilitated. The mother of the addict is often the best ally of health care professionals trying to provide care to the addict and her child. Countless grandmothers have taken on the obligation of raising their addicted daughter's child. This certainly blurs generational boundaries as grandmothers try to assist their children and their children's children, but it is a practical solution to a problem that is otherwise insurmountable. Addicted babies need a host of services, and these services are costly. Because cocaine-addicted babies are a recent phenomenon, no one knows what the cost will be in the future, once they start school. Programs are being offered, but many are based on expedience rather than long-range planning.

A number of child advocates are concerned about the children of crack-addicted mothers who are moved from one care facility to another and have no opportunity to form the attachments that are essential to normal emotional development. One expert warns that if the process of moving a child from home to home occurs over and over again, children may give up forming attachments at all because the pain of repeated loss is so great. The predicament of these children is complicated by debate about the rights of children versus the rights of parents to have their children returned to them. State and federal laws require health care professionals to document in the courts cases of child abandonment, neglect, or abuse, and to strive to provide enough social services to keep children and parents together if at all possible (Morgan, 1990).

The Adolescent Drug Addict

Abuse of alcohol and other substances is widespread in the adolescent and young adult population. The reasons for drug abuse in this age group are varied. The young person's perception of drug use by parents, peers, and prominent persons is a very important factor. From parents, peers, and the media, young people learn that drugs enable them to escape the humdrum world of home, school, or work. Unhappily, social and experimental drug use leads to addiction, for which an insufficient number of programs are available. For the young addict, as for any drug-dependent person, a residential treatment program is recommended. Here addicts live together after going through withdrawal. Most of these drug programs emphasize education, group confrontation, and commitment. Vocational counseling, legal assistance, full family participation and lengthy aftercare are part of the total program.

Therapeutic Guidelines

Programs for drug addicts stress confrontation, but this technique is more useful if it takes place between addicts. For most addicts this is more acceptable than confrontation by members of the "straight" world.

In formulating a treatment plan for the young drug addict, assessment of parental drug use and of family dynamics need to be included. Parents should be asked what they know about their child's drug habits, their reaction to this knowledge, and their relationship with the addicted child. Significant information from parents about a child's behavioral changes, academic standing, and peer relationships provides data that are useful in providing care.

When the addict is an adolescent, the health care team should exert great effort not to deal with her as if she is a bad person. The concept of "tough love" has been advocated in recent years for parents dealing with rebellious youngsters. This is described as a willingness of parents to do whatever is necessary to bring the child face to face with the implications of his actions. Parents should not try to be reliable rescuers, but at the same time they should protect the addict from actions that are dangerous or potentially fatal, such as overdosing or engaging in drug peddling. When parents stand idly by without intervening in the self-destructive actions of an addicted child, they may be motivated by rage toward the child. Tough love means setting limits without adding extreme consequences to the situation. Parents of addicts need help in finding a balance between constantly rescuing and giving up on the addict. Like the health care team, parents should neither exaggerate nor minimize the seriousness of drug abuse. Specific parental tactics are described in the following section.

Families of Drug Addicts

Families of drug addicts have received scant attention in the past, but this is beginning to change. Alexander and Dibb (1977) in an early study report how an addict's family perpetuates drug abuse. Families in their sample impeded addicts' autonomy by encouraging them to rely on parents as problem solvers. Not only were parents willing to rescue, make decisions, and solve problems, they also interfered with the addicts' efforts to develop skills and initiative. In doing this, parents condoned their child's manipulation by accepting it as normal behavior for addicts. At the same time, parents held addicts in low regard and thought them different from themselves. Overall, parental reactions fostered passivity, irresponsibility, and low self-esteem in addicted offspring.

When drug abuse and addiction make their appearance in adolescence, family dynamics can be crucial in the treatment program. The prototype family of an addict is often a system where one parent is very involved with the addict, while the other is uninvolved, punitive, or absent. Usually, but not always, the overinvolved parent is of the opposite gender. At times the overinvolvement of one parent is extreme enough to include incest. More often, however, the drug addict serves other family functions, such as reducing tension between parents by being a channel into which marital discontent is detoured. Addiction may be the sole issue that holds parents together even though they may not agree on how to deal with the addict.

Adolescence is a time when parents must face the prospect of losing their child to outsiders. The addiction to drugs is a destructive solution to the question of individuation and separation. It enables the addict to separate by achieving an identity distinct from that of other family members; yet it makes it possible for the family and the addict to remain closely connected. Stanton (1979) coined the term *pseudoindividuation* for the contradictory behavior of drug addicts who use addiction to depart from the family of origin yet remain bound to it in countless ways.

Having a schizophrenic child in the family may keep parents together by giving them a problem to share that does not threaten the marital relationship, and having a drug-addicted child may perform the same function. For the drug-dependent offspring, this may extend addiction beyond adolescence into adulthood. There is evidence that stability in the family of origin is meaningful to addicts, most of whom maintain close ties up to and past 30 years of age (Stanton et al., 1982). Attachment between addicts and their families of origin transcends class, although class differences may cause variations in addict and parent behavior. Middle-class addicts who live elsewhere and adopt a countercultural life-style return periodically to escape crises of one kind or another. They may be met with recrimination but seldom with parental rejection. Lower-class families may have fewer resources to place at the disposal of the addict, but their actions attest to the same kind of connectedness. This is shown by the behavior of grandmothers who continue to help children who are addicts and take on the task of rearing grandchildren whom the addict has abandoned. Many addicts maintain the illusion of separating from their families of origin and joining a peer group subculture. However, they continue to be part of their family of origin, which simultaneously disapproves of and accepts them.

Addicts who marry or live with a sexual partner are part of two family systems, the family of origin and the newer nuclear family they have established. Textor (1987) believes that therapy that concentrates on an addict's marriage and ignores the family of origin is rarely successful. In response to intervention that overlooks the family of origin and deals only with the marriage, the addict often leaves the spouse and returns to the parental roof. In trying to overcome addiction, the person in treatment almost always insists that parents are more helpful than a spouse or other partner. In many instances the parents of the addict did not grant wholehearted permission for the marriage or cohabiting relationship to succeed. The implicit message from the parents is that if the addict encounters problems with the partner, it is always possible to return to the parental hearth. Although this message sounds solicitous, it also reveals the ambivalence of parents who say they want the addict to be like everyone else but are prepared to help in any circumstances.

Interesting interactions are reported by clinicians observing interactions between a male addict's mother and his wife (Stanton et al., 1982). In some cases there is virtually no communication between the two. Even when they encounter each other face to face, they seldom speak. In the second type of interaction, the addict's wife seems to be tolerated by the mother but is undermined in subtle ways. For example, the mother might "accidentally" reveal the wife's shortcomings to the addict; such revelations might range from criticism of the wife's spending to disclosures of her sexual indiscretions. The third type of interaction consists of an unspoken alliance between mother and wife in which both women act like a pair of young mothers responding to the addict as if he were a wayward child. They both engage in helpful gestures, are indulgent toward the addict, and display attitudes of amused and condescending tolerance when the addict's incompetence is revealed.

The intensity of the addict's connection to the original family may prevent the formation of age-appropriate relationships with girlfriends and boyfriends during adolescence, and with spouses and offspring later on. Drug addiction may offer addicts a way of dealing with interpersonal problems and sexual anxieties. It is quite likely that some addicts avoid or retreat from interpersonal and sexual relationships through their attachment to the chosen chemical substance. The drug itself, with its ritual of preparation and administration, may be an erotic experience. Certainly many addicts use colorful, sexual terminology when speaking of various aspects of the drug experience. For evidence one has only to recall the street names given to certain drugs by users—dollies, perkies, lords, hot shot, to name a few. The same can be said of alcoholics who refer to liquor by feminine names, such as Amber or Rose. Alcoholism group leaders have heard members refer to whiskey as "the woman who never fails you" and the "sweetheart who never lets you down." Many illegal substances such as opiates reduce the sex drive by providing another sort of high, and the depressant alcohol may increase desire but impair performance. In time, addiction to any chemical substance produces physiological inroads that have negative sexual effects. By substituting some chemical substance for a real-life sexual partner, the addict can experience orgastic sensations without being unfaithful to a wife or a mother, and without risking interpersonal commitment.

Therapeutic Guidelines

During the decades of the 1960s, 1970s, and 1980s, individual psychotherapy with drug addicts proved ineffective, even when combined with such adjuncts as residential treatment, methadone maintenance, and crisis intervention. There continue to be high rates of recidivism among addicts who initially responded to treatment. Textor (1987) explains that clinicians find during the period of improvement that an addict's family of origin seems to suffer various crises in which parents become depressed and contentious. Some parents may contemplate divorce or report troubling symptoms in siblings of the addict. This interpersonal process constitutes a reactive deterioration in which the addict's recovery threatens family unity and the addict's relapse restores family equilibrium. These clinical observations have led to closer attention to dynamics in addicts' families of origin and in their marital families.

A family model recommended to health care professionals working with addicts incorporates strategies applied at the level of the individual, the family, and the social group (Textor, 1987). On the individual level the first step is withdrawal to abstinence status. This may be accomplished in a hospital, in an outpatient facility, or, ideally, in the home where the addict and family members share the experience. Regardless of the setting where detoxification takes place, responsibility for undergoing withdrawal and staying drug-free rests with the addict.

All addicts, even those in their 30s and 40s, need help in accomplishing the critical tasks of adolescence, which they have not yet achieved successfully. They need guidance in learning how to control their own lives and actions. Assertiveness training, role play, role modeling, and relaxation techniques are all means of learning self-control and self-management. Addicts need to be taught to face the realities of life instead of avoiding realities through drugs. Peak experiences induced by drugs must be replaced by relationships and social skills that reduce the interpersonal anxiety that contributes to addiction. The purpose of drug treatment is not only to keep addicts drug-free but to prepare them for adulthood. Thus individuation and separation from the family of origin are among the treatment objectives.

A family approach to drug treatment includes all members of the family of origin, not just the addict. The family is considered dysfunctional in some way, with the addict's behavior a manifestation of the dysfunction. This approach cuts through the blaming and scapegoating that may be present. Because one parent is apt to be overinvolved and the other underinvolved, some clinicians advise giving the less involved parent the task of helping the addict through detoxification and of keeping drug-abusing companions at a distance. Because the parents and the siblings of drug addicts may themselves abuse alcohol or other substances, a family approach requires them to confront their own actions in this regard. Huberty and Huberty (1983) write:

> Because of the high incidence of parental and sibling substance abuse, we ask all members in therapy to abstain from all mood altering substances. In addition to detecting otherwise hidden parental and sibling drug or alcohol abuse, such an agreement removes the double standard attached to the drug user in therapy. (p. 98)

Asking all members to abstain from mind-altering substances gives parents and siblings insight into the feelings of addicts who are dealing with peer pressure and everyday stress without chemical crutches. Concentrated attention is removed from the addict and focused on the system. In sessions, family members are instructed to speak directly to one another, not to or through the therapist. They are encouraged to argue and disagree openly with one another, and to revive in the session disputes that arose at home instead of trying to describe them to the therapist.

Usually the marriage of the addict's parents needs to be strengthened by improving marital communication and reducing distances between the partners. It is often helpful to comment on the mutual support each partner needs from the other, and to reinforce the idea that the parents are indeed partners in charge of the family system. To help parents relate as partners, homework can be given, such as asking them to set aside special time for the two of them, either to discuss in a compatible way the events of the day or to engage in a recreational activity they both enjoy. As the addict starts to improve, dissension between the parents may increase because they are less distracted by the addict's behavior. At this point therapeutic efforts should be directed toward "detriangling" the addict. There are several ways to do this, depending on the structure and patterns of the family. Strengthening connections between siblings and reducing the overinvolvement of one of the parents reinforces subsystem and generational boundaries.

The parent who is of the same sex as the addict is usually more detached and should be more central in the family. By promoting more involvement with the addict by this parent, the protectiveness, rescuing, and growth-inhibiting actions of the other parent are moderated. When the distant parent becomes more involved with the addict, there is less tendency on his or her part to stand apart and criticize. As the distant parent draws closer to the addict and the overinvolved parent becomes less active, opportunity arises for the clinician to restructure the family so that the parents move closer to each other and begin to operate as a team. If interventions establish generational boundaries and functional subsystems, it is easier for the addict to move from adolescence to adulthood. Restructuring lessens separation anxiety on the part of parents and the addict alike.

Family work with addicted persons generally centers on the family of origin. For married or cohabiting addicts, however, problems in the relationships within their families of procreation must also be addressed. Parents of addicts need help in accepting the partners of their addicted offspring. Equally important is the need to establish clear boundaries between the family of origin and the family of procreation so that all participants perceive themselves as distinct systems. Marital patterns between the addict and the spouse or cohabiting partner often replicate patterns carried over from the family of origin. Emphasizing boundaries between the two families gives the clinician freedom to explore roles and habits present in the family of origin and to point out the transfer of the same patterns to the newer family system. Unless dynamics present in the family of origin are examined and moderated, dysfunctional replication in the newer family cannot be adequately understood by the parents, the addict, and the partner.

On a social level, family therapy for addicts must include relationships both within and outside the drug culture. Addicts in treatment should be protected from peers who are still using drugs, but group sessions with other recovering addicts are helpful. Positive peer experiences replace negative ones; separation from the family of origin and personal autonomy are encouraged by comparing similar experiences of other addicts. Multifamily meetings are offered in many treatment programs to aid parents and children of addicts. These groups provide education about drugs, reduce family alienation, and promote ongoing change. Clinicians working with addicts are opposed to simple rescue operations but are willing to contact officials in school or the workplace in order to improve addicts' relationships with authority figures. What the clinician undertakes is to mitigate destructive influences in the life of addicts by intervening at the level of the individual, the family, and the larger social order, using strategies that propel addicts toward the maturity that they and their parents have avoided.

Brief Catalogue of Recommended Strategies for Families of Addicts

- Include as many family members as possible in treatment.
- Try to recruit a family member as sponsor or advocate for the addict.
- Listen to families express what they want and need from treatment, and their perceptions of "normal" family life.
- Adjust treatment goals to the objectives and capabilities of the family.
- Emphasize how every family member will benefit by treatment; acknowledge stresses families have experienced in dealing with the addict.
- Anticipate and deal with the resistance of members to participating in the meetings, and their fear of change in the family system.
- Avoid blaming the family or any particular member for the addict's problems.
- Identify all family members as potentially helpful in decision making and problem solving.
- Help the addict and family members establish a support network such as multifamily meetings in a drug treatment program, or attending Narcotics Anonymous in the company of the addict.
- Offer psychoeducation programs to teach families about drug treatment and improve their understanding of addiction.
- Be specific about what is expected of family members and about the purpose of therapy sessions in which they are included.

Source: Adapted from Wermuth and Scheidt (1986).

CLINICAL EXAMPLE: DRUG ABUSE AS A FAMILY ISSUE

Tom is a 24-year-old single male. He lives in the parental home and has had problems with alcohol and other drugs since age 15. A high school dropout, he began using marijuana in school, quickly proceeded to experiments with other drugs such as bennies (amphetamines) and speed (methamphetamine). He tried a few common opiates like codeine and morphine, then became addicted to heroin. By the time he was 19 he was in methadone maintenance treatment, a program used for heroin addiction. He remained with this program until age 21, when he took to using cocaine. He was arrested twice for possession and spent time in jail. His other problems were exacerbated by chronic use of alcohol, usually wine or beer because these were cheaper. By age 24 he had been in two treatment programs. After that he spent three months in a halfway house and was drug-free for a year.

Assessment

Recently Tom was referred to a drug rehabilitation program in a mental health center. This occurred after a four-day hospitalization for an acute reaction to crack cocaine. His return to cocaine was in the aftermath of the loss of his girlfriend, who had left him for another man. This use of cocaine was a violation of his five-year probation period. Because he had been drug-free and regularly employed for a time, he was referred to an inpatient drug unit rather than sentenced to incarceration.

In his family of origin Tom is the youngest of four children, the second son in a single-parent lower-class family headed by his mother. His oldest sibling, a brother, Henry, was killed in a motorcycle accident when Tom was 14 years old. At the time of his death Henry was 21 years old. Of the remaining siblings, the oldest is Anna, who is 28 years old and married, with two small children. Sara, the younger sister, is 26 years old and attends a hairdressing school.

Tom's father, who was also alcoholic, was a day laborer who deserted the family when Tom was 8 years old. Two years after his desertion the family heard that he had died in another city when he tried to jump from a moving freight train after hitching a ride. Tom's mother worked as a cleaning woman. When her children were small she was intermittently on public assistance. She is now quite ill with a heart condition and unable to work. Although the family suffered economic hardships, there are memories of some good times. The father was not abusive, and Tom recalls going on outings with him before he deserted the family.

Tom's mother is a strong, nurturing person who attends an evangelical church regularly. In previous years she had kept the family together and provided stability for her children. She leaned heavily on Henry, her oldest son, and considered him the man of the house in the absence of his father. Henry's reaction was to become unruly, join a reckless peer group, and subsequently lose his life in the motorcycle accident. Tom had loved and admired his older brother and was devastated by his death. In retrospect, it appears that Tom was probably depressed as a teenager, although this was never recognized. He had begun skipping school in response to peer pressure. It is likely that in response to his feelings of depression, he turned to alcohol and drugs for relief.

Planning

At the drug rehabilitation program to which he was referred, Tom had several intake interviews. Specific attention was paid to the loss of his girlfriend and its meaning for him at this stage of his life. Interviews were arranged with his mother to assess her current physical condition as well as her relationship with Tom. Tom's sisters were also contacted and invited to join some family sessions. The older sister was protective of her brother, but the younger one expressed disgust with Tom for breaking his probation. The older sister was maternal in her attitude toward Tom, whereas the younger sister seemed angry with him.

The mental health team recommended referral to an inpatient drug/ alcohol rehabilitation program, and this was followed.

Intervention

Apparently the loss of his girlfriend stirred up for Tom his memories of the traumatic loss of his father and his brother. In family meetings it became evident that for Tom the dark shadow of loss and death hung over the family. The seriousness of his mother's heart condition posed yet another threat of loss. Tom's individual and family therapists met several times with Tom, his mother, and two sisters. His brother-in-law whom Tom liked, and his two nephews, aged 2 and $3^1/_2$, were included whenever possible. Interestingly, the two little boys had been named John and Henry, respectively, after their deceased grandfather and uncle. Actually, the family proved to be more close-knit than had originally been thought by the health care professionals who were involved.

Like Tom, the family members had not completely worked through the loss of a father and a brother. With help they came to realize that they could grieve together and comfort one another. Tom's behavior was interpreted as his customary response to loss rather than a character defect. A full medical workup was suggested for mother, and a meeting with her physician and adult family members was scheduled. If mother's condition warranted it, a daily home health aide would be made available, which was a great relief for Tom and his sisters. Tom's former boss was contacted. Because Tom was a dependable employee when he worked as a presser in a dry cleaning establishment, his boss was willing to take him back. Tom planned to return to work as soon as possible.

The inpatient drug rehabilitation program that Tom attended offered new support for him and his family. After discharge, outpatient follow-up care was available for Tom, as well as monthly family meetings if they wished to attend.

Evaluation

Using a family approach erased much of the stigma attached to Tom and kept him within the family unit. Because he remained a fragile and lonely person, he needed to feel that he was still accepted by his family. As a result of their involvement, family support and reassurance replaced peer pressure. Although he continued to be vulnerable, the prognosis for Tom to remain drug-free is good. His use of alcohol may continue because this is more socially acceptable than drug addiction. However, the strengths that existed within Tom's family were utilized on his behalf, and family commitments were strengthened.

CLINICAL EXAMPLE: A FAMILY APPROACH TO DRUG ADDICTION

The Morgan household consists of Douglas, his wife Marjory, and their 3-year-old grandson, Dougie. Douglas and Marjory are a middle-aged couple who are the parents of three grown children, none of whom live at home. Their older son is married and the father of three children, and their daughter is married but has no children. Their youngest child, Greg, is unmarried and has his own apartment. Greg is 23 years old, unemployed, and currently being treated for multiple drug addiction at an outpatient program offered by a nearby community mental health center. Greg states that he no longer uses cocaine or heroin; he is more evasive when asked about marijuana or alcohol use. Although he has his own apartment, Greg returns often to his parents' home for meals and to see Dougie, who is his only child. Greg and Dougie's mother were not married, and she was not interested in raising the child. Custody was awarded to Greg, but Dougie has been cared for by his grandmother almost since his birth. He is a bright, agreeable child, much loved by his grandparents and by his father.

Greg and Marjory argue a great deal about Greg's friends, his joblessness, and his drug habits, which Marjory continues to view with suspicion. Caring for Dougie is another subject on which Greg and his mother fiercely disagree. Marjory is willing to have Greg visit the child in her home but refuses to permit the child to stay in Greg's apartment. She objects strenuously to Greg's friends and accuses them of using the apartment as a "hangout" for their questionable activities. Dougie has been taught to call his grandparents Mama and Papa; he calls his father Uncle Greg.

Douglas is looking forward to retiring from work as a maintenance man. He is far quieter than Marjory but is devoted to her. He smokes cigarettes and drinks alcohol in moderation, except on weekends when he tends to become "pickled," to use Marjory's word. Douglas has trouble sleeping at night, and his family physician recently prescribed an antianxiety drug to be taken at bedtime.

Assessment

The Morgan family tends to reshape reality to suit their own purposes. Marjory is a loving grandmother, but she distorts the relationship that actually exists between her husband, herself, and her grandson. She is comfortable being an indulgent mother figure for Dougie and a critical authority figure for Greg. In obscuring generational boundaries, she ignores the legitimate needs of her husband, who foresees retirement in a household where there is little consideration for him.

Greg is trying to abstain from using hard drugs, but he finds it difficult. He finds an ally in his older brother and visits him often. The two brothers are in agreement that their mother is a "hard" woman. They feel sorry for their father because he is under Marjory's thumb; they see him as a fretful, lonely man. Greg's brother is annoyed that Dougie is growing up without knowing who his father is, but he counsels Greg to be patient, find employment, and try to recover Dougie when the child is older. Greg sees the wisdom in this advice but believes that it would be easier to stay off drugs if he had Dougie with him all the time.

Planning

The Morgan family showed some resistance to being seen as a group. Greg's sister, who was newly married, refused to participate at all. His older brother was more than willing to attend, and his father agreed without much hesitation. Marjory wondered what the point was of having family meetings, but said she would do almost anything to help Greg.

The family therapist noted that Marjory was totally engrossed with her grandson and was determined to prevent Greg from enacting the role of father. She was locked into an adversarial relationship with Greg that overlooked his valiant struggle to be drug-free and mocked his desire to be a father to Dougie. On a conscious level she hoped that Greg would succeed in building a good life for himself, but on a deeper level she knew that his rehabilitation meant that she would see less of her adored grandson. She insisted that Greg was incapable of looking after his son even for a weekend, and she used the pretext of meals, naps, and daily routines to curtail any time they spent together.

Intervention

The dynamics of this family were apparent to the therapist, who saw that the crux of the problem was Marjory. In the first session a suggestion was made that Dougie begin to address his father as Daddy and his grandparents as Grandma and Grandpa. When Marjory objected that this might upset the child, she was told that the truth would be less upsetting now than it might be later on, especially if the child learned the truth from outsiders. The child's grandfather and his uncle strongly supported the suggestion, and their response brought tears to Greg's eyes.

Marjory's careful attention to the child's health and welfare were praised, and the therapist agreed that Greg was probably not yet ready to take full responsibility for such a young child. It was possible for Greg to begin taking some of the child care off Marjory's shoulders. This could be done gradually, with Marjory acting as a teacher for Greg since she had already proved herself in this area.

With some direction and permission, Douglas was able to talk about his forebodings around retirement and his belief that Marjory would be unwilling to join him in some of the activities he had planned. At one point Douglas was able to say to his wife, "You're not a saint and you don't always have to be a full-time mother once Greg gets on his feet."

Greg's brother proved to be a constructive force in the family meetings. He could say things to his mother that she would not accept from anyone else, accusing her of being a mother hen who needed a chick to cluck over, but adding that she had some other grandchildren who wanted to share the attention lavished on Dougie. He added further that he would like his own children to spend more time with Dougie but that he hesitated to arrange this because of the lies surrounding the boy.

Evaluation

Access to his son is a powerful motivator for Greg. He has broken with some of his more deviant companions and has asked his mother to visit him frequently so that she can see how acceptable the household now is for Dougie. The little boy now calls his father and grandparents by their real titles, and accepted the change without a qualm. Greg is taking vocational aptitude tests and plans to enter a job training program. His drug counselor credits the family meetings with helping Greg abstain from drugs. Greg's brother and his family are extremely helpful. They show Greg almost every day that it is possible to enjoy family life and to provide for a wife and children, all without the use of drugs. Marjory continues to be very attached to Dougie, but he is becoming interested in playing games with his youthful father and his cousins. For the present Dougie still lives with his grandparents, except when they take a trip. At such times he stays with his father. Marjory and Greg agree that current arrangements will continue until Dougie is in school or until his father marries. The most appreciative family member is Greg's father, who enjoys his wife's greater interest in him and is able to tell her this.

SUMMARY

Alcohol abuse is a form of drug abuse, but in this chapter a distinction is made between problem drinking and other forms of substance abuse. Considerable research has been devoted to developing a profile of a typical alcoholic, but without notable success. There are, however, certain conflicts operating in alcoholics that influence their general behavior as well as patterns of drinking. The preferred defense mechanism of alcoholics is denial, and it is a defense shared by family members. The family of an alcoholic usually tries to appear normal to outsiders; this often leads to rescue behaviors that prevent the alcoholic from experiencing the consequences of drinking. The rescuer of an alcoholic is usually an enabler as well, who makes it possible for the alcoholic to continue drinking. In families of alcoholics the spouse and often the children become codependents. This means that their behaviors, attitudes, and decisions are controlled by the problem drinker. The consequences to the spouse and especially to the children are enormous. Adult children of alcoholics suffer lasting damage. They tend to become chronic reacters rather than spontaneous interacters, and they often have trouble with interpersonal relationships. Despite the trauma they endured in their family of origin, adult children of alcoholics remain connected to parents. Family members need counseling both when the alcoholic is sober and when drinking resumes. A recovering alcoholic may not always be welcomed by a family that has adjusted to a problem drinker. The spouse and the children need help in realigning the family to make a place for the sober alcoholic.

Special needs of the male alcoholic, the female alcoholic, the adolescent alcoholic, and the elderly alcoholic are described in the chapter. Therapeutic guidelines are suggested for each of the foregoing groups.

Drug abuse occurs in all levels of society and at all ages. Most drug abusers never come to the attention of health professionals, but manage to function after a fashion. Reinforcers of drug abuse include the pleasureable effects of the drug itself, the appeal of the peer group, and eventually the fear of the discomfort of withdrawal and abstinence. Users of illegal drugs often enter treatment reluctantly, in response to family, employer, or legal insistence. Treatment is complicated by their manipulation and their reluctance to endure much discomfort. Sometimes an addict will go through withdrawal merely to lower the amount of drug needed to produce the desired effect. An addict who chooses substances that are outside the law is apt to be more deviant, reckless, and provocative than an alcoholic.

Family therapy for drug addicts is receiving increased attention, partly because other therapeutic approaches have not been very successful. Drug abuse and addiction often appear during adolescence, when the critical task for the individual is separation and individuation and the critical task for the family is launching the children. Addiction to drugs can be a destructive solution to the problem of separation. It permits the addict to forge an identity different from that of other family members, while also keeping the family and the addict closely connected. Some addicts establish separate households but return repeatedly to the parental home, even after they marry. In many cases the parents of an addict are not enthusiastic about the spouse and they aggravate problems in the marriage. The addict's parental family represents a system in which one parent is very involved with the addict, while the other is uninvolved, punitive, or absent.

The purpose of family work with addicts is not just to keep them drug-free but to prepare them for adulthood. Strengthening the marriage of the parents encourages the overinvolved parent to free the addict. This is facilitated by inducing the less involved parent to become more central in the family. Participation of the addict's siblings is another way to reinforce generational boundaries and sibling subsystems.

Special characteristics of the adult drug addict, the female drug addict, and the adolescent drug addict are included in the chapter, followed by therapeutic guidelines applicable to each.

REFERENCES

Alexander, B. K., & Dibb, G. S. (1977). "Interpersonal Perception in Addict Families." *Family Process*, 16(1): 17–28.

Allan, C. A., & Cooke, D. J. (1985). "Stressful Life Events and Alcohol Misuse in Women: A Critical Review." *Journal of Studies in Alcohol*, 46(2): 147–153.

Anderson, R. C., Anderson, K. E., & Smith, A. O. (1986). "Effects of Alcohol Consumption During Pregnancy." *American Association of Occupational Health Nurses Journal*, 38(1): 88–91.

Bennett, G., Vourakis, C., & Woolf, D. S. (1983). *Substance Abuse: Pharmacological Development and Clinical Perspectives*. New York: Wiley.

Brown, S. (1988). *Treating ACOAS: A Developmental Perspective*. New York: Wiley.

Brown, S., & Beletsis, S. (1986). "The Development of Family Transference in Groups for ACOAS." *International Journal of Group Psychotherapy*, Winter: pp. 97–144.

Busch, D., McBride, A. B., & Bonaventura, L. M. (1985). "Chemical Dependency in Women." *Journal of Psychosocial Nursing*, 24(1): 26–30.

Davies, J. L. (1989). "Altered Patterns of Societal Adjustment." In E. H. Janosik & J. L. Davies (Eds.), *Psychiatric Mental Health Nursing*. Monterey, CA/Boston: Jones and Bartlett.

Eels, M. A. (1986). "Interventions with Alcoholics and Their Families." *Nursing Clinics of North America*, 21: 493–503.

Franks, L. (1985). "A New Attack on Alcoholism." *New York Times Magazine*, October 20, pp. 47–50, 61–69.

Frishman, R. (1989). "Innocent Drug Abuse Casualties." *Democrat and Chronicle*, Rochester, New York, September 17, p. 21A.

Gulino, C., & Kaden, M. (1986). "Aging and Reactive Alcoholism." *Geriatric Nursing*, 7(20): 148–151.

Hansen, J. A. (1989). "Female Addicts Overwhelm Rescue Efforts with Cries for Help." *Democrat and Chronicle*, Rochester, New York, September 17, p. 21A.

Huberty, D. J., & Huberty, C. E. (1983). "Drug Abuse." In M. R. Textor (Ed.), *Helping Families with Special Problems*, New York: Aaronson.

Kaplan, H. I., Freedman, A. M., & Sadock, B. J. (1980). *Comprehensive Textbook of Psychiatry*, 3rd ed. (Vol. 2). Baltimore, MD: Williams and Wilkins.

Kaufman, E. (1986). "The Family of the Alcoholic Patient." *Psychosomatics*, 27(5): 347–360.

Lewis, S., & Feldman, T. B. (1989). "The Patient with Drug Dependence." In S. Lewis, R. Grainger, W. A. McDowell, R. J. Gregory, & R. L. Messner (Eds.), *Manual of Psychosocial Interventions: Promoting Mental Health in Medical-Surgical Settings*. Philadelphia: W. B. Saunders.

Lewis, S., McDowell, W. A., Gregory, R. J., & Messner, R. L. (1989). "The Patient with Alcoholism." In S. Lewis, R. Grainger, W. A. McDowell, R. J. Gregory, & R. L. Messner, *Manual of Psychosocial Interventions: Promoting Mental Health in Medical-Surgical Settings*. Philadelphia: W. B. Saunders.

Morgan, T., (1990). "Addicted Parents' Children Pose Foster Care Challenge." *New York Times*, October 19, p. B3.

Nathan, P. E. (1983). "Failure in Prevention: Why We Can't Prevent the Devastating Effects of Alcoholism and Drug Abuse." *American Psychologist*, 38(4): 459–467.

Parker, D., & Harford, T. (1988). "Alcohol Related Problems, Marital Disruption, and Depression Symptoms among Adult Children of Alcohol Abusers in the United States." *Journal of Studies in Alcohol*, 49(3): 265–268.

Smith, D. E., & Wesson, D. R. (1985). *Treating the Cocaine Abuser*. Center City, MN: Hazeldon Foundation.

Stanton, M. D. (1979). "Family Treatment Approaches to Drug Abuse Problems: A Review." *Family Process*, 18(3): 251–280.

Stanton, M. D., Todd, T. C., & Associates. (1982). *The Family Therapy of Drug Abuse and Addiction*. New York: Guilford Press.

Steiner, C. (1974). *Games Alcoholics Play*. New York: Ballantine.

Tesson, B. M. (1990). "Who Are They: Identifying and Treating Adult Children of Alcoholics." *Journal of Psychosocial Nursing*, 28(9): 16–21.

Textor, M. R. (1987). "Family Therapy with Drug Addicts: An Integrated Approach." *American Journal of Orthopsychiatry*, 57(4): 495–507.

Wentzel, M. (1989). "Drug Mom." *Democrat and Chronicle*, Rochester, New York, September 17, p. 21A.

Wermuth, L., & Scheidt, S. (1986). "Enlisting Family Support in Drug Treatment." *Family Process*, 25(1): 25–33.

Wortitz, J. (1983). *Adult Children of Alcoholics*. Hollywood, FL: Health Communications.

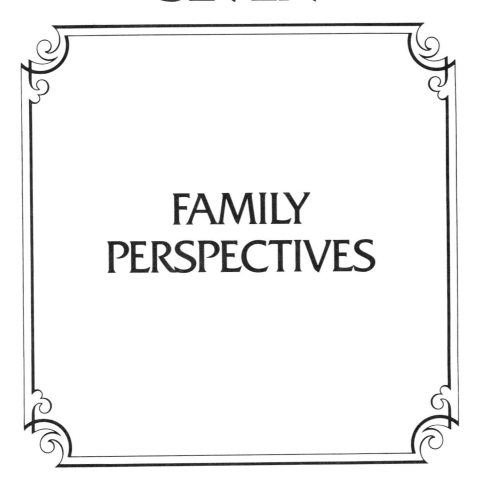

PART
SEVEN

FAMILY
PERSPECTIVES

CHAPTER FOURTEEN

Family Perspectives:
The Healthy Family

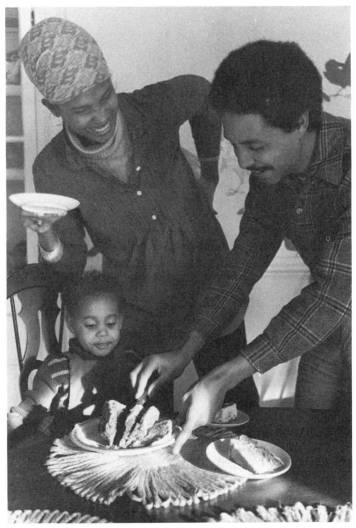

© 1991 Jerry Howard/POSITIVE IMAGES

*Look to your health; and if you have it, praise God,
and value it next to a good conscience; for health is the
second blessing that we mortals are capable of; a blessing that money cannot buy.*

Izaak Walton

In the mental health field, health care professionals are geared toward identifying problems and dysfunction, and even to putting labels on apparently pathologic behaviors. Many health care workers are really not sure how to define healthy family functioning and usually think that families are "normal" when they embrace values and beliefs that are similar to the health care worker's own. Defining what is "normal" is an extremely complex and difficult task. The medical model, with its emphasis on the diagnosis and treatment of disease, has often overlooked cultural influences that influence manifestation of "normal" and "abnormal" behavior. A family evaluation should include a description of the family's strengths, its healthy coping patterns, and should relate these to the family's life cycle, ethnic background, and cultural heritage. This chapter attempts to expand the definition of healthy or "normal" family functioning. Table 14.1 provides an outline of how the major models of family therapy view normal family functioning (Walsh, 1982). The chapter begins with a glimpse of how early studies of the family focused on severely disturbed family groups to the exclusion of what was "healthy" or "normal." The chapter then addresses significant early research attempts to explore healthy family relationships (Lewis et al., 1976). This same group, along with Beavers and Hampson (1990), has revised its measurement scales on family *competence* and family *style*, and these are reported on in considerable detail.

Brief descriptions of the research of others on the assessment of healthy family functioning continues with the McMaster Model of Normal Family Functioning, which has been in use for over twenty years. Unique studies of healthy communication in families at risk to develop psychopathology (Fisher, 1980; Wynne et al., 1982) are reported on. Beavers's discussion of the attributes of healthy couples (1985) is reviewed. Hansen's experience (1981) of *living* with three normal families is presented. The role of cultural influences in assessing normality in families' relationships is emphasized. Finally, a few guidelines for the health care professional in assessing a family's strengths are offered. A summary concludes the chapter's contents.

[456]

TABLE 14.1. Major Models of Family Therapy

Model of Family Therapy	Characteristics of Normal Family Functioning
Structural: Minuchin Montalvo Aponte	1. There are set and clear boundaries. 2. Strong parental coalition is present. 3. There is encouragement of individual growth. 4. Adaptation to both internal (developmental) and external (environmental) requirements is present.
Strategic: Haley Milan team	1. There are easily understood rules about family hierarchy. 2. Adaptability to change is present. 3. There are many available options for problem solving and life cycle transitions.
Behavioral-social exchange: Liberman Patterson Alexander	1. Rewards are for conforming behavior. 2. Nonconforming behavior is not rewarded. 3. Benefits outweigh the burdens or sacrifices. 4. Give and take among family members is on a long-term basis.
Psychodynamic: Ackerman Boszormenyi-Nagy Framo Lidz Meissner Paul Stierlin	1. Parental roles and responsibilities are well defined and sex linked. 2. There are well-defined generation boundaries. 3. Relationships are based on present realities and not past projections.
Family systems therapy: Bowen	There is a clear definition of self and a balance between the intellectual and emotional aspects of the personality.
Experiential: Satir Whitaker	1. Value is placed upon self-esteem. 2. Communication is explicit, concise, and honest. 3. There is a link to the larger system of community and society, which is open and optimistic. 4. There are many elements of family structure and shared family experiences.

Source: Adapted from Walsh (1982).

FAMILY RESEARCH PRIOR TO STUDIES ON THE HEALTHY FAMILY

Some of the formal systematic studies of the *family* had their early beginnings in the 1940s at the Yale Psychiatric Institute, which had contact with relatives of hospitalized schizophrenic patients. Lidz, Fleck, and Cornelison

(1965) studied 17 families with a schizophrenic offspring. Wynne and Singer (1963) also were pioneers in clinical research on schizophrenics' families; they focused on structure and communication patterns rather than content, and wrote about family transactions and types of schizophrenic thought disorders. In the early research on family systems, none of the methods focused on healthy families. What was healthy in families was assumed to be what was *not* dysfunctional. This fact was noted by Lewis and colleagues (1976) of the Timberlawn Foundation in Dallas, Texas, who embarked on a study of psychological health in family systems. One of their primary motivations was a search for preventive methodologies in the mental health field. The review of their work in this chapter will focus on the development and description of their measurement scales rather than on their treatment strategies.

EARLY STUDIES ON HEALTHY FAMILY FUNCTIONING

The family competence instrument known as the Beavers-Timberlawn Family Evaluation Scales was initially developed in 1972 and was used in the Timberlawn Research Foundation's early study of healthy families (Lewis et al., 1976). Assessing a family's competence gives direct attention to the family's coping strengths. These scales have since been revised and now appear as the Beavers Interactional Scales of (I) Family Competence and (II) Family Style. To understand family competence and strength, one needs to recognize a family's structure and relationships. The assessment of the intimately related dimension *family style* is essential to plan effective therapeutic intervention (Beavers & Hampson, 1990). These two sets of comprehensive measurements are given the detailed attention that they merit here. Their development has historical significance in the family therapy field in that they represent a careful, systematic study that not only *defines* healthy family functioning, but also offers the health care professional a blueprint for assessing healthy family functioning in a clear and orderly fashion.

The areas covered by the Family Competence scale are summarized in the following outline.

Family Competence

I. *Structure of the Family*
   A. *Overt power:* Who addresses whom, and who directs the exchange among the family members. This dimension is measured on a scale of five levels, from chaos to egalitarian interactions.
   B. *Parental coalition:* All of the various theories of family health give paramount importance to the strength and quality of the parental

dyad. This dimension is measured on a scale of five levels, from parent–child coalition to strong parental coalition.

C. *Closeness:* In this subscale, the clarity of interpersonal boundaries is considered on five levels, from amorphous, vague, and indistinct boundaries among family members, to closeness with distinct boundaries among members. In Eriksonian terms, in order to be intimate, one must first be an autonomous, separated person (Erikson, 1963). The lowest point of the scale is represented by Bowen's description of the undifferentiated family ego mass (Bowen, 1978), discussed earlier in this text.

II. *Mythology:* This subscale deals with the reality perception of the family, varying from congruent to incongruent. Again, there are five levels on which to rate the family. The rating is focused on the degree of difference between the observer's perception of family qualities and how the *family* actually views itself descriptively. For example, a family may say they are "loving and caring," yet their interactions reveal they ignore and distance each other. The rating here would be (4) or (5), depending on the degree of disparity.

III. *Goal-directed negotiation:* This subscale assesses the family's ability to negotiate problem situations. There are five steps in the scale, from extremely efficient to extremely inefficient. Inefficiency is represented by an inability to focus on the task or problem and an inability to discuss openly and directly the differences that have led to the problem.

IV. *Autonomy:* There are three parts to this subscale, each of which has five levels of rating:

A. *Clarity of expression* has to do with the degree to which family members are allowed or encouraged to express their own ideas and feelings, which is, of course, closely related to boundary issues. Can the family provide a safe environment for persons to express their ideas and feelings?

B. *Responsibility:* Related to the degree to which family members take responsibility for their own past, present, and future behavior, both inside and outside the family relationships.

C. *Permeability:* Has to do with the degree to which the family members are open and receptive to the self-statements of each other and to the statements from others outside the family circle. This relates to the "open" and "closed" family systems of Virginia Satir (1972).

V. *Family affect:* There are four parts to this subscale, each with five levels for rating:

A. *Range of feeling:* Has to do with the limits of "width" of expressed emotions in the family, from direct expression of a wide range of feelings to little or no expression of feelings.

B. *Mood and tone:* Relate to openness and optimism versus cynicism and pessimism. The five ratings go from affection and humor to cool politeness, to open hostility, to depression, to hopeless pessimism.

    C. *Unresolvable conflict:* Covers the condition of chronic underlying conflict versus the ability to resolve disagreements. In almost all families there are issues of difference and disagreement. The rater must note the effectiveness of the family members in negotiating conflicts. There may be severe impairment in the ability to resolve problems or, at the other end of the scale, little or no unresolvable conflict.

    D. *Empathy:* This subscale refers to the joining and sharing of feelings among family members, an accurate perception and understanding of a person's emotional responses. Family members are either consistently empathic, or on the opposite end of the scale, grossly inappropriate with regard to feelings.

VI. *Global health–pathology scale:* In addition, health care workers have available the global rating scale with ten levels for assessment, from most dysfunctional to healthiest. Beavers and Hampson specify that this is a subjective summary, which represents the overall impression of the structure, communication, affect, and effectiveness of the family system. Each family encountered by the health care professional will show relative strengths and weaknesses, areas of greater and lesser competence, which are necessary to evaluate in order to plan appropriate therapeutic interventions.

The second of the Beavers and Hampson comprehensive measurements referred to earlier is the assessment of the family's *style.* A family's style has to do with characteristic ways of relating and interacting among family members, particularly in the areas of dependency, conflict, closeness and separateness, social presentation, assertion and aggression, and the expression of positive and negative feelings. In order to assess a family's style, the Beavers group has developed a series of eight subscales, each with five rating levels:

1. Dependency needs
2. Adult conflict
3. Proximity
4. Social presentation
5. Expression of closeness
6. Assertive/aggressive qualities
7. Expression of positive and negative feelings
8. Global centripetal/centrifugal style

In describing family systems, the terms *centripetal force* and *centrifugal force* have been used. By definition, a centripetal force attracts toward the center, or axis, around which it rotates; movement is diverted inward. Centrifugal force repels away from the axis; movement is directed outward. According to the Beavers and Hampson style scales, a *centripetal rating* for a family means that the family emphasizes looking inward to the family for gratification of emotional needs. In their research, this style appears more in middle- and upper-class families, who pride themselves on making a "good" appearance to the outside world; they prescribe somewhat inflexible role-related status for family members. In the extreme, control is maintained by dependency and guilt manipulation; the father's authority is overtly un-challenged. For the most part, feelings are internalized and not expressed openly.

In contrast, a centrifugal rating means that the family has tenuous external boundaries, family members look outside the family for satisfac-tion, and offspring are pushed out too early. Styles may shift normally as the family moves in the family life cycle. For example, in the early years of child rearing, a centripetal style promotes nurturance and caretaking, whereas the centrifugal style adapts to the family's need to help the adoles-cent move out gradually into the outside world. Any family style that remains inflexible signifies a decreased competence in a family system's operation.

Beavers and Hampson describe further clinical family groupings of severely dysfunctional, borderline, midrange, adequate, and optional fami-lies and draw connections between the health/competence dimension and the stylistic dimension.

In the health/competence scale developed by Beavers and Hampson (1990), severely dysfunctional and borderline families had poor boundaries and unclear chaotic communication. They lacked focus and were full of despair, cynicism, and ambivalence. There was much distancing, depres-sion, and outbursts of rage. On the healthy side, the adequate or optimal families revealed relatively clear boundaries; were able to negotiate around conflicts for the most part; showed respect, warmth, and humor; and exer-cised control over emotions.

THE McMASTER MODEL OF NORMAL FAMILY FUNCTIONING

Another significant method of assessing family functioning is the McMaster model of family functioning, in use for over twenty years (Epstein et al., 1982). It is based on systems theory and does not cover all aspects of family functioning; rather, it focuses on those areas that have the most impact on the emotional and physical health or the problems of family members. The dimensions of family functioning are as follows (rating scales were devel-oped for each of these areas):

- Problem solving
- Communication
- Roles: Allocation and accountability
- Affective responsiveness
- Affective involvement
- Behavior control

Briefly described, the following postulates are presented. Effective families solve most problems efficiently and easily; as family functioning becomes less effective, problem solving becomes less systematic. Toward the

---

TABLE 14.2. Table of Assessment Scales

Family Competence Scale (Beavers & Hampson)
I. Structure of the family
   A. Overt power
   B. Parental coalition
   C. Closeness
II. Mythology
III. Goal-directed negotiation
IV. Autonomy
   A. Clarity of expression
   B. Responsibility
   C. Permeability
V. Family affect
   A. Range of feeling
   B. Mood and tone
   C. Unresolvable conflict
   D. Empathy
VI. Global health/pathology scale

Family Style Scale (Beavers & Hampson)
1. Dependency needs
2. Adult conflict
3. Proximity
4. Social presentation
5. Expression of closeness
6. Assertive/aggressive qualities
7. Expression of positive and negative feelings
8. Global centripetal/centrifugal style

McMaster's model: Dimensions of Family Functioning
I. Problem solving
II. Communication
III. Roles: Allocation and accountability
IV. Affective responsiveness
V. Affective involvement
VI. Behavior control

lower end of the normal functioning scale, communication around problems becomes less clear and direct. With regard to roles, at the healthy end of the scale, the allocation of roles does not overburden anyone, and role accountability is clear. On the affective responsiveness scale, at the healthy end, the family is capable of expressing a full range of emotions. It is suggested that cultural variability must be considered. In the section on affective involvement, empathic involvement is considered optional for healthy functioning. Family functioning becomes less effective as families move in either direction away from empathic involvement. Flexible behavior control is the most effective style of behavior control and chaotic control the least effective on the McMaster scale.

Table 14.2 provides an outline of the Beavers and Hampson and McMaster assessment scales.

STUDIES OF WYNNE AND FISHER

Lyman Wynne and his group (1982) state that healthy communication in families promotes healthy adjustment in offspring and provides a model for the children to develop the cognitive ability to attend, focus, remain task-oriented, and communicate thoughts and feelings directly and clearly. This group finds provocative results in their study of communication patterns in families where children were at risk to develop psychopathology. They learned that healthy communication patterns can and do exist between parents in these at-risk families. When the parents can communicate in a structured, easy, and task-appropriate manner, their children seem to be regarded as socially and academically competent. In a sample where a parent in each family had a serious mental illness that in the past had required psychiatric hospitalization, the children revealed a wide range of *healthy* as well as deviant levels of functioning, as assessed in the setting of school (Fisher, 1980).

ATTRIBUTES OF HEALTHY COUPLES

The healthy family is committed to the care and nurturance of its members, to the promotion of their happiness, and to their developing a strong sense of self and purpose. Healthy parents usually mean a strong marital dyad. Based on research and clinical study, Beavers (1985) writes about the attributes of the healthy marital couple. The following is a summary of his findings about the beliefs and characteristics of these couples.

- Healthy couples believe that human beings are limited and finite; they do not possess the "unchallengable truth." They consider truth and subjective reality to be relative, not absolute.

- Healthy couples believe that human encounters are usually rewarding.
- They believe that people's motives are basically benign.
- Healthy couples have clear personal boundaries and can distinguish between one person's feelings and those of another.
- Healthy couples respect each other's individuality and autonomy; separateness is not seen as a threat or an area for competition.
- They believe that human behavior is usually the result of many variables rather than a single cause.
- Healthy partners respect each other's perceptions, even if they differ. Ideally, they can fight and negotiate without the one up–one down position. Only with true equality are risk taking and dialogue possible, and the achievement of intimacy.
- Almost all couples quarrel and can momentarily lose a sense of reasonable dialogue and clear boundaries. When emotions are calmer, healthy couples can redefine boundaries and come to a mutually agreed-on resolution.
- Healthy couples are aware of their own history with their families of origin and can relate to it with some perspective and a sense of humor.
- Most healthy couples focus on present life tasks rather than dwelling on misfortunes or conflicts in the past.

HANSEN'S STUDY OF LIVING WITH NORMAL FAMILIES

Another unique study of "normal" families took place in the mid-1960s and is worthy of mention. Hansen, a student of the noted family therapist Virginia Satir, lived for one week apiece with three "normal" families. Her work, which describes her experience and findings, was published posthumously and edited by a colleague, Jules Riskin. In Hansen's study (1981), the three families met the following criteria: (1) The parents gave no report of behavior that indicated psychiatric problems, (2) the children had adjusted adequately in school, and (3) the parents were satisfied with their family relationships. No striking contradictions are noted in Hansen's observations. The goals of the exercise were (1) to compare the particular differences in each family's patterns of interaction, (2) to look for causes of these differences, and (3) to learn whether the findings could be useful to the families or to those who assisted them. Only the significant conclusions about the more functional families are reported here.

Hansen accompanied the family to various activities outside the home, visited the children's schools, and spoke with their teachers. All dinner conversations were taped. Regarding the three families studied, Hansen found that one was a "superior" family, another was an "above average" family, and the third was a "below average" family. The following is a summary of her significant findings.

1. A smoother, more relaxed rhythm appears to facilitate a healthy adjustment more than a jerky, tense rhythm. *Rhythm* is defined as the totality of interactional patterns that are repetitive and pervasive. Rhythm provides an indicator of how successfully the family is functioning.
2. It is important to have an overall pattern in addressing a problem; the sooner it is approached, the better.
3. It appears possible to have a "functional family" with the marital relationship given a lower priority than the parental and parent–child relationship.
4. A couple have less reason to discuss openly or fight when they have high spontaneous agreement. A couple who have a rule against expressing anger may use indirect means for dealing with their feelings. They also may suffer from some lack of closeness and may experience a dullness in their relationship.
5. In the most functional family, there is the least use of authoritarianism and threats of punishment, although it was clear the parents were in charge. The parents tend to use more persuasion and humor, to treat the children with the same kind of respect they ask for themselves.

In the more functional families:

6. Parents do not feel guilty or reluctant about limiting the children when they become too demanding.
7. The directives are clear, with reminding, follow-up, and consistency, and the directives are met.
8. The parents appear to assume that the child will spontaneously grow by himself and grow in a way that will please the parents. They do not feel the need to "make" the child grow, because they believe it is within the child's capability as an innate wish *and* need to survive.
9. The siblings appear to get along well together and to help each other.
10. The parents are genuinely interested in their children and have adequate time for them, listen to them at a deep level, and arrive at realistic expectations of them.

THE ROLE OF CULTURE IN ASSESSING NORMALITY IN FAMILIES' FUNCTIONING

Health care professionals attempting to define what is "normal" or "healthy" in family functioning must not ignore cultural influences on human behavior. A culture may determine whether behavior is normal or abnormal and whether behavioral symptoms are labeled "pathological." Symptoms may differ from one ethnic group to another.

The subject of ethnicity often brings out strong emotional feelings, and discussions about ethnic influences on individuals and families can become polarized and judgmental. It is usual for people to fear and reject that which they do not understand and that which is not in their own realm of experience (McGoldrick, 1982). In order to plan appropriate and effective therapeutic interventions, the health care professional needs to understand a family's behavior in relationship to its ethnic background and cultural belief systems. The health care professional will need to struggle with his or her own inevitable subjectivity in order to recognize the limitations of his or her own *and* any other belief system. (For a more comprehensive study of the influence of cultural beliefs and ethnicity on family systems, see Chapter Four.)

HEALTHY FAMILIES: GUIDELINES FOR THE HEALTH CARE PROFESSIONAL

1. Look through a wide-angle lens when you evaluate a family: Look for some signs of strength for healthy functioning, no matter how small.
2. Remember, even in severely dysfunctional, chaotic families there may be some signs of strength. For example, the father of a schizophrenic son may be a college professor and have a stable work history.
3. A poor, homeless, single-parent mother may have a well-functioning set of values for her children, who have never been in trouble with the law.
4. Does the family have a set of beliefs to which they adhere? Are these beliefs congruent with their religion, culture, and ethnic origin?
5. Certain behaviors are normative when considered in the context of a family's life cycle stage. For example, a sick 85-year-old man may think a lot about illness and death. Is this abnormal? In itself, of course not! If he takes to his bed every day, broods endlessly, and does not eat, then this behavior is considered to be that of a seriously depressed old person.
6. To assess a family's strengths, keep your questions simple. For example, does the family provide adequate food, clothing, and shelter? Are there wage earners who have a stable work history?
7. *Everyone* has biases about what is healthy or normal in family functioning and what is not. Be aware of yours. Identify or name your own predisposed point of view.
8. Above all, be aware of your own ethnic heritage and the cultural belief systems in your family of origin, particularly with respect to men's and women's roles, parent–child relationships, and expectations around education and the work ethic.

Table 14.3 lists some terms often associated with healthy family functioning and with family dysfunction.

	TABLE 14.3. Terms Often Associated with Healthy Family Functioning and with Family Dysfunction	
Healthy Families		Dysfunctional Families
empathy		suppression
respect		blame
acceptance		coercion
individuation		rigidity
optimism		hurtful
openness		dominance
humor		scapegoat
spontaneity		distortion
support		closed
trust		vagueness
warmth		pessimism
affection		grudge, revenge
assurance, encouragement		distrust
success		invasiveness
growth		confusion, chaos
resolution		attack
competence		defensiveness
strength		amorphous
coping		dismissal
integration		undermining
happiness		contradictory
joy		accusation
will power		failure
steadiness		incompetence
effectiveness		disordered
durability		disturbed
energy		hopelessness
toughness		helplessness
substantiality		disruption
		depression, sadness

SUMMARY

This chapter on healthy families attempts to define what is healthy or "normal" family functioning. Table 14.1 shows how the major models of family therapy view normal family functioning: the structural, strategic, behavioral-social exchange, psychodynamic family systems and experiential models (Walsh, 1982). The chapter discusses how the early studies of family functioning began with severely dysfunctional families, with no attempt to define what was healthy or functional. Some of these early studies began with a detailed analysis of families with a schizophrenic offspring, at the Yale Psychiatric Institute, with Lidz, Fleck, and Cornelison (1965). Lewis and his group in Dallas, Texas, recognized this lack and embarked on a longitudinal study of healthy family functioning. The early support was by the Timberlawn Foundation, with the publication in 1972 of the book *No Single Thread: Psychological Health in Family Systems.* This group, with Beavers et al., has continued its research endeavors and has developed measurement scales that measure family *competence* and family *style*, two important aspects in defining a healthy functioning family system. The relationship between the health/competence dimension and the stylistic dimension was described on page 461. The family *competence* scale describes the structure of the family, the mythology, the goal-directed negotiation, the autonomy, and the family affect, and has a global health–pathology scale at the end. Each of the scales mentioned has subscales to aid further in clarifying the dimension of functioning. The family *style* scale looks at dependency needs, adult conflict, proximity issues, social presentation, *expression* of closeness, assertive-aggressive qualities, and the expression of positive and negative feelings. It also concludes with a global rating scale. The terms centripetal force and centrifugal force are defined in family function terms.

The McMaster model of normal family functioning has been used for over twenty years (Epstein et al., 1982). It does not cover all aspects of family functioning but, rather, focuses on the following dimensions of family functioning: problem solving, communication, roles (allocation and accountability), affective responsiveness, affective involvement, and behavior control.

The studies of Wynne et al. (1982) and Fisher (1980) found healthy family communication patterns in families where children were at risk to develop psychopathology. Even in families in which a parent had been hospitalized for a serious mental illness, the children revealed a wide range of *healthy* as well as disturbed levels of functioning, as assessed in the school. They learned that when parents in these families can communicate in a well-structured, flexible, and task-appropriate manner, the children could be socially and academically competent.

Beavers (1985) discusses the attributes of healthy couples who hold certain beliefs about human interaction. For example, healthy couples assume that people's motives are usually benign, and human encounters are usually rewarding. Healthy couples respect each other's differences, and competition/power struggles are either nonexistent or at a very low plane. Mostly, healthy couples can be objective about themselves and their early relationships and have a sense of humor.

Hansen records a special research experience: She lived with three different "normal" or healthy families for one week each and drew interesting conclusions about the encounters. She described a relaxed "rhythm" in interactional patterns that seems to facilitate a healthy adjustment, in contrast to a "jerky" rhythm. She observed that more functional families, who least used authoritarianism and punishment, but consistently reminded and followed through, had children who obeyed without rebellion and defiance. Parents who respected their children's feelings got respect in return. Healthy parents expected that their children would grow up spontaneously and autonomously on their own and did not need rigid controls or strict directives.

The role of culture must not be overlooked in evaluating a family's functioning. It is important to know the cultural beliefs and values of a family, as these influence feelings and behavior. A culture determines what is considered normal or abnormal, and behavioral symptoms may differ from one ethnic group to another.

In conclusion, the most important guideline for the health care professional as he or she attempts to assess whether a family's functioning is healthy or not is to be aware of one's own *biases* about what is normal. The health care professional needs first of all to be aware of the influence of his or her own cultural heritage, ethnic origins, and family of origin's belief systems about family relationships—all of which define *for us* what is healthy and "normal" or what is "abnormal" or pathological.

In summary, healthy families have both strengths and vulnerabilities. Healthy family members love, fight, vie with each other within the family group, and resolve difficulties in one way or another. Healthy families struggle with internal and external issues that affect them. A healthy family protects its generation boundaries and promotes the need for privacy without condoning the kind of secrets that may breed resentment. Usually, there is joy, passion, and commitment to each other in healthy families, as well as compassion for humankind and a commitment to the social world and community beyond the boundaries of the family unit.

REFERENCES

Beavers, W. R. (1985). *Successful Marriage: A Family Systems Approach to Couples Therapy*. New York: W. W. Norton.

Beavers, W. R., & Hampson, R. B. (1990). *Successful Families: Assessment and Intervention*. New York: Norton.

Bowen, M. (1978). *Family Therapy in Clinical Practice*. New York: Aronson.

Epstein, N. B., Bishop, D. S., & Baldwin, L. M. (1982). "McMaster Model of Family Functioning: A View of the Normal Family." In F. Walsh (Ed.), *Normal Family Processes*. New York: Guilford Press.

Erikson, E. H. (1963). *Childhood and Society*, 2nd ed. New York: W. W. Norton.

Fisher, L. (1980). "Child Competence and Psychiatric Risk: 1. Model and Method." *Journal of Nervous and Mental Diseases*, 168: 323–331.

Hansen, C. (1981). "Living in with Normal Families." *Family Process*, 20(1): 53–75.

Lewis, J. M., Beavers, W. R., Gossett, J. T., & Phillips, V. A. (1976). *No Single Thread: Psychological Health in Family Systems*. New York: Brunner/Mazel.

Lidz, T., Fleck, S., & Cornelison, A. R. (1965). *Schizophrenia and the Family*. New York: International Universities Press.

McGoldrick, M. (1982). "Normal Families: An Ethnic Perspective." In F. Walsh (Ed.), *Normal Family Processes*. New York: Guilford Press.

Satir, V. (1972). *Peoplemaking*. Palo Alto, CA: Science and Behavior Books.

Walsh, F. (Ed.). (1982). *Normal Family Processes*. New York: Guilford Press.

Wynne, L. C., Jones, J. E., & Al-Khayyal, M. (1982). "Healthy Family Communication Patterns: Observations in Families 'At Risk' for Psychopathology." In F. Walsh (Ed.), *Normal Family Processes*. New York: Guilford Press.

Wynne, L. C., & Singer, M. T. (1963). "Thought Disorder and Family Relations of Schizophrenics." *Archives of General Psychiatry*, 9: 191–206.

GLOSSARY

Abuse
Actions that mistreat, injure, or threaten the self or others; drug abuse inflicts injury on the self; child abuse inflicts injury on children.

Accommodation
Process of reorganizing information already known in order to include new information; adjusting to reality and unfamiliar experiences.

Achieved role
Role conferred because of special skills or attributes of an individual; sometimes referred to as assumed role.

Acrophobia
Extreme fear of heights.

Acting out
Discharging tension by responding to the present situation as if it were a previous situation when the response was initiated.

Adaptation
Response to change within the organism or outside its boundaries; adaptation requires mobilization of the organism in addition to processes of assimilation.

Addiction
Dependency, physical or psychological, on alcohol or other substances.

Adjustment
Modification of various aspects of the self in order to cope with the demands of daily life.

Affect
An emotional or feeling state.

Aggression
Actions performed in order to gratify the need to excel, achieve, compete, and/or separate from the group; aggressive actions may be positive or negative in nature.

Agitation
Extreme restlessness and excitability.

Agoraphobia
Extreme fear of open spaces.

Akathisia
Sensations of restlessness and unease; often caused by reactions to psychotropic medication.

Alienation
Loss or lack of relationships with others.

Altruism
Concern for the well-being of others without regard for personal gain.

Alzheimer's disease
Degenerative neurological disorder characterized by loss of mental powers, disorientation, and motor impairment; thought to be congenital in nature.

Ambivalence
Conflict resulting from simultaneous feelings of being attracted and repelled by the same object, action, or goal; often expressed in approach–avoidance behavior.

Amnesia
Loss of memory for events within a certain period of time; may be temporary or permanent.

Amniocentesis
Drawing of amniotic fluid from the amniotic sac of a pregnant woman in order to examine fetal cells for chromosomal abnormalities; Down's syndrome, among other disorders, may be diagnosed in utero through this diagnostic technique.

Anaclitic separation
Loss of the mother or mother figure by the infant during the first year of life, often resulting in developmental deficits and/or indications of depression.

Anhedonia
Inability to experience pleasure or joy.

Anomie
Absence or loss of meaningful relationships with other individuals or groups; absence or loss of social norms and values.

Anorexia nervosa
Refusal of individuals to eat because of psychological factors such as distorted body image or control issues; may result in extreme emaciation and even death.

Anxiety
Vague sense of apprehension or dread originating within the individual; may be communicated to other persons through the process of empathy; may not necessarily be generated by identifiable external stimuli.

Apathy
Lack of feeling, interest, or initiative.

Ascribed role
Role conferred because of status, age, gender, or position and not because of attribute or qualities within the control of the individual.

Assertiveness
Ability to express one's needs, goals, or preferences appropriately and effectively in interpersonal transactions.

Assimilation
Process of integrating new information or experience into what is already known and understood.

Ataxia
Deficient muscular coordination causing difficulty in walking.

Autism
Preoccupation with private, self-determined thoughts or actions without concern for reality or objective standards shared with others.

Autism (primary)
Disorder of childhood characterized by language deficits and inability to relate to others.

Autonomic nervous system
Part of the nervous system that supplies internal organs; is subdivided into the sympathetic and parasympathetic nervous systems.

Autonomy
Self-determination and self-reliance; the sense of being individual and independent.

Aversion therapy
Form of behavior modification in which a painful stimulus is linked to a pleasurable stimulus, thus causing dislike (aversion) for the stimulus previously associated with pleasure.

Behavior modification
Therapeutic modality utilizing stimulus and response conditioning in order to alter dysfunctional patterns of behavior.

Biofeedback
Use of electrical devices to monitor autonomic physiological processes in order to produce relaxation and reduce tension.

Biogenic amines
Organic substances that serve as transmitters or monitors of neural impulses.

Bipolar disorder
Disturbance of mood and affect in which at least one manic episode can be identified; may or may not be characterized by depressive episodes.

Bisexual
Individual who is sexually attracted to both males and females.

Blocking
Difficulty in communicating because channels of thought are obstructed or interrupted for emotional reasons.

Body image
Internalized impressions and attitudes of an individual regarding one's physical self.

Bonding
Attachment of a parent to an infant; any process in which individuals make a mutual commitment.

Brief psychotherapy
Short-term therapy that usually focuses on the restoration of functioning and providing emotional support.

Burnout
Reaction to stressful occupational conditions in which workers feel exhausted and depleted; often expressed behaviorally through anger, apathy, depression, or detachment.

Bulimia
Alternating episodes of overeating (binge eating) followed by deliberate, self-induced vomiting.

Castration
Injury or trauma to the genitals; in broader terms, a threat to the masculinity or femininity of individuals.

Catatonia
State of muscular rigidity and inflexibility, often accompanied by symptoms such as tremor, excitability, or stupor.

Cathexis
Psychoanalytic term used to describe a bond or attachment.

Central nervous system
Neural structures of brain and spinal cord.

Circumstantiality
Communication pattern in which tangential, trivial details are given; usually the purpose is to lower the anxiety of the narrator.

Claustrophobia
Extreme fear of being confined in a small space.

Client advocacy
Process in which professionals, paraprofessionals, and clients themselves attempt to improve the quality of care and protect the rights of persons receiving care.

Cognition
The act, process, or result of knowing, learning, or understanding.

Cohesion
Conditions of attraction among group members, and between individual members and the group as a whole.

Coitus
Sexual intercourse between persons of opposite sexes.

Coma
Deep stupor or loss of consciousness.

Commitment
Hospitalization that was not sought by the client but was arranged by family members, legal or medical officers when the client was considered a clear danger to the self or others.

Compulsion
An irrational, repetitive act that must be performed in order to control rising anxiety.

Concordance
Trait or disorder in one person that occurs in others, usually family members.

Concreteness
Use of literal statements instead of abstract or symbolic forms of communication.

Confabulation
Filling in lost memory gaps with manufactured details.

Confidentiality
Responsibility of professionals to disclose no information about clients except to participating colleagues, and then only with the knowledge and consent of the client.

Conflict
Discomfort (anxiety) experienced by persons torn between a wish for something and fear of the consequences if the wish is gratified; a clash between opposing intrapersonal or interpersonal forces.

Confrontation
Communication designed to help others engage in reflection and self-examination of their motives and behaviors.

Congruence
Agreement between verbal and nonverbal levels of communication.

Consensual validation
Process of ensuring that the message sent is the same as the message received in order to correct distortion or misinterpretation.

Consultation
A collaboration model in which persons with special expertise deal indirectly with clients by working with persons directly responsible for care.

Context
Setting and circumstances in which an event or transaction occurred.

Contract
Agreement between client and profession concerning therapeutic goals and regimen; usually developed collaboratively.

Conversion reaction
Transformation of anxiety-producing thoughts and feelings into somatic symptoms; previously termed a hysterical reaction.

Coping
Efforts directed toward managing and solving various problems, events, and stressors.

Correlation
Establishing of relationships between variables; correlation shows connec-

tions but not cause-and-effect relationships between variables.

Countertransference
Activation in care providers of inappropriate feelings for the client, usually originating in the previous experience of the care provider.

Covert
Concealed, masked, not openly manifest.

Crisis
Periods of vulnerability and/or disorganization that have the potential for growth and maturation.

Crisis intervention
Therapeutic intervention designed to restore functioning at or above pre-crisis levels, usually time limited in nature.

Critical task
Developmental milestone that involves the acquisition and mastery of specific behaviors and competence.

Culture
Sum of the customs, habits, and traditions of a particular ethnic or social group.

Data base
Sum of information collected from which to make inferences, develop hypotheses, assess needs, and evaluate outcomes.

Day hospital
Facility offering a therapeutic program for clients who attend during the day and return home at night; a form of partial hospitalization.

Decompensation
Disorganization of the personality or ego during periods of overwhelming stress.

Defense mechanisms
Unconscious, intrapsychic processes used to reduce anxiety and emotional conflict.

Deinstitutionalization
Return to community living of persons previously hospitalized for long periods; a movement emphasizing community aftercare rather than institutional care for clients.

Déjà vu
A sense that a new occurrence or experience has transpired in the earlier life of the individual; a sense of having experienced new events previously.

Delinquency
Legally prohibited actions committed by a juvenile or minor.

Delirium
Impairment of mental processes to the extent of confusion and disorientation, usually caused by a specific agent or stressor.

Delirium tremens
Withdrawal state of alcoholism characterized by tremors, hallucinations, and occasionally convulsions; a reaction to abstinence or reduced ingestion of alcohol.

Delusion
False, fixed belief maintained despite the absence of factual or corroborating evidence.

Dementia
Absence, impairment, or reduction of cognitive and intellectual abilities.

Dementia praecox
Outmoded term once applied to schizophrenia.

Denial
Refusal to acknowledge the reality of certain events, thereby protecting the individual from the unwelcome recognition of such events.

Dependency
Tendency to rely on others.

Depersonalization
Feelings of unreality and disconnection from the self occurring as a result of personality disorganization.

Depression
Psychological state characterized by dejection, lowered self-esteem, hopelessness, helplessness, indecision, and rumination.

Desensitization
Reduction of intense reactions to various stimuli by repeatedly exposing the individual to the stimuli in milder forms.

Detoxification
Elimination of a toxic agent from the body via natural physiological processes or with the aid of medical and nursing measures.

Deviance
Noncompliance with norms established and upheld by the group.

Discrimination
Ability to differentiate and respond differently to two or more stimuli.

Disengagement
Interactional process characterized by withdrawal; often the withdrawal is reciprocal, as in the case of interactions between the elderly and society or in family situations where members maintain distance between each other.

Disorientation
Confusion and impaired ability to identify time, place, and person.

Displacement
Transfer of emotion or behaviors activated by one person or event to an unrelated person or event; substituting one target of emotions or behavior for another target.

Dissociative reactions
Protective mechanism that protects the self from awareness of anxiety-producing stimuli; amnesia, somnambulism, fugue, and multiple personality are examples of dissociative reactions.

Double bind
Communication in which a positive command is followed by a negative command; the recipient cannot obey both commands and therefore feels confused and trapped.

Down's syndrome
Form of mental retardation associated with chromosomal abnormalities.

Drive
Psychoanalytic term describing instinctual urges and impulses arising from biological and psychological needs; the id component of personality is the repository of instinctual drives.

Drug dependence
Physiological and/or psychological dependence on a chemical substance.

Dyad
Two-person group.

Dynamic formulation
Synthesis of a client's traits, values, behaviors, and conflicts for the purpose of explaining, understanding, and helping the client.

Dynamics
Interactive forces within the individual, usually unconscious, that are manifested in thoughts, feelings, behavior, and symptomatology.

Dyslexia
Impaired ability to read.

Dyspareunia
Painful sexual intercourse; occurs in both sexes but more often in women.

Dystonia
Muscle spasms of the face, head, neck, and back; usually an acute side effect of antipsychotic medication.

Ego
Psychoanalytic term describing the aspect of the personality that mediates between the demands of the id and those of the superego; the aspect of the personality that deals with reality.

Ego dystonic
Thoughts, feelings, impulses, acts that are unacceptable to the ego and therefore produce anxiety; ego alien is an alternative term.

Ego ideal
The internalized image of the self as one would like to be.

Ego syntonic
Thoughts, feelings, impulses, acts that are acceptable to the superego and therefore do not produce anxiety.

Electroconvulsive therapy (ECT)
Therapeutic seizures, tonic and clonic in nature, produced by means of electric current applied to the temporal areas under controlled conditions.

Electroencephalogram (EEG)
Graphic record of the electrical activity of the brain obtained by means of electrodes applied to areas of the head.

Empathy
Ability to understand the feelings of others and respond sensitively to their perceptions of experience.

Enmeshment
Maladaptive pattern of overinvolvement and intensity seen in families.

Epidemiology
Study of the distribution of physical and mental disorders in a given population.

Episodic
Tendency of events, conditions,

symptoms, and disorders to abate and recur intermittently.

Etiology
Systematic study of the cause of disorders.

Ethnocentrism
Belief that one's own group, race, or culture is superior to any other.

Eugenics
Utilization of selective breeding methods for the purpose of improving the species.

Euphoria
Exaggerated sense of well-being and pleasure.

Exogenous
Originating in external sources or causes.

Extended family
All persons related by birth, marriage, or adoption.

Extinction
Gradual disappearance of a conditioned response; occurs when the response is no longer reinforced.

Family therapy
Treatment modality focused on relationships within the family system.

Fantasy
Unrealistic mental images based on conscious or unconscious wish fulfillment.

Feedback
Process by which functioning is monitored, corrected if necessary, and maintained if appropriate.

Fetal alcohol syndrome
Fetal irregularities such as low body weight and cardiac and other abnormalities caused by alcohol ingestion during pregnancy.

Fetish
An object or a part of the body to which sexual significance or meaning is attached.

Fixation
Attachment to immature levels of thinking and acting instead of progressing developmentally.

Flashback
Recurrence of an experience, often drug-induced, without further use of the substance; memory traces of intense experiences that continue to intrude on the individual and cause emotional discomfort.

Flight of ideas
Rapid movement from one topic to another in response to stimuli from outside and from within the individual.

Forensic psychiatry
The branch of psychiatry that deals with legal issues surrounding mental disorders.

Free association
Psychoanalytic technique in which the client (analysand) communicates whatever thoughts come to mind without interference from the therapist (analyst) or the client.

Frustration
Curtailment of gratification by conditions of external reality or by internal controls.

Genitalia
Reproductive organs, particularly the external structures.

Genetics
Science of heredity.

Geriatrics
Study and treatment of disorders associated with aging.

Gerontology
Study of the aging process.

Grief
Mourning as a response to loss, actual or imagined, of a meaningful person, object, or situation.

Grief work
The process of reacting to loss in which anger, denial, and idealization of what was lost may play a part before detachment and restitution can occur.

Group
Collection of three or more persons who are interdependent to some extent and share meaningful interaction.

Group therapy
Treatment modality that involves several persons in the same session and utilizes interpersonal group behaviors to produce corrective or supportive interactions.

Guilt
Sense of culpability and self-blame due to transgressions against one's internalized values and principles.

Habeus corpus
Right of persons who are detained involuntarily to a legal hearing held to determine whether the detainment should continue.

Hallucination
False sensory perception in the absence of any external stimuli.

Hallucinogen
Substance producing a temporary psychotic state in which contact with and perceptions of reality are impaired.

Helplessness
Belief on the part of individuals that they cannot help themselves.

Homeostasis
Tendency of organisms to maintain balance by preserving a constant internal environment.

Homosexuality
Sexual attraction for or preference for persons of the same gender as oneself.

Hopelessness
Belief on the part of individuals that no one can help them.

Hostility
Impulses or urges directed toward the destruction of a person or object.

Hyperactivity
Behavior characterized by high energy expenditure and excessive activity; accelerated motor activity, emotional lability, and flight of ideas may be present.

Hyperventilation
Rapid respiration due to high levels of anxiety.

Hypochondriasis
State of exaggerated concern for one's physical well-being in the absence of actual physiological problems.

Hysteric
An individual who deals with anxiety by means of self-dramatization, excitability, and attention seeking behavior.

Id
Component of the personality that is present at birth and is the repository of drives and instincts, according to psychoanalytic theory.

Ideas of reference
Belief that certain events or objects have a special meaning or significance for oneself.

Ideology
A belief system.

Identification
Process in which the attributes and traits of another are adopted and made part of oneself.

Identity
Sense of selfhood that makes possible and sustains an integrated, consistent personality structure.

Illusion
Misinterpretation of a sensory stimulus.

Impotence
Failure to achieve or maintain an erection.

Incest
Sexual relationships between persons related biologically or by marriage, other than a husband and wife.

Individuation
A developmental process in which a person separates from others and develops a unique, distinct identity.

Inferiority complex
Intense, generalized feelings of inadequacy that influence the way an individual behaves and relates to others.

Inhibition
Control or restraint imposed on an unacceptable impulse, thought, or action; usually but not always self-imposed.

Insanity
A synonym for mental disorder or psychosis; rarely applied by professionals except in legal matters.

Integrity
Commitment to honesty, ethics, and values in various aspects of life.

Intellectualization
Use of rationalization to avoid uncomfortable insight or awareness.

Intelligence quotient
Mental age of an individual multiplied by 100 and divided by the chronological age; an arbitrary measure obtained by standardized intelligence tests.

Interpersonal
Arising or generated between two or more persons.

Intrapsychic
Arising, generated, or residing within the self.

Isolation
Separation of thoughts or ideas or actions from their emotional aspects.

Judgment
Ability to predict the consequences of an action and modify one's behavior accordingly; ability to make rational decisions based on cognition and reality.

Labeling
Consigning an individual to a category or classification based on behavior patterns, personality configuration, or psychiatric diagnosis.

Lability
Changeable and poorly controlled emotional states.

Latent
Describing an inactive or dormant condition that nevertheless has the potential for becoming active or manifest.

Lesbian
Female homosexual; female with a sexual preference for other females.

Lethality
Degree or extent of suicide potential; the likelihood or probability that an individual will commit suicide.

Libido
Psychoanalytic term applied to instinctual energy; usually denotes sexual drive or energy.

Limit setting
Actions that encourage others to respect rules and norms; consequences attached to failure to adhere to rules and norms.

Magical thinking
Belief that thinking about a possible occurrence can make it happen; a primitive, immature form of thinking.

Malingering
Conscious, deliberate feigning or exaggeration of disability or incapacity.

Malpractice
Failure of a professional to adhere to established practice standards of a discipline.

Mania
State of accelerated activity, mental and physical; generally thought to be a maladaptive defense against depression.

Manipulation
Exertion of indirect control or influence over the actions of others in order to obtain one's own purpose.

Masochism
Gratification obtained by experiencing pain, abuse, or humiliation from others; usually applied to deviant sexual actions.

Masturbation
Gratification obtained by self-stimulation of the genitals.

Maturation
Progress resulting from development and/or heredity rather than learning.

Maturational crisis
Developmental episode in which life transitions occur and the individual is vulnerable to disequilibrium.

Milieu
Immediate environment, physical and social, in which individuals function.

Milieu therapy
Treatment modality that uses all aspects of the environment, physical and social, in order to promote adaptive change.

Mourning
Psychological and physiological response of individuals to loss; a necessary process involving gradual renunciation of what was lost followed by the ability to form new attachments.

Negative reinforcement
Behavior modification procedure that induces change by removing aversive conditions after a certain response occurs, thus increasing the probability of obtaining the response.

Negativism
Refusal to cooperate or follow directions; exhibiting behaviors contrary to what is desired or expected.

Norm
A standard of behavior upheld by a family, group, or community.

Nuclear family
Two-generational family consisting of parents and their offspring, natural or adopted; family of procreation established by the parental dyad.

Obesity
Excess weight that exceeds accepted standards by more than 20 percent.

Occupational therapy
A therapeutic method involving planned, purposeful activity in which tangible products or discernible goals are accomplished.

Operant conditioning
Behavior modification that changes behavior by manipulating stimuli and the consequences of reactions to stimuli.

Orientation
Awareness of time, place, and person.

Overload
Sensory input or performance demands that are beyond the tolerance or capacity of the individual.

Overt
Open, direct, unconcealed.

Panic
Severe disorganization caused by intense anxiety; characterized by cognitive, emotional, and behavioral distortion.

Paranoia
Extreme suspiciousness of others; usually related to use of the defense mechanism projection, whereby anxiety-producing thoughts and feelings are disowned by the individual and attributed to other people.

Passive-aggressive
Describing behavior employed to express hostility and aggression indirectly.

Perception
Individualistic process of viewing, comprehending, and interpreting the world and one's own experiences.

Personality
Accumulated configuration of traits, attributes, behaviors, qualities, and attitudes that characterize the individual.

Perversion
Deviation from what is considered normal and acceptable by the majority.

Phallic
Pertaining to the penis.

Phobia
Extreme, irrational fear of certain objects or circumstances.

Primary prevention
Measures used to promote health and reduce the incidence of disorder or dysfunction by opposing causative agents.

Primary process
Primitive, infantile thought processes that seek instant outlets; in psychoanalytic theory, those thought processes controlled by id forces.

Projection
Attribution of blame or responsibility for one's own acts and feelings to other people.

Pseudohostility
Family dissension that avoids genuine sources of conflict.

Pseudomutuality
Family harmony that is superficial and maintained at the expense of one or more family members.

Psychic determinism
Psychoanalytic axiom that human behavior is neither random nor accidental but is determined by preceding experiences and events.

Psychoanalysis
A form of therapy utilizing techniques of free association and exploration of the unconscious level of mental activity. Theoretical and therapeutic approach that explores anxiety-producing events of early life. Through the defense mechanism of repression, the memory of such events becomes unconscious. The purpose of psychoanalysis is to bring repressed material into conscious awareness so that it may be dealt with adaptively.

Psychodrama
Use of dramatization under professional direction to help clients act out life experiences before an audience of peers who offer constructive alternative suggestions for coping.

Psychodynamic
Pertaining to the causes and consequences of behavior and experience, with attention to underlying motivation, conscious and unconscious.

Psychogenic
Psychological in origin.

Psychomotor retardation
Slowed motor activity, often seen in depressed persons.

Psychopathology
Study of the causes and nature of abnormal behavior; in general, the study of psychiatric disorders.

Psychosis
Dysfunction in which the ability to recognize reality, communicate, and relate to others is seriously impaired, resulting in reliance on maladaptive defenses and an inability to cope with life.

Psychosurgery
Surgical intervention for psychiatric disorders, usually involving neural pathways or areas of the brain.

Psychotherapy
Measures and interventions employed to offer support and/or modify maladaptive behavior; may include identification of problems troubling the client, goal setting, and negotiation of a therapeutic regimen.

Psychotropic
Having an effect on the mind.

Rape
Sexual intercourse with a minor (statutory rape); sexual intercourse without the consent of the partner (forcible rape).

Rapport
Shared understanding and harmony between two people based on mutual trust.

Rationalization
Utilization of socially acceptable reasons to justify actions, thoughts, or feelings that might be unacceptable to the self or others.

Reaction formation
Control or eradication of unacceptable ideas or impulses by engaging in opposite forms of behavior or attitudes.

Reality
The world as it actually is; the external world as opposed to the internal world of daydreams and fantasy.

Reality principle
Psychoanalytic concept applied to the gradual development of ability to delay gratification and modify one's desires in accordance with the demands of society and external reality.

Reality testing
An essential ego function that enables the individual to distinguish internal stimuli from external stimuli; differentiating subjective from objective experience.

Reality therapy
A treatment approach that employs existential concepts of responsibility, self-determination, and progress toward goals.

Recidivism
Recurrence of delinquency or criminality despite punishment, incarceration, or treatment.

Reflection
Communication technique in which ideas or feelings expressed by one person are verbalized by the other in order to clarify meaning and encourage amplification.

Regression
Retreat to less mature levels of thought and action in an attempt to deal with stressful or anxiety-producing situations.

Relaxation therapy
Utilization of consciously induced states of relaxation in order to reduce tension and various maladaptive responses to stress.

Repression
Removal of unpleasant, anxiety-producing thoughts, desires, or memories from conscious awareness.

Resistance
Tendency to maintain maladaptive patterns of thinking and behaving despite therapeutic intervention.

Reversal
Behavior in which instinctual feelings are expressed by opposing actions.

Role
A set of behavioral expectations associated with an individual's status and functions in the family, group, or community.

Sadism
Gratification obtained by inflicting pain, abuse, or humiliation on others; usually applied to sexually deviant acts.

Scapegoat
An individual who is the target of aggression from others but who may not be the actual cause of hostility or frustration in others.

Schism
A term applied to families characterized by severe conflict and dissension.

School phobia
Aversion to school often generated by fears of separation from parents; also known as school avoidance behavior.

Secondary gain
Additional gain or reward such as attention derived from any illness or disability.

Secondary prevention
Measures designed to reduce the prevalence of dysfunction and disorders through early detection and adequate care.

Secondary process
Rational, mature thought processes considered to be under the control of the ego.

Security operations
Any behavior employed to increase psychological comfort and reduce anxiety; may be conscious or unconscious.

Self-actualization
Process of reaching one's full potential.

Self-awareness
Recognition of what one is experiencing and how one is reacting.

Self-concept
Sum of an individual's knowledge and beliefs about the self and its relation to the physical and social environment.

Self-differentiation
Extent to which the individual preserves a sense of identity and separateness from the group.

Self-esteem
Feelings held by individuals regarding their own worth and value.

Self-fulfilling prophecy
A phenomenon in which expectations shape and maintain behavior, events, and interpersonal transactions.

Separation anxiety
Apprehension generated by loss or fear of loss of the mothering person; subsequent loss of significant persons or objects may reactivate separation anxiety.

Shaping
Form of behavior modification in which any behaviors resembling the desired goal are rewarded (reinforced); eventually only the closest approximate behaviors are rewarded; finally only the desired behavior is rewarded.

Sibling rivalry
Competition between brothers and sisters for recognition and affection.

Sick role
Set of behaviors, privileges, and obligations expected from persons designated as being ill.

Significant others
Essential persons, often but not always related to the individual, who are meaningful and sources of support for the individual.

Situational crisis
Disturbed equilibrium that develops as a result of the impact of a specific event.

Socialization
Process of acquiring the values, attitudes, and behaviors considered appropriate in a particular culture.

Stereotype
Generalization of how members of a particular group or category are likely to look or act.

Stress
Any situation or condition requiring adjustment on the part of the individual, family, or group.

Stressor
A stimulus, event, or experience that demands changed or new behavior; usually stressors require expenditure of considerable energy, thus arousing alarm and mobilization responses.

Sublimation
Conscious transformation of unacceptable drives and impulses into socially acceptable behavior in order to satisfy the drive or impulse.

Successive approximation
See Shaping.

Suicide
Self-inflicted death.

Superego
Psychoanalytic term describing that aspect of the personality that monitors thoughts and actions; comparable to the conscience or internal censor.

Suppression
Conscious inhibition or control of certain desires, thought, or emotions.

Symbol

The representation of an idea or concept by means of an object, sign, or signal that conveys connotative and denotative meanings.

Sympathetic nervous system

That part of the autonomic nervous system that is activated by stressful conditions, actual or perceived.

Syndrome

Grouping or cluster of symptoms that represent the usual clinical manifestations of a disorder.

System

Set of interrelated components defined by boundaries, interdependent and interacting in such a manner that any stimulus affecting one component affects every other component, as well as acting on the system as a whole.

Undoing

Performance of activities designed to atone for errors or misdeeds, thereby canceling them.

Violence

Expression of aggressive impulses by acting destructively toward others.

Withdrawal

Behaviors adopted to avoid interacting with others.

NAME INDEX

Abramowitz, I. A., 344, 348
Ackerman, N. 209
Alers, J. O., 133
Alexander, B. K., 438
Alexandrowicz, D. R., 161
Al-Khayyal, M., 456
Allan, C. A., 414
American Psychiatric Association, 163, 274, 344, 359
Alvirez, D., 138
Anderson, A., 378
Anderson, K. E., 414
Anderson, R. C., 414
Anderson, W. P., 367–368
Aroian, K. J., 142
Astrachan, A., 7
Atkin, E., 217, 219
Auerback, S., 285

Baldwin, B., 158, 168
Baldwin, L. M., 461, 468
Bales, R. F., 83–85, 107
Baltes, P. B., 35
Barocas, H. A., 161
Barringer, F., 252
Barzini, L., 110
Bateson, G., 51–52, 344
Bauer, B. G., 367–368
Bauer, K., 282
Beavers, R. W., 456, 458, 460–463, 468
Beck, A. T., 360
Beigler, E., 273
Beletsis, S., 420
Belkin, L., 255–256
Bell, A., 273, 275, 281–282, 296
Bell, N. W., 5
Belsky, J., 177–179
Bennett, G., 429
Benson, S., 182
Berger, R. M., 285–286

Berman, C., 182
Berman, L. B., 327–328
Bernardo, S., 104
Bernier, S. L., 278, 307, 313
Berren, M. R., 156
Bettelheim, B., 159–160, 168
Biddle, E. A., 106
Bigner, J. J., 282–284, 296
Bishop, D. S., 461, 468
Bjornsten, O. J., 244, 254
Blessing, P. J., 106
Blos, P. 209
Bohannon, P., 197
Bonaventura, L. M., 144
Bovard, E. W., 162
Boyd, J. H., 357–358
Boyd, J. L., 343
Boyd-Franklin, N., 125, 129
Bowen, M., 40–46, 64, 75–76, 80, 132, 227, 233, 235, 459
Bozett, F. W., 280, 282–285, 289, 296
Bradley, L. A., 319
Briar, K. H., 153–154
Brice, J., 131
Brody, E., 193
Brown, J. L., 276
Brown, S., 418–420
Browne, A., 393
Bruch, H., 366–367
Brumberg, J. J., 365–366
Brunnquell, D., 177
Burgess, A. W., 158–168
Burish, T. G., 319
Busch, D., 414

Carlson, G. A., 315
Cain, A., 78
Cancro, R., 354
Carrera, M., 273
Carter, E. A. (Betty), 32, 209, 210, 393

SUBJECT INDEX

Acute physical illness, 303–306
  family role factors in, 304
  health care professional's role in, 305
  impact on families, 304–306
  therapeutic guidelines, 330
AIDS (acquired immune deficiency
    syndrome), 311–314
  considerations for the health care
    professional, 311–312
  guidelines for working with, 314
  impact on patient's parents, 313
  services needed for persons with,
    314
Alcohol and alcoholism
  alcohol and society, 408–411
  the alcoholic family, 417–418
    children of alcoholics, 418–420
    residual behaviors of adult chil-
      dren of alcoholics, 420
    therapeutic guidelines, 420–423
  defined, 409
  the elderly alcoholic, 416
    therapeutic guidelines, 416–417
  the female alcoholic, 413–414
    therapeutic guidelines, 414
  the male alcoholic, 409–411
    therapeutic guidelines, 411–413
  the teenage alcoholic, 415
    therapeutic guidelines, 415
Applied family theory, 68–96

Black American family, 124–131
  education in, 126–127
  historical background, 124–125
  impact of slavery on, 124–125
  male-female relationships, 124–125,
    129
  prejudice and discrimination against,
    128
  role flexibility in, 125–126
  role of women, 130
  strength of, 125
  unemployment in, 125, 127

Changing attitudes regarding sexual be-
    havior, 251–252
Child abuse, 380–386
  characteristics of the abusing parent,
    381–382
  child sexual abuse, 383–386
    consequences of, 384
    contribution of the child, 382–383
    contribution of the nonabusing
      parent, 382
    definitions seen in historical per-
      spective, 380–381
    incest patterns, 383–386
    incidence of, 381
  legal issues, 386
  single-parent child abuse, 386
  therapeutic guidelines, 387
Childhood illnesses, 321–330
  birth defects, 322
  childhood disorders, long-term, 323
  chronic illness, 321–330
    financial burden of, 325
    impact on parents, 324–329
    impact on siblings, 329–330
  handicapped or disabled children,
    323–324
  impact on the child, 322–324
  legal issues: implications of with-
    holding treatment, 324–325
  support groups for families, 333
Childless couples, 175–176
Chinese American family, 116–121
  attitudes toward authority, 117–118
  attitudes toward the elderly, 118
  attitudes toward the health care sys-
    tem, 120